CLINICAL GASTROENTEROLOGY

Series Editor
George Y. Wu
University of Connecticut Health Center, Farmington, CT, USA

For further volumes:
http://www.springer.com/series/7672

Nancy Reau • Fred F. Poordad
Editors

Primary Liver Cancer

Surveillance, Diagnosis and Treatment

※ Humana Press

Editors
Nancy Reau
Medical Center, Center for Liver Disease
The University of Chicago
Chicago, IL
USA

Fred F. Poordad
Chief, Hepatology
Cedars-Sinai Medical Center
Professor of Medicine
David Geffen School of Medicine at UCLA
Los Angeles, CA
USA

ISBN 978-1-61779-862-7   ISBN 978-1-61779-863-4 (eBook)
DOI 10.1007/978-1-61779-863-4
Springer NewYork Heidelberg Dordrecht London

Library of Congress Control Number: 2012932614

Printed on acid-free paper

Humana Press is a brand of Springer
Springer is part of Springer Science+Business Media (www.springer.com)

Preface

The incidence of hepatocellular carcinoma is rising in many countries due to the aging population of individuals infected with viral hepatitis as well as the obesity epidemic. Ideally, care of the patient with HCC involves many disciplines including gastroenterology, hepatology, radiology, oncology, surgery, and the primary care physician. The patient affected by liver cancer is a management challenge as the degree of liver function has direct implications in both diagnostic and therapeutic avenues. The field is quickly evolving as a result of new drug development as well as diagnostic and interventional technologies.

This issue of clinics in gastroenterology is a multidisciplinary endeavor, written by expert clinical scientists who not only care for liver cancer patients but will also impact the future of the care they provide.

We begin with an appraisal of the epidemiology and natural history of hepatocellular carcinoma. Drs. Woreta, Hamilton, and Koteish alert the reader to the increasing role HCC will play in health care and its many faces of presentation. Without an understanding of who is at risk to develop the malignancy and how it may present patients will be found at a time when options are limited by advanced disease. Drs. Chowdhury and Satoskar cover the difficult task of identifying which individuals are appropriate for screening and what to use for surveillance. Once a lesion of concern is found, Drs. Thomas, Otto, Giusto, and Jakate discuss the radiologic and pathologic features of liver cancer. However, equally important is identifying what is not a primary hepatoma. This task is beautifully orchestrated by Drs. Wesson and Cameron. Although typically not considered a pediatric affliction, HCC is the second most common malignant liver tumor in children. Drs. Sokollik, Gupta, and Ling review the care of the pediatric patient.

The management of a patient with HCC is dependent on tumor characteristics, the individual's hepatic function, and available therapeutics. Because these management decisions are multidisciplinary, a universal language is imperative. Drs. Bunchorntavakul, Hoteit, and Reddy review the systems used to stage liver tumors. Drs. Nissen and Annamalai clarify liver anatomy and function from a therapeutic perspective. And Drs. Susnow, Baker, and Kulik evaluate therapeutic modalities, including resection, local-regional and systemic therapies, as well as liver transplantation.

Unfortunately, HCC recurrence is a reality. Drs. Chandok and Marotta discuss the prevention and management of recurrent HCC, and Drs. Dharel and Lau review primary HCC prevention.

Lastly, the arsenal of therapeutic and diagnostic options is exploding. Drs. Pillai, Fimmel, Dhanasekaran, and Cabrera highlight the technologies that are in development.

We are grateful for the dedication and work of our authors in bringing this edition to life. They invested time and energy, and this has resulted in a comprehensive multidisciplinary collection of the current knowledge on the management of hepatocellular carcinoma.

We would also like to thank Daniel Dominguez for his patience and efforts in helping coordinate this work.

Chicago, IL, USA   Nancy Reau
Los Angeles, CA, USA   Fred F. Poordad

Contents

Contributors

Alagappan Annamalai, MD Department of Surgery, Comprehensive Transplant Center, Cedars-Sinai Medical Center, Los Angeles, CA, USA

Talia B. Baker, MD Department of Transplantation Surgery, Feinberg School of Medicine, Northwestern University, Chicago, IL, USA

Chalermrat Bunchorntavakul, MD Division of Gastroenterology and Hepatology, Department of Medicine, University of Pennsylvania, Philadelphia, PA, USA

Roniel Cabrera, MD, MS Division of Gastroenterology, Hepatology and Nutrition, Section of Hepatobiliary Diseases, University of Florida, Gainsville, FL, USA

Andrew M. Cameron, MD, PhD Department of Surgery, The Johns Hopkins Hospital, Baltimore, MD, USA

Natasha Chandok, MD Division of Gastroenterology, University of Western Ontario, London, ON, Canada

Po-Hung Chen, MD Division of Gastroenterology and Hepatology, The Johns Hopkins Hospital, Baltimore, MD, USA

Reezwana Chowdhury, MD Georgetown Transplant Institute, Georgetown University Hospital, Washington, DC, USA

Renumathy Dhanasekaran, MD Department of Medicine, University of Florida, Gainsville, FL, USA

Narayan Dharel, MD Liver Center, Division of Gastroenterology, Department of Medicine, Beth Israel Deaconess Medical Center, Harvard Medical School, Boston, MA, USA

Claus J. Fimmel, MD Division of Gastroenterology, Hepatology and Nutrition, Loyola University Medical Center, Maywood, IL, USA

Deborah Giusto, MD 4Path Pathology Services, Justice, IL, USA

Abha Gupta, MD, MSc, FRCPC Division of Hematology/Oncology, Department of Paediatrics, University of Toronto, The Hospital for Sick Children, Toronto, Canada

James P. Hamilton, MD Division of Gastroenterology and Hepatology, Department of Medicine, The Johns Hopkins University School of Medicine, Baltimore, MD, USA

Maarouf Hoteit, MD Division of Gastroenterology and Hepatology, Department of Medicine, University of Pennsylvania, Philadelphia, PA, USA

Shriram Jakate, MD, FRCPath Department of Pathology, Rush University Medical Center, Chicago, IL, USA

Ayman Koteish, MD Department of Medicine, The Johns Hopkins Hospital, Baltimore, MD, USA

Laura Kulik, MD Departments of Hepatology and Transplantation Surgery, Feinberg School of Medicine, Northwestern University, Chicago, IL, USA

Daryl T. Lau, MD, MSc, MPH Liver Center, Division of Gastroenterology, Department of Medicine, Beth Israel Deaconess Medical Center, Harvard Medical School, Boston, MA, USA

Simon C. Ling, MBChB, MRCP Division of Gastroenterology, Hepatology and Nutrition, Department of Paediatrics, University of Toronto, The Hospital for Sick Children, Toronto, Canada

Paul Marotta, MD, FRCPC Division of Gastroenterology, University of Western Ontario, London, ON, Canada

Nicholas N. Nissen, MD Department of Surgery, Comprehensive Transplant Center, Cedars-Sinai Medical Center, Los Angeles, CA, USA

Center for Liver Diseases and Transplantation, Los Angeles, CA, USA

Aytekin Oto, MD Department of Radiology, University of Chicago, Chicago, IL, USA

Anjana A. Pillai, MD Emory University Hospital, Division of Digestive Diseases, Emory Transplant Center, Atlanta, GA, USA

K. Rajender Reddy, MD Division of Gastroenterology and Hepatology, Department of Medicine, University of Pennsylvania, Philadelphia, PA, USA

Hospital of the University of Pennsylvania, Philadelphia, PA, USA

Rohit Satoskar, MD Georgetown Transplant Institute, Georgetown University Hospital, Washington, DC, USA

Christiane Sokollik, MD Division of Gastroenterology, Hepatology and Nutrition, Department of Paediatrics, University of Toronto, The Hospital for Sick Children, Toronto, Canada

Nate Susnow, MD Division of Gastroenterology, University of Washington, Seattle, WA, USA

Stephen Thomas, MD Department of Radiology, University of Chicago, Chicago, IL, USA

Russell N. Wesson, MD Department of Surgery, The Johns Hopkins Hospital, Baltimore, MD, USA

Tinsay A. Woreta, MD, MPH Division of Gastroenterology and Hepatology, Department of Medicine, The Johns Hopkins University School of Medicine, Baltimore, MD, USA

Chapter 1
Hepatocellular Carcinoma: Etiology and Natural History

Tinsay A. Woreta and James P. Hamilton

Hepatocellular carcinoma (HCC) is the most common type of primary liver cancer, accounting for ~85% of all cases [1]. Overall, it is the fifth most common cancer worldwide, representing about 5.7% of all new human cancer cases [2]. It also ranks as the third leading cause of cancer-related death in the world [2]. The number of deaths per year due to HCC is almost identical to its incidence, which highlights the poor prognosis and aggressive nature of the cancer [2]. The goal of this chapter is to review the epidemiology, etiologic associations, and natural history of HCC, which poses a significant public health problem in many countries around the world.

Incidence of HCC

Geographic Distribution

Recent estimates indicate that each year, there are more than 600,000 new cases of HCC that occur worldwide [2]. The incidence of HCC varies widely by geographic region, mainly due to the association of HCC with specific risk factors which differ in prevalence around the world. The highest age-adjusted incidence rates of the disease occur in Eastern and Southeast Asia and Central and Western Africa, where the incidence ranges from 21 to 48 cases per 100,000 men/year [2, 3]. The geographic regions with the lowest incidence rates include Northern Europe, Australia and New Zealand, and North and South America, where the incidence is <10 cases per 100,000 men/year (Fig. 1.1) [2, 3]. More than 80% of cases of HCC occur in developing countries, with China alone accounting for greater than >50% of cases [2].

T.A. Woreta, MD, MPH • J.P. Hamilton, MD (✉)
Division of Gastroenterology and Hepatology, Department of Medicine,
The Johns Hopkins University School of Medicine, Baltimore, MD, USA
e-mail: jhamil16@jhmi.edu

N. Reau and F.F. Poordad (eds.), *Primary Liver Cancer: Surveillance, Diagnosis and Treatment*, Clinical Gastroenterology, DOI 10.1007/978-1-61779-863-4_1,
© Springer Science+Business Media New York 2012

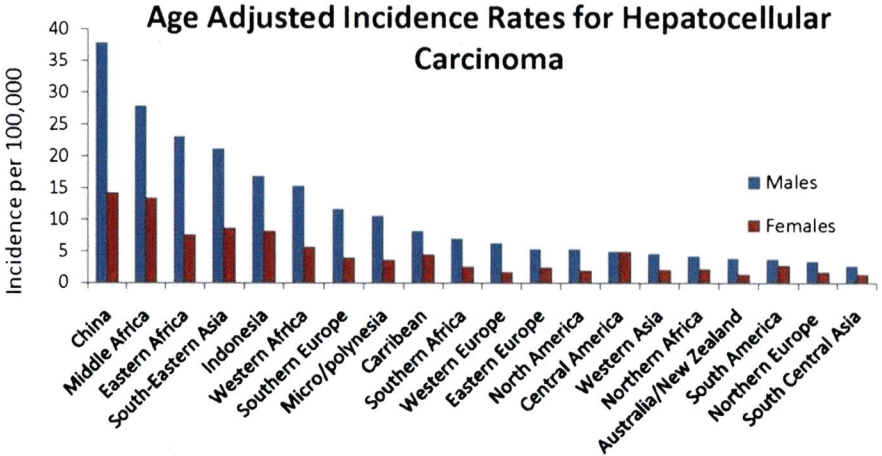

Fig. 1.1 Age-standardized incidence rates for liver cancer. Adapted from Parkin et al. [2]

In the last few decades (1980–2010), there has been a trend toward decreasing incidence rates of HCC in some areas with high incidence rates, such as Hong Kong, Shanghai, and Singapore [4]. This is likely due to the advent of strategies designed to prevent the transmission of hepatitis B. In contrast, increasing incidence rates have been observed in several developed countries, including the United States, Canada, Australia, Italy, France, and The United Kingdom [4]. Since the mid-1980s, the incidence of HCC in the United States has been rising rapidly, with a doubling of the age-adjusted incidence rates in the past two decades [5, 6]. According to data from the Surveillance, Epidemiology and End Results (SEER) program of the National Cancer Institute, the average age-adjusted rate of HCC increased from 1.4 per 100,000 persons during 1975–1977 to 3 per 100,000 persons during 1996–1998 [6]. Analysis of more recent data from 2001 to 2006 from the SEER program and the Center for Disease Control's National Program of Cancer Registries determined that the average incidence rate of HCC was 3 per 100,000 persons, with an increase from 2.7 per 100,000 persons in 2001 to 3.2 in 2006 [7]. The increase in incidence in HCC in North America and Western Europe is related to the rising incidence of important etiologic factors, such as hepatitis C and obesity, discussed below.

Variation by Ethnicity and Race

The incidence of HCC among populations in the United States varies greatly by ethnic origin and race. A population-based study examining the incidence of HCC from 1992 to 2004 found that the highest incidence rates occur among Asians, with a rate more than four times higher than that of Caucasians (11 vs. 2.6 per 100,000 persons/year) and nearly twice that of white Hispanics (11 vs. 6.8 per 100,000 persons/year) [8]. In another more recent population-based study, the incidence rates were found to be 7.8 per 100,000 persons among Asians/Pacific Islanders and 4.2 per 100,000 among blacks compared to 2.6 per 100,000 among whites [7]. Studies of immigrant populations have shown that liver cancer incidence rates are higher in Asian men born in Asia than their descendants born in the United States. However, Asian Americans still have higher rates than US white men [9]. Such studies highlight the role of both environmental and genetically determined risk factors in the etiopathogenesis of HCC.

Gender and Age Distribution

In most regions of the world, the incidence of HCC is 2–4 times higher among men compared to women [2]. The overall gender ratio is more pronounced in high-risk areas, where the male to female ratio may be as high as 8:1 [10]. In the USA, the incidence rates for men and women between 2001 and 2006 were 5 and 1.3 per 100,000 persons, respectively [7]. The reason for this gender disparity is not fully understood, but may partly be due to differences in the prevalence of risk factors between sexes.

The age distribution of HCC varies by incidence. In most high-risk areas, such as Southeast Asia, the rates of liver cancer increase after age 20 and peak at the age of 50 years and above. HCC may present at a younger age in African blacks, with chronic hepatitis B infection, family history of liver cancer, HIV coinfection, and exposure to aflatoxin accounting for the majority of cases in younger patients [11–13]. In low-risk countries, there tends to be a steady increase with age, with the highest rates occurring among individuals ages 75 years and older [3]. The differences in the incidence of HCC with respect to age are likely related to similar regional differences in the age of acquisition of certain risk factors, such as infection with viral hepatitis. For example, in high-risk areas, many individuals are infected with hepatitis B at birth or early in childhood; thus, the incidence of HCC peaks 20–50 years after acquisition of the hepatitis B virus. In low-risk areas, a majority of at-risk patients acquire risk factors such as hepatitis C or heavy alcohol use in early adulthood, resulting in a maximum rate of HCC 20–50 years later, or in their 70s. This epidemiologic evidence indicates that similar to other cancers, the pathogenesis of HCC is slow and insidious and requires decades of exposure to etiologic agents before the diagnosis of HCC is made.

Etiology and Risk Factors

A variety of risk factors for the development of HCC have been clearly identified, which has shed light into its etiology and provided the basis for prevention campaigns and surveillance strategies for early detection. In 80% of cases, HCC develops in a cirrhotic liver, and cirrhosis is the strongest independent risk factor for

HCC, irrespective of etiology [14]. The most common risk factors are hepatitis B (HBV) and hepatitis C (HCV) infections, which account for more than 80% of HCC cases worldwide [15]. Another important cause in Asia and sub-Saharan Africa is exposure to aflatoxin B1, which is produced by the frequent contamination of grains and legumes by *Aspergillus* species in those regions. Other risk factors include alcohol, tobacco, iron overload including genetic hemochromatosis, obesity, diabetes mellitus, nonalcoholic fatty liver disease (NAFLD), stage 4 primary biliary cirrhosis, and alpha-1 antitrypsin deficiency [13].

Cirrhosis

Cirrhosis is the single most important risk factor for the development of HCC, irrespective of etiology. About 70–90% of cases of HCC occur in patients with underlying cirrhosis [16]. Almost all cases that arise in noncirrhotic livers are associated with chronic hepatitis or aflatoxin. The annual incidence of HCC in individuals with compensated cirrhosis is about 3–4% [17]. Among those with established cirrhosis, the main predictors of HCC risk include male gender, age, elevated serum alpha-fetoprotein (AFP) levels, disease severity, and high liver cell proliferation activity [17, 18]. Patients with cirrhosis secondary to HBV, HCV, or hereditary hemochromatosis (HH) have the highest risk of developing HCC. The cumulative probability of HCC in individuals with HH and established cirrhosis was estimated to be 30% over 10 years, which is 200 times higher than the risk in the general population [19].

Nonalcoholic fatty liver disease is an emerging cause of cryptogenic cirrhosis and an increasingly recognized cause of underlying liver disease in patients with HCC. Epidemiologic studies have shown that obesity and diabetes mellitus are risk factors for HCC, which may, in part, be due to the association with NAFLD [20, 21]. Finally, cirrhosis secondary to primary biliary cirrhosis, Wilson's disease, and autoimmune hepatitis are associated with an increased incidence of HCC, but the risk is substantially lower than that associated with cirrhosis due to the above-mentioned causes [22].

Hepatitis B

Worldwide, ~400 million people have chronic hepatitis B infection, the majority of whom live in Asia and Africa. Epidemiologic and experimental studies have provided robust evidence for the association of chronic HBV infection with HCC. Accordingly, there are strong geographic correlations between the incidence of HCC and the prevalence of chronic HBV infection [10]. A study in Taiwan demonstrated that the risk for HCC in men chronically infected with HBV was 102 times greater than the risk in the uninfected [23]. In a study of native Alaskan men who were chronically infected with HBV, the annual incidence of HCC was found to be 387 per

100,000 men [24]. The lifetime risk of HCC in infected men is estimated to be between 10% and 25%, while the risk in infected woman is lower [15].

Among those with chronic HBV (aka "carriers"), the risk of HCC increases with duration of infection. In many developing countries in Asia and Africa where HBV is endemic, the majority of infections are acquired during the perinatal period or during very early childhood [25]. Studies have shown that HBV carriers born to HBV-infected mothers have an increased risk of HCC compared to other HBV carriers, which is likely related to a longer duration of infection [23]. Thus, in high-risk countries, HCC is not a rare occurrence at ages 20–35 years [3]. This is in contrast to the situation in countries with a relatively low incidence of HCC, where most HBV infections are acquired in adulthood through sexual contact, intravenous drug use, blood transfusions, or invasive medical procedures. The carcinogenic potential of neonatal infection with HBV was illustrated by experimental studies involving the woodchuck hepatitis virus model, which parallels human HBV infection. Inoculation of newborn woodchucks with woodchuck hepatitis virus led to chronic infection with the virus and HCC within 3 years [26].

Severity of liver disease is also a key determinant of risk of HCC among individuals infected with HBV. The annual risk for HCC among chronic carriers [i.e., hepatitis B surface antigen (HBsAg) positive] ranges from 0.3% to 0.6%. The risk increases to 1% in patients with chronic hepatitis and 2–6.6% in cirrhotic patients [1]. The risk of HCC appears to be higher in chronic carriers who are also hepatitis B e antigen (HBeAg) positive. A prospective study of more than 11,000 Taiwanese men followed for 10 years revealed that the relative risk of HCC was 60.2 times (95% confidence interval, 35.5–102.1) greater in men positive for both HBsAg and HBeAg and 9.6 times (95% confidence interval, 6.0–15.2) greater among those positive for HBsAg alone, when compared to men who were negative for both antigens [27]. Another large prospective study performed in Taiwan found that the incidence of HCC increased directly with the serum level of HBV DNA in a "dose–response" relationship, with a cumulative incidence rate of 1.3% for individuals with HBV DNA levels of <300 copies/ml and 14.9% for those with HBV DNA levels of one million copies/ml and greater [28]. In addition to viral load, genotype C HBV infection is associated with increased risk of HCC [29]. Other factors which increase the risk of HCC among chronic carriers of HBV include male gender, age, family history, alcohol abuse, tobacco use, aflatoxin exposure, coinfection with hepatitis C or D virus, and core promoter mutations (T1762/A1764) [30, 31].

The implementation of universal vaccination programs against hepatitis B has led to a decrease in the incidence of chronic HBV infection and the subsequent development of HCC worldwide. Studies from Taiwan have shown that after introduction of a universal infant vaccination program against HBV in 1984, the incidence of HCC among children ages 6–14 years declined from 0.7 per 100,000 children between 1981 and 1986 to 0.57 between 1986 and 1990 and to 0.36 between 1990 and 1994 [32]. Several meta-analyses have shown that successful treatment of chronic HBV infection with antiviral therapies and subsequent reduction in detectable viral load also significantly decreases the risk of HCC [33, 34].

Hepatitis C

Chronic hepatitis C infection is one of the most important risk factors for HCC in developed countries including the United States, many countries in Europe, and Japan. Worldwide, there are about 170 million people with chronic HCV infection, with 3–4 million new infections occurring each year [15]. In contrast to other Asian countries, in Japan, HCV infection accounts for 80–90% of all cases of HCC [35]. In the United States, HCV accounts for about one-third of HCC cases [36]. The rising incidence of HCC in the United States and Europe in recent decades is thought to be largely due to the concomitant increase in the prevalence of longstanding HCV infection [36].

Before the identification of HCV in 1989, Okuda et al. hypothesized that a non-A, non-B virus accounted for a significant proportion of HCC in Japan based on the fact that the incidence of HCC had doubled despite a reduction in HBV-associated HCC [37]. This hypothesis was verified when assays for detection of HCV antibodies were discovered [38]. Subsequent prospective data on patients in Japan and elsewhere confirmed that HCC can result from long-term infection with HCV [39]. In almost all cases, the development of cirrhosis precedes the diagnosis of HCC [15].

In a meta-analysis of 32 case–control studies, the estimated risk of HCC was found to be 17-fold greater in individuals with chronic HCV infection compared to HCV-negative individuals [40]. Similar to chronic HBV infection, the duration and severity of liver disease are crucial determinants of the risk for developing HCC in those with chronic HCV infection. The annual risk of developing HCC was 0.4% in HCV carriers with abnormal ALT values, 1.7% in those with chronic active hepatitis, and 2.5% in those with compensated cirrhosis [1]. Another prospective study showed that the annual incidence of HCC increased with degree of hepatic fibrosis, from 0.5% in patients with little or no fibrosis to 7.9% among those with advanced fibrosis [39]. In addition to coinfection with HBV, other factors associated with increased risk of HCC in HCV include alcohol abuse, diabetes mellitus, obesity, and male gender [41, 42]. Coinfection with human immunodeficiency virus (HIV) is also associated with more rapid progression of liver disease and increased risk of HCC in patients with chronic HCV infection [43].

The majority of HCV infections are acquired in adulthood, mainly as a result of exposure to contaminated blood products or intravenous drug abuse. Unfortunately, there is no current vaccine available against HCV. Prevention efforts are thus based on preventing transmission by transfusion of contaminated blood products and nosocomial infections as well as targeting high-risk populations [44]. Treatment with interferon, ribavirn, and directly-acting antivirals to prevent the progression of chronic infection to advanced cirrhosis has been shown to significantly decrease the risk of HCC, especially among patients who achieve sustained virologic response [39]. It is important to recognize that patients with HCV-induced cirrhosis who have cleared the virus remain at risk for HCC, albeit at lower rates than HCV cirrhotics with detectable viral loads [45].

Aflatoxin

Aflatoxin B1 is a mycotoxin produced by strains of *Aspergillus flavus* and related fungi. It is a common contaminant of corn, peanuts, and soybeans in many countries in Asia and sub-Saharan Africa, where warm environmental conditions and methods of food storage can result in large quantities of aflatoxins in the food supply [1]. Humans are exposed by ingestion of contaminated grains, legumes, or animals fed with contaminated cereals. Aflatoxin B1 is highly mutagenic and, once ingested, is metabolized to an active epoxide intermediate that has been shown to covalently bind to and damage DNA [46]. A specific mutation at the third base of codon 249 of the tumor suppressor gene TP53 has been found in HCC from individuals living in areas in Africa and China with high levels of dietary exposure to aflatoxin [1]. In animal models, rats treated with aflatoxin B1 developed HCC in a dose-dependent manner [22].

Globally, the incidence of HCC parallels the prevalence of aflatoxin-contaminated food products [1]. A nested case–control study of 18,000 men in Shanghai revealed a relative risk for HCC of 3.8 (95% confidence interval, 1.2–12.2) among men with only aflatoxin biomarkers detected. The risk of HCC increased to 8.5 (95% confidence interval, 2.8–26.3) among chronic HBV carriers and skyrocketed to 60.1 (95% confidence interval, 6.4–561.8) among those with both aflatoxin and HBV exposure [47]. Thus, this environmental carcinogen appears to act synergistically with chronic HBV infection to increase the risk of HCC. In a study of men with chronic HBV infection in Qidong, China, aflatoxin exposure, which was measured by the aflatoxin metabolite M1 in pooled monthly urine samples, increased the relative risk for HCC 3.3-fold (95% confidence interval, 1.2–8.7) [48]. In many areas of the world where aflatoxin exposure is common, chronic HBV infection is also endemic, which highlights the importance of HBV vaccination in these regions and public health efforts to reduce aflatoxin exposure by preventing contamination of food products.

Alcohol

Alcohol abuse is a major risk factor for the development of HCC in western countries. The mechanism by which alcohol increases HCC risk is not well understood. Although there are associations between heavy alcohol use and some cancers, there is little direct evidence that alcohol has carcinogenic properties [1]. However, long-standing alcohol abuse can lead to cirrhosis, which is a predisposing factor for HCC. Studies have shown that alcohol abuse is a risk factor for HCC independent of hepatitis B or C infection, although higher levels of intake are likely needed for HCC development in the absence of infection [49]. The relationship between alcohol consumption and the risk of HCC appears to be dose dependent. Furthermore, there appears to be a synergistic effect of alcohol abuse with either HBV or HCV infection [49].

Table 1.1 summarizes the primary etiologic risk factors for HCC.

Table 1.1 Risk factors for hepatocellular carcinoma

Chronic viral hepatitis (HCV, HBV)

Toxins (alcohol, aflatoxin)

Metabolic liver disease (hereditary hemochromatosis)

Cirrhosis of any etiology

Diabetes mellitus*

Obesity*

* Diabetes and obesity are additional risk factors in the setting of cirrhosis

Molecular Pathogenesis

There is increasing evidence that the development of HCC, similar to most other cancers, is a multistep process involving a number of different genetic and epigenetic alterations that eventually leads to the malignant transformation of hepatocytes [50, 51]. The genetic changes appear to be complex and may occur over decades, which may partly explain the difficulty in elucidating the sequential molecular changes that lead to HCC. Furthermore, there appears to be a great deal of genetic heterogeneity among tumors, even among different tumor nodules in the same patient. This likely reflects the heterogeneity of etiologic factors, which contribute to HCC development, and suggests that a common unifying pathway for hepatocarcinogenesis may not exist.

Regardless of the etiologic agent, malignant transformation of hepatocytes is thought to occur through a pathway of continuous hepatocyte injury and regeneration which takes place in the setting of chronic inflammation over many years. This leads to increased stem cell proliferation, hepatocyte turnover, and accumulation of genetic and epigenetic changes that allow hepatocytes to expand in a clonal fashion, leading to dysplastic nodules and the development of liver cancer (Fig. 1.2) [52, 53]. Such genomic alterations may include chromosomal rearrangements, activation of cellular oncogenes, and inactivation of tumor suppressor genes [50]. This may occur in conjunction with defective DNA mismatch repair, telomerase activation, and induction of growth and angiogenic factors [50]. Chronic viral hepatitis, alcohol abuse, and metabolic liver diseases such as HH are thought to act mainly through this indirect pathway of chronic liver injury, resultant oxidative stress, and inflammation [50].

Hepatitis B infection may also directly cause HCC through integration of its DNA into the genome of infected hepatocytes. HBV is a member of a family of oncogenic viruses known as hepadnavirus. Integrated HBV sequences have been detected in HCC cell lines and 80% of HBV-associated HCC [54]. The integration sites are often located in genes which play an important role in cell signaling and regulation of growth, leading to a selective growth advantage of infected cells and tumor development. The genetic aberrations observed as a result of HBV integration include inverted duplications, deletions, amplifications, and chromosomal translocations [16]. This results in an increase in host chromosomal instability, inactivation of tumor suppressor genes, and production of oncogenic proteins [16].

Pathway of Hepatic Neoplasia

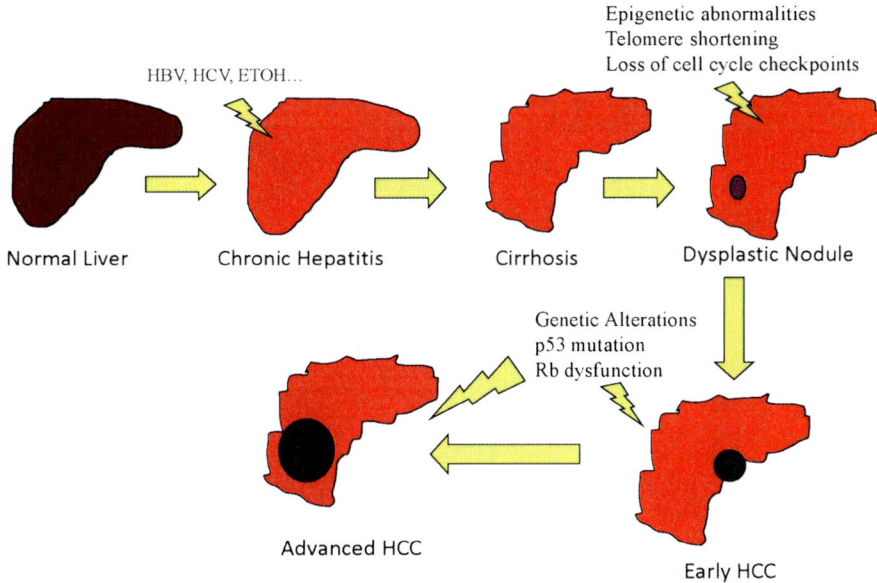

Epigenetic abnormalities
Telomere shortening
Loss of cell cycle checkpoints

HBV, HCV, ETOH...

Normal Liver   Chronic Hepatitis   Cirrhosis   Dysplastic Nodule

Genetic Alterations
p53 mutation
Rb dysfunction

Advanced HCC

Early HCC

Fig. 1.2 Pathway of hepatic neoplasia. An etiologic agent such as hepatitis C (HCV) infects the liver leading to injury and inflammation. Chronic hepatitis leads to fibrosis and cirrhosis. Epigenetic alterations develop, leading to the clonal proliferation of hepatocytes into dysplastic nodules. Further cell turnover and injury lead to genetic abnormalities and full-blown carcinoma. *Rb* retinoblastoma

Furthermore, the X protein of the hepatitis B genome has been shown to interfere with the expression of tumor suppressor genes which in turn leads to inhibition of the important pro-apoptotic protein TP53 [55].

Unlike HBV, the HCV RNA virus is unable to integrate into the genome of its host cell due to the absence of reverse transcriptase activity. The fact that HCC develops after many years of chronic infection and is almost always preceded by progression to cirrhosis provides support for the paradigm of chronic liver injury, leading to cell death, regeneration, cirrhosis, and development of HCC [50]. However, recent studies have shown the HCV may also directly lead to the malignant transformation of hepatocytes. The core protein of HCV and the NS3 protease protein have been shown to have oncogenic potential [50]. The development of HCC in individuals with HCV infection without cirrhosis, although rare, has been reported, and provides support for this possibility [56].

Advances in molecular biology including the ability to perform genome wide analysis of gene expression has led to the identification of a host of genetic and epigenetic alterations and signaling pathways that play a role in HCC pathogenesis. Almost 30% of HCC cases have mutations in the p53 gene. Mutations in genes that disrupt the canonical WNT-β catenin signaling pathway, the activation of which regulates specific oncogenes, are also common [52]. The Raf/Ras/Erk pathway is almost ubiquitously activated in advanced liver cancer as a result of increased signaling from growth factors such as epidermal growth factor (EGF), hepatocyte growth factor (HGF), and insulin-like growth factor (IGF) [57]. Angiogenesis, as in most cases of human cancer, plays a crucial role and is mediated by the activation of various pathways including vascular endothelial growth factor receptor (VEGFR) and platelet-derived growth factor receptor (PDGFR) [58, 59]. The understanding of the molecular basis of HCC pathogenesis has led to the discovery of therapies for HCC directed against novel molecular targets. For example, sorafenib is a multikinase inhibitor of VEGFR2, PDGFR, Raf-1, B-Raf, and other molecules and has been shown to have a survival benefit and delay tumor progression in patients with advanced HCC [60].

Natural History and Prognosis

A few decades ago, the prognosis of HCC was universally dismal, with the majority patients dying within 1 year of diagnosis [61]. The implementation of surveillance programs targeting high-risk populations such as chronic HBV carriers and individuals with cirrhosis has led to the detection of HCC at earlier stages when potentially curative treatments are an option. In developed countries, 30–40% of patients are now being diagnosed at such early stages [62]. A study in Hong Kong showed that patients in whom HCC is diagnosed by regular screening with AFP testing and/ or ultrasonography have a significantly smaller tumor size, lower serum AFP levels, and a lower prevalence of multifocal disease, portal vein infiltration, and distant metastases compared to patients presenting with symptomatic disease [63]. Thus, a higher proportion of patients who underwent screening were eligible for curative resection compared to symptomatic patients (26.8% vs. 7.9%, respectively) [63].

HCC is detected as a multinodular tumor in half of the patients with compensated cirrhosis undergoing surveillance [64]. A multinodular pattern is more common in patients with multiple etiologic risk factors [65]. Multinodular HCC may represent either primary tumors of multifocal origin or intrahepatic metastases from a primary tumor [1].

During its early stages, HCC tends to be clinically indolent. The median doubling time for small tumors is highly variable, ranging from only 1 month to 20 months [1]. A study by Okazaki found that the median doubling time for small tumors, defined as a size <4.5 cm in diameter, was 6 months, with a positive correlation existing between tumor doubling time and survival length [66]. Given the variability in tumor doubling time, tumor size alone does not predict disease course. For example, 40% of tumors <2 cm in size have evidence of microscopic venous invasion, which is a surrogate for the presence of metastatic disease [67]. Characteristics of HCC which are associated with more aggressive disease include large tumor size (>6 cm), poorly differentiated histology, lack of fibrous capsule, and early vascular invasion [16].

HCC has a strong propensity for vascular invasion and metastasis. An autopsy study of 490 cases of HCC in Sweden found that 56% of cases had evidence of vascular invasion [68]. Metastases were commonly observed to the lymph nodes, lungs, and skeleton. Rare but important sites of metastases are the adrenal glands and brain. The presence of metastases was associated with vascular invasion, multinodular disease, bilobar involvement, and poorly differentiated histology [68]. A retrospective review of 347 patients with HCC in the United States who had undergone a workup for metastatic disease found that 42% of patients had evidence of thoracic, abdominal, or bone metastases [69]. Again, the strongest predictors of metastatic disease identified by logistic regression analysis were poorly differentiated histology, multilobular spread, and tumor size of ≥ 5 cm [69].

Unfortunately, the majority of patients with HCC are still diagnosed at advanced stages when surgery is no longer an option for treatment. At this stage, patients may be symptomatic with jaundice and abdominal pain. The prognosis for symptomatic HCC is dismal, with a median survival of <6 months from the onset of symptoms and no survival benefit from treatment [70].

Staging

The prognosis of HCC is determined by a combination of factors including tumor status, underlying liver function, and performance status [1]. Tumor status is defined by the size of the main nodule and number of nodules. A number of staging classification systems which incorporate these variables have been used to predict the prognosis for HCC, none of which have been universally adopted. Such staging systems are used to guide treatment selection as they strongly predict treatment outcome.

The tumor node metastasis (TNM) staging system widely used in oncology does not accurately predict survival in patients with HCC, in whom underlying liver function also plays a critical role in determining outcome. The Okuda staging system, devised by Okuda et al. in 1985, was the first widely accepted system to predict prognosis which incorporates tumor size and severity of hepatic impairment [61]. The variables in this model which assess hepatic function are the presence of ascites and serum levels of albumin and bilirubin. The median survival of untreated patients with Stages 1, 2, and 3 disease was 8 months, 2 months, and 0.7 months, respectively [61].

Newer prognostic scoring systems have been developed that incorporate additional variables, such as the presence of vascular invasion and metastases, which more accurately predict survival in patients with HCC. The Cancer of the Liver Italian Program (CLIP) system allocates points to four variables that affect prognosis: Child–Pugh stage, tumor morphology, serum AFP levels, and the presence of portal vein thrombosis (Table 1.2) [71]. A validation study revealed median survival times of 31, 27, 13, 8, and 2 months for CLIP Stages 0, 1, 2, 3, and 4–6, respectively [72].

Table 1.2 Cancer of the Liver Italian Program (CLIP) staging system

Scores	Tumor morphology	Child–Pugh	AFP (µg/dl)	Vascular invasion
0	Single nodule of liver <50%	A	<400	No
1	Multinodular of liver >50%	B	>400	Yes
2	Massive	C		No

Adapted from Gallo et al. [71]

Table 1.3 Barcelona Clinic Liver Cancer (BCLC) staging classification

Staging	Performance status	Tumor stage	Child–Pugh
(A) Early	0	Single <5 cm Three nodes<3 cm	A&B
(B) Intermediate	0	Large/multinodular	A&B
(C) Advanced	1–2	Vascular invasion Extrahepatic spread	A&B
(D) End-stage	3–4	Any of above	C

Adapted from Llovet et al. [70]

The Barcelona Clinic Liver Cancer (BCLC) Group staging classification consists of four stages based on tumor stage (which incorporates tumor size and the presence of vascular invasion or extrahepatic spread), Child–Pugh class, performance status, and the presence of constitutional symptoms (Table 1.3) [70]. Characterization of patients according to such stages allows for selection of the best possible treatment options for patients. Patients with early stage (A) disease have small, asymptomatic tumors and experience a significant survival benefit from curative therapies such as surgical resection or transplantation. Intermediate stage (B) patients have asymptomatic, multinodular disease, while advanced stage (C) patients have symptomatic tumors, vascular invasion, or extrahepatic spread. Such patients may be candidates for palliative treatments or enrollment in randomized clinical trials of experimental therapies including sorafenib and/or transarterial chemoembolization (TACE). Patients with end-stage (D) disease have very poor survival, and only symptomatic treatment is indicated given the lack of any survival benefit from current therapies [70].

Conclusions

Hepatocellular carcinoma is the most common malignant tumor of the liver and represents a major global public health problem. The incidence of the disease varies widely by geography, ethnicity, and gender because of its association with well-defined risk factors which differ in prevalence around the world. Infection with hepatitis B and C virus leading to chronic hepatitis and cirrhosis is the leading cause worldwide and accounts for more than 80% of all cases of HCC. Prevention efforts including implementation of HBV vaccination programs and reduction of dietary aflatoxin exposure in developing countries can substantially reduce the incidence and mortality of the disease. The rise in HCC incidence in developed countries such as the United States due to the increase in Hepatitis C infection highlights the need for efforts to prevent Hepatitis C transmission by targeting high-risk groups and preventing the use of contaminated blood products. The molecular pathogenesis of HCC is not fully understood, but appears to involve multiple complex genetic and epigenetic changes that occur over decades in the setting of chronic liver injury and regeneration. A better understanding of the steps in hepatocarcinogenesis can lead to novel molecular-targeted therapies. The overall survival of patients with HCC remains poor, as many patients present with advanced stages of the disease when curative treatment is not available. Important determinants of prognosis include characteristics of the tumor (including size, presence of vascular invasion, and histology) and the patient's underlying liver function.

References

1. Columbo M. In: Sorrell MF, Schiff ER, Maddrey WC, editors. Diseases of the liver. Philadelphia: Lippincott Williams & Wilkins; 2003. pp. 1378–91.
2. Parkin DM, et al. Global cancer statistics, 2002. CA Cancer J Clin. 2005;55(2):74–108.
3. Bosch FX, et al. Primary liver cancer: worldwide incidence and trends. Gastroenterology. 2004;127(5 Suppl 1):S5–16.
4. McGlynn KA, et al. International trends and patterns of primary liver cancer. Int J Cancer. 2001;94(2):290–6.
5. El-Serag HB, Mason AC. Rising incidence of hepatocellular carcinoma in the United States. N Engl J Med. 1999;340(10):745–50.
6. El-Serag HB, et al. The continuing increase in the incidence of hepatocellular carcinoma in the United States: an update. Ann Intern Med. 2003;139(10):817–23.
7. Hepatocellular carcinoma—United States, 2001–2006. MMWR Morb Mortal Wkly Rep, 2010. 59(17):517–20.
8. Wong R, Corley DA. Racial and ethnic variations in hepatocellular carcinoma incidence within the United States. Am J Med. 2008;121(6):525–31.
9. Rosenblatt KA, Weiss NS, Schwartz SM. Liver cancer in Asian migrants to the United States and their descendants. Cancer Causes Control. 1996;7(3):345–50.
10. Bosch FX, Ribes J, Borras J. Epidemiology of primary liver cancer. Semin Liver Dis. 1999;19(3):271–85.
11. Kew MC. Hepatocellular carcinoma in African Blacks: Recent progress in etiology and pathogenesis. World J Hepatol. 2010;2(2):65–73.
12. Umoh NJ, et al. Aetiological differences in demographical, clinical and pathological characteristics of hepatocellular carcinoma in the Gambia. Liver Int. 2011;31(2):215–21.
13. Bruix J, Sherman M. Management of hepatocellular carcinoma: an update. Hepatology. 2011;53(3):1020–2.
14. Colombo M, Berr F, Bruix J, Hauss J, Wands J, Wittekind C. In: Berr F, Bruix J, Hauss J, Wittekind C, Wands J, editors. Risk groups and preventive strategies. Malignant liver tumors: basic concepts and clinical management (Falk Symposium). Kluwer Academic Publishers BV and Falk Foundation; 2003. pp. 67–74.
15. McGlynn KA, London WT. Epidemiology and natural history of hepatocellular carcinoma. Best Pract Res Clin Gastroenterol. 2005;19(1):3–23.

16. But DY, Lai CL, Yuen MF. Natural history of hepatitis-related hepatocellular carcinoma. World J Gastroenterol. 2008;14(11):1652–6.
17. Donato MF, et al. High rates of hepatocellular carcinoma in cirrhotic patients with high liver cell proliferative activity. Hepatology. 2001;34(3):523–8.
18. Colombo M, et al. Hepatocellular carcinoma in Italian patients with cirrhosis. N Engl J Med. 1991;325(10):675–80.
19. Niederau C, et al. Survival and causes of death in cirrhotic and in noncirrhotic patients with primary hemochromatosis. N Engl J Med. 1985;313(20):1256–62.
20. Calle EE, et al. Overweight, obesity, and mortality from cancer in a prospectively studied cohort of U.S. adults. N Engl J Med. 2003;348(17):1625–38.
21. Adami HO, et al. Excess risk of primary liver cancer in patients with diabetes mellitus. J Natl Cancer Inst. 1996;88(20):1472–7.
22. Colombo M, Sangiovanni A. Etiology, natural history and treatment of hepatocellular carcinoma. Antiviral Res. 2003;60(2):145–50.
23. Beasley RP. Hepatitis B virus. The major etiology of hepatocellular carcinoma. Cancer. 1988;61(10):1942–56.
24. McMahon BJ, et al. Hepatitis B-related sequelae. Prospective study in 1400 hepatitis B surface antigen-positive Alaska native carriers. Arch Intern Med. 1990;150(5):1051–4.
25. Gacic-Dobo M, et al. Global progress toward universal childhood hepatitis B vaccination, 2003. MMWR Morb Mortal Wkly Rep. 2003; 52(36):868–70.
26. Popper H, et al. Hepatocarcinogenicity of the woodchuck hepatitis virus. Proc Natl Acad Sci USA. 1987;84(3):866–70.
27. Yang HI, et al. Hepatitis B e antigen and the risk of hepatocellular carcinoma. N Engl J Med. 2002;347(3):168–74.
28. Chen CJ, et al. Risk of hepatocellular carcinoma across a biological gradient of serum hepatitis B virus DNA level. J Am Med Assoc. 2006;295(1):65–73.
29. Yu MW, et al. Hepatitis B virus genotype and DNA level and hepatocellular carcinoma: a prospective study in men. J Natl Cancer Inst. 2005;97(4):265–72.
30. Raoul JL. Natural history of hepatocellular carcinoma and current treatment options. Semin Nucl Med. 2008;38(2):S13–8.
31. Liu CJ, et al. Role of hepatitis B viral load and basal core promoter mutation in hepatocellular carcinoma in hepatitis B carriers. J Infect Dis. 2006;193(9):1258–65.
32. Chang MH, et al. Universal hepatitis B vaccination in Taiwan and the incidence of hepatocellular carcinoma in children. Taiwan Childhood Hepatoma Study Group. N Engl J Med. 1997;336(26):1855–9.
33. Sung JJ, et al. Meta-analysis: treatment of hepatitis B infection reduces risk of hepatocellular carcinoma. Aliment Pharmacol Ther. 2008;28(9):1067–77.
34. Papatheodoridis GV, et al. Incidence of hepatocellular carcinoma in chronic hepatitis B patients receiving nucleos(t)ide therapy: a systematic review. J Hepatol. 2010;53(2):348–56.
35. El-Serag HB, Rudolph KL. Hepatocellular carcinoma: epidemiology and molecular carcinogenesis. Gastroenterology. 2007;132(7):2557–76.
36. Davila JA, et al. Hepatitis C infection and the increasing incidence of hepatocellular carcinoma: a population-based study. Gastroenterology. 2004;127(5):1372–80.
37. Okuda K, et al. Changing incidence of hepatocellular carcinoma in Japan. Cancer Res. 1987;47(18):4967–72.
38. Kiyosawa K, et al. Interrelationship of blood transfusion, non-A, non-B hepatitis and hepatocellular carcinoma: analysis by detection of antibody to hepatitis C virus. Hepatology. 1990;12(4 Pt 1):671–5.
39. Yoshida H, et al. Interferon therapy reduces the risk for hepatocellular carcinoma: national surveillance program of cirrhotic and noncirrhotic patients with chronic hepatitis C in Japan. IHIT Study Group. Inhibition of Hepatocarcinogenesis by Interferon Therapy. Ann Intern Med. 1999;131(3):174–81.
40. Donato F, Boffetta P, Puoti M. A meta-analysis of epidemiological studies on the combined effect of hepatitis B and C virus infections in causing hepatocellular carcinoma. Int J Cancer. 1998;75(3):347–54.

41. Hassan MM, et al. Risk factors for hepatocellular carcinoma: synergism of alcohol with viral hepatitis and diabetes mellitus. Hepatology. 2002;36(5):1206–13.
42. Ohki T, et al. Obesity is an independent risk factor for hepatocellular carcinoma development in chronic hepatitis C patients. Clin Gastroenterol Hepatol. 2008;6(4):459–64.
43. Garcia-Samaniego J, et al. Hepatocellular carcinoma in HIV-infected patients with chronic hepatitis C. Am J Gastroenterol. 2001;96(1):179–83.
44. Llovet JM, Burroughs A, Bruix J. Hepatocellular carcinoma. Lancet. 2003;362(9399):1907–17.
45. Morgan TR, et al. Outcome of sustained virological responders with histologically advanced chronic hepatitis C. Hepatology. 2010;52(3):833–44.
46. Scaife JF. Aflatoxin B(1): Cytotoxic mode of action evaluated by mammalian cell cultures. FEBS Lett. 1971;12(3):143–7.
47. Ross RK, et al. Urinary aflatoxin biomarkers and risk of hepatocellular carcinoma. Lancet. 1992;339(8799):943–6.
48. Sun Z, et al. Increased risk of hepatocellular carcinoma in male hepatitis B surface antigen carriers with chronic hepatitis who have detectable urinary aflatoxin metabolite M1. Hepatology. 1999;30(2):379–83.
49. Donato F, et al. Alcohol and hepatocellular carcinoma: the effect of lifetime intake and hepatitis virus infections in men and women. Am J Epidemiol. 2002;155(4):323–31.
50. Moradpour D, Wands JR. Molecular pathogenesis of hepatocellular carcinoma in hepatology: a textbook of liver disease. In: Zakim D, Boyer TD, editors. Philadelphia: Saunders; 2003. pp. 1333–54.
51. Hamilton JP. Epigenetic mechanisms involved in the pathogenesis of hepatobiliary malignancies. Epigenomics. 2010;2(2):233–43.
52. Minguez B, et al. Pathogenesis of hepatocellular carcinoma and molecular therapies. Curr Opin Gastroenterol. 2009;25(3):186–94.
53. Mishra L, et al. Liver stem cells and hepatocellular carcinoma. Hepatology. 2009;49(1):318–29.
54. Brechot C, et al. Presence of integrated hepatitis B virus DNA sequences in cellular DNA of human hepatocellular carcinoma. Nature. 1980;286(5772):533–5.
55. Chung TW, et al. Hepatitis B Virus X protein modulates the expression of PTEN by inhibiting the function of p53, a transcriptional activator in liver cells. Cancer Res. 2003;63(13):3453–8.
56. De Mitri MS, et al. HCV-associated liver cancer without cirrhosis. Lancet. 1995;345(8947):413–5.
57. Calvisi DF, et al. Ubiquitous activation of Ras and Jak/Stat pathways in human HCC. Gastroenterology. 2006;130(4):1117–28.
58. Chiang DY, et al. Focal gains of VEGFA and molecular classification of hepatocellular carcinoma. Cancer Res. 2008;68(16):6779–88.
59. Villanueva A, et al. Genomics and signaling pathways in hepatocellular carcinoma. Semin Liver Dis. 2007;27(1):55–76.
60. Villanueva A, Toffanin S, Llovet JM. Linking molecular classification of hepatocellular carcinoma and personalized medicine: preliminary steps. Curr Opin Oncol. 2008;20(4):444–53.
61. Okuda K, et al. Natural history of hepatocellular carcinoma and prognosis in relation to treatment. Study of 850 patients. Cancer. 1985;56(4):918–28.
62. Bruix J, Llovet JM. Prognostic prediction and treatment strategy in hepatocellular carcinoma. Hepatology. 2002;35(3):519–24.
63. Yuen MF, et al. Early detection of hepatocellular carcinoma increases the chance of treatment: Hong Kong experience. Hepatology. 2000;31(2):330–5.
64. Fasani P, et al. High prevalence of multinodular hepatocellular carcinoma in patients with cirrhosis attributable to multiple risk factors. Hepatology. 1999;29(6):1704–7.
65. Benvegnu L, et al. Evidence for an association between the aetiology of cirrhosis and pattern of hepatocellular carcinoma development. Gut. 2001;48(1):110–5.
66. Okazaki N, et al. Evaluation of the prognosis for small hepatocellular carcinoma based on tumor volume doubling time. A preliminary report. Cancer. 1989;63(11):2207–10.
67. Tsai TJ, et al. Clinical significance of microscopic tumor venous invasion in patients with resectable hepatocellular carcinoma. Surgery. 2000;127(6):603–8.

68. Kaczynski J, Hansson G, Wallerstedt S. Metastases in cases with hepatocellular carcinoma in relation to clinicopathologic features of the tumor. An autopsy study from a low endemic area. Acta Oncol. 1995;34(1):43–8.
69. Si MS, et al. Prevalence of metastases in hepatocellular carcinoma: risk factors and impact on survival. Am Surg. 2003;69(10):879–85.
70. Llovet JM, Bru C, Bruix J. Prognosis of hepatocellular carcinoma: the BCLC staging classification. Semin Liver Dis. 1999;19(3):329–38.
71. Gallo C, et al. A new prognostic system for hepatocellular carcinoma: A retrospective study of 435 patients. Hepatology. 1998;28:751–5. doi: 10.1002/hep.510280322.
72. Farinati F, et al. How should patients with hepatocellular carcinoma be staged? Validation of a new prognostic system. Cancer. 2000;89(11):2266–73.

Chapter 2
Surveillance for Hepatocellular Carcinoma

Reezwana Chowdhury and Rohit Satoskar

Background

Screening for cancer has become an integral part of medicine. Screening is a public health service in which members of a defined population are offered a test to identify individuals who are likely to benefit from further testing or treatment aimed at reducing the risk of a disease or its complications. Surveillance, on the other hand, is the continuous monitoring of disease occurrence using the screening test within an at-risk population to achieve the same goals as screening [1].

The ultimate goal of a cancer screening program is to reduce site-specific mortality. The benefits of screening should outweigh the costs before the use of a given test is promoted [1]. Ideally, screening will help to reduce morbidity and mortality by detecting asymptomatic disease or disease precursors and thereby allowing early treatment initiation in the natural history of a disease. Numerous screening tests have been investigated throughout the years, and many are now part of standard practice. These tests include the Papanicolaou test for cervical cancer, mammography for breast cancer, and colonoscopy for colorectal cancer. These methods have been shown to detect asymptomatic, treatable, early-stage disease and affect mortality [1]. On the other hand, if there is no effective treatment or if the disease is too rapidly progressive, then there is no value in screening [1]. If patients benefit from treatment before the onset of symptoms, then survival improvements should be associated with the gain in lead time compared to those diagnosed after the onset of symptoms. If there is no survival advantage and if life expectancy is not extended beyond when death would occur without early detection, then there is only the appearance of greater survival. This is referred to as lead time bias and serves as a major pitfall in many studies of screening and surveillance methods. In addition,

R. Chowdhury, MD • R. Satoskar, MD (✉)
Georgetown Transplant Institute, Georgetown University Hospital, Washington, DC, USA
e-mail: Rohit.S.Satoskar@gunet.georgetown.edu

N. Reau and F.F. Poordad (eds.), *Primary Liver Cancer: Surveillance, Diagnosis and Treatment*, Clinical Gastroenterology, DOI 10.1007/978-1-61779-863-4_2,
© Springer Science+Business Media New York 2012

Table 2.1 Recommendations for HCC surveillance in high-risk patients [2–5]

American Association for the Study of Liver Diseases (AASLD)	European Association for the Study of the Liver (EASL)	Asian Pacific Association for the Study of the Liver (APASL)	National Comprehensive Cancer Network (NCCN)
Ultrasound every 6 months	Ultrasound and AFP every 6 months	Ultrasound and AFP every 6 months	Ultrasound and AFP every 6 months

there are potential harms associated with screening such with perforation from a colonoscopy or unnecessary concern and anxiety over a lesion that may be detected on mammography. In addition, the specificity and sensitivity of all currently available screening tests are less than 100%, producing false-positive result and false-negative results, respectively. Therefore, it is important to screen populations which are considered at risk for the disease in question.

The World Health Organization has set criteria for a cancer screening program. First, the disease for which screening is being recommended should be an important health problem. Second, there should be an identifiable target population who is at risk for disease. Third, treatment of the occult disease should offer advantages compared with treatment of symptomatic disease. Fourth, the screening test should be affordable and must achieve an acceptable level of accuracy. Finally, the test must be acceptable to the target population and to health-care professionals, and standardized recall procedures should be used for when an abnormality is identified [1].

The utility of screening for hepatocellular cancer has been debated for many years and further fueled by the paucity of randomized controlled trials that show a clear benefit. However, despite this, HCC surveillance is widely applied to at-risk individuals and is currently recommended by most professional societies (Table 2.1).

Importance of HCC as a Health Problem

Hepatocellular carcinoma (HCC) is the fifth most common solid tumor worldwide and accounts for 5.6% of all cancers [6]. The incidence of HCC has been rising since the early 1980s, and it is now the third leading cause of cancer-related mortality. In the USA, an estimated 18, 910 liver cancer deaths are expected in 2010 according to the American Cancer Society [7]. There is geographic variation in the incidence of liver cancer around the world and is highest in Mongolia with an age adjusted rate of 116.6 cases per 100,000 person–years for men and 74.8 cases per 100,000 person–years for women [8]. Eighty percent of cases are found in developing countries, with highest rates in Asia and sub-Saharan Africa [9]. These rates mirror the rates of chronic viral hepatitis [10]. Over the past two decades, the incidence of HCC has increased in the USA and continues to rise particularly in white middle-aged men most likely due to chronic HCV infection [11, 12].

At-Risk Population

In all areas of the world, the incidence is higher in males than females, with ratios varying from 1.4 to 3.3. The most common risk for development of HCC is cirrhosis, with annual risk for between 1% and 8%. In fact, more than 80% of HCCs arise in patients with cirrhosis of the liver [13]. In addition, the risk of developing HCC also varies according to the cause of chronic liver disease. Based on a theoretical cohort study, the current AASLD guidelines suggest that screening should be employed in cirrhotics when risk of HCC exceeds 1.5% per year [14, 15].

Chronic HBV

Chronic hepatitis B infection accounts for 52.3% of all HCC worldwide, and approximately 40% of patients with chronic HBV that develop HCC are not cirrhotic. The incidence of HCC in chronic HBV as a whole ranges from 0.26% to 0.5% per year, and these individuals are 100 times more likely to develop HCC than those who are uninfected [16, 17]. In patients with chronic HBV and cirrhosis, the incidence may be as high as 2.8% per year [18]. Aside from the presence of cirrhosis, factors which affect risk of HCC in chronic HBV include family history of HCC, ethnic background, HBV DNA level, HBV genotype, and presence of HBV mutants. The Risk Evaluation of Viral Load Elevation and Associated Liver Disease/ Cancer-Hepatitis B Virus (REVEAL-HBV) trials study a prospective cohort of patients in Taiwan with chronic HBV who were recruited to a community-based cancer screening program. In this population, incidence of HCC increased in a dose response-dependent relationship as HBV viral load at entry increased. Cumulative incidence of HCC in patients with HBV DNA > one million copies/mL was 14.9% at the end of the 13th year of follow-up [19, 20]. Additional data from this group also shows that patients with HBV genotype C and precore or basal core promoter mutations are at higher risk of developing HCC [21]. The age at which an individual acquires HBV and the rate of active viral replication affect the age at which an individual develops HCC.

In a study comparing HBV carriers from Haimen City, China, and Senegal, West Africa, HCC mortality appeared higher in Haimen City than in Senegal, 878 vs. 68 per 10^5 person–years. There was a dramatic difference in HBV DNA levels at varying ages. In the Senegalese group, 14.5% were HBV DNA positive in their 20s, and this declined with each decade of age to 3.3%, 2.9%, and 0% thereafter. In the Chinese group, there was a higher prevalence of HBV DNA-positive males (29.4%) in their 1920s, and there was no consistent reduction seen per decade. The authors concluded that the prolonged maintenance of productive virus infection in Chinese carriers compared with Senegalese carriers might explain the higher risk of HCC in Chinese carriers [22]. This provides some further evidence that prolonged exposure to high HBV viral loads can influence HCC risk. In addition, environmental factors such as exposure to carcinogens, diet, and lifestyle factors such as alcohol consumption, cigarette smoking, genetic and ethnic differences, and mode of transmission of HBV can affect one's risk of HCC and can make it difficult to compare cancer risk among different ethnicities.

The incidence of HCC in hepatitis B carriers also differs according to race. Asian women and men without cirrhosis who are considered chronic carriers without active replication or necroinflammation still appear to have an increased risk of HCC [2]. This does not appear to be as true of patients of Caucasian descent and may be related to the duration of infection. In addition, African patients with HBV seem to be at higher risk of developing HCC at a younger age. Based on cost-effectiveness studies, guidelines recommend that Asian men with chronic HBV in the absence of cirrhosis should undergo surveillance for HCC starting at age 40 and women at age 50. Africans with chronic HBV may develop HCC at an even younger age, and most recommend institution of screening from age 20 [23]. Regardless of age, however, all HBV carriers with underlying cirrhosis should be screened for HCC.

Data from the REVEAL-HBV group provides further insight into the HCC risk for individuals of Asian descent who are considered to be inactive HBV carriers. One thousand nine hundred and thirty-two patients who were seronegative for HBV e antigen, had serum levels of HBV DNA < 10,000 copies/mL and did not have cirrhosis, HCC or elevated serum levels of ALT were classified as inactive carriers, and compared to 18, 137 patients were HBsAg negative and negative for HCV with similar clinical features. Cox regression models were used to determine the risk of liver-related death and HCC. The mean follow-up was 13.1 years, and the annual incidence rates of HCC and liver-related death were 0.06% and 0.04% for inactive HBV carriers. The rate was 0.02% for both liver-related death and HCC for controls. The hazard ratio for carriers of inactive HBV compared to controls was 4.6 for HCC and 2.1 for liver-related death. This supports the theory that even inactive Asian HBV carriers have a higher risk of HCC and liver-related death compared with individuals who are not infected with HBV [24].

Newer studies have attempted to develop scores or nomograms to better define the risk of HCC in patients with chronic HBV. As part of REVEAL-HBV, study cohorts were allocated for model derivation and validation. Previously confirmed independent risk predictors—sex, age, family history of HCC, alcohol consumption habit, serum ALT level, HBeAg serostatus, serum HBV DNA level, and HBV genotype—were used in three regression models. Risk scores were created based on the regression coefficient from these models and were then used to predict an individual risk of HCC over 5- and 10-year periods. Overall risk was then depicted by nomogram and validated. In each of the models, either HBeAg seropositivity or HBeAg seronegativity with high viral load (HBV DNA level ≥ 100,000 copies/mL) and genotype C infection had the highest risk scores. These data show that the easy-to-use nomograms based on noninvasive clinical characteristics can accurately predict the risk of HCC in patients with HBV and may help determine who should be screened [25]. Other risk scores have been developed based on retrospective data from smaller study populations but are not well validated. Yuen et al. also examined various risk factors including gender, HBV viral load, HBeAg/Ab status, as well as core and precore mutations, age, and presence of cirrhosis to predict risk of HCC. The study found that age, HBV viral load, core mutations, cirrhosis, and male gender appeared to be independent risk factors for development of HCC. The risk score had a sensitivity of 84% and specificity of 76% in predicting the 5- and 10-year risks for development of HCC [26].

Chronic HCV

Liver disease from chronic HCV infection accounts for 20% of all HCC. In the USA, an epidemic of HCV infection began in the 1960s and peaked in the 1980s with the highest risk of infection occurring in the people 20–30 years old [27, 28]. While most HCC occurs in patients with HCV in the presence of cirrhosis, there are also documented cases of HCC development in HCV patients without cirrhosis. Data from HALT-C showed that this 5-year cumulative risk of developing HCC with bridging fibrosis was 4.1% [29]. The yearly incidence of HCC in compensated cirrhotics is between 2% and 8%. A study by Sun et al. [30] showed that patients with hepatitis C and cirrhosis who have achieved viral clearance on therapy should continue to undergo surveillance. A more recent study published by Singh et al. [31] showed that HCV patients with cirrhosis who had SVR with therapy had a relative risk for HCC of 0.35 vs. nonresponders. However, 5% of the patients who did achieve SVR still developed HCC in long-term follow-up. Therefore, although the risk is decreased in patients with SVR, the authors of the study still continue to recommend regular surveillance. However, patients who clear HCV prior to developing cirrhosis have a very low likelihood of developing HCC and may not warrant surveillance.

Patients with HIV and either HBV or HCV are also at increased risk for HCC. In a large retrospective study conducted at the Veterans Administration Hospital, coinfection of HIV and HCV increased the risk of HCC fivefold compared to monoinfected patients with HIV and increased the risk of cirrhosis by 10–20-fold [32]. Current guidelines recommend entering coinfected patients with HBV/HCV and HIV using similar criteria for monoinfected patients with HCV or HBV [2]. Other risk factors for HCC in patients with chronic HCV include alcohol consumption, older age at infection, and the presence of porphyria cutanea tarda [33, 34].

Alcoholic Liver Disease

Alcohol intake is clearly a well-recognized cause of chronic liver disease and cirrhosis. It has been suggested that alcohol might be involved in the pathogenesis of HCC through a direct genotoxic pathway in addition to an indirect mechanism via cirrhosis [35].

Donato et al. investigated the association of alcohol use and risk of HCC. The study included patients hospitalized in Brescia, Italy, between 1995 and 2000.

Four hundred and sixty-four patients with a first diagnosis of HCC were compared to a control group of 686 subjects who had no underlying liver disease. The authors found that there was a linear increase in HCC risk with increasing intake of alcohol at >60 g of alcohol use/day even without underlying HBV or HCV. In addition, the odds ratio of HCC was increased twofold for each hepatitis virus infection for subjects who drank >60 g/day [35]. While the cohort was mostly men, there was no gender-based difference for risk of HCC with greater than 60 g of alcohol use. In a separate single center study, heavy alcohol consumption contributed to 32% of all HCCs, and there was synergy between heavy alcohol use, viral hepatitis, and diabetes in terms of increasing HCC risk [36].

NAFLD

Obesity is a risk factor for chronic liver disease and liver fibrosis without any other underlying etiology [37]. In a retrospective cohort study conducted in Paris, survival and complications in overweight cirrhotics were compared to normal-weight patients with either HCV-related or cryptogenic cirrhosis. While severity of liver disease did not differ between the overweight and lean groups, survival was decreased among the overweight group. In addition, a similar proportion of patients developed HCC in the overweight and HCV groups highlighting the carcinogenic potential of obesity-related cirrhosis. In addition, cirrhosis was detected later in life in overweight patients and at a more decompensated state compared to patients with HCV indicating a need for recognizing obesity as a cofactor for advanced liver disease and death [38].

As obesity continues to rise in the USA and the Western world, the incidence of cancer will continue to rise [39]. In a single center prospective study conducted in University of Michigan, 105 patients presenting with HCC were studied. The most common etiology of liver disease was HCV (51%) followed by cryptogenic cirrhosis (29%). Half of the patients with cryptogenic cirrhosis had features associated with nonalcoholic fatty liver disease (NAFLD). Patients who underwent surveillance had smaller tumors and were more likely to be eligible for surgical treatment with better median survival. The patients who had cryptogenic cirrhosis were less likely to have undergone HCC surveillance and had larger tumors. NAFLD accounted for at least 13% of the HCC cases [40]. The authors of this study concluded that the incidence of HCC in the USA may continue to rise even if the HCV epidemic levels off because of the increasing prevalence of NAFLD. This also highlights the current impact of NAFLD in the USA in terms of HCC risk.

A prospective study conducted at the Veteran Affairs hospital examined the risk of diabetes and chronic nonalcoholic liver disease [41]. 173,643 patients with diabetes and 650,620 without diabetes who were hospitalized in VA facilities between 1985 and 1990 were followed through 2000. Patients with known concomitant liver disease were excluded. The Kaplan–Meier survival analysis showed a significantly higher cumulative incidence of HCC among patients with diabetes compared to patients without diabetes (2.39 vs. 0.87 per 10,000 person–years, respectively, $p < 0.0001$). The conclusions from this study showed that diabetes more than doubled the risk of chronic liver disease and HCC. The risk was highest among patients with more than 10 years of follow-up. The study further supports the association between diabetes, chronic liver disease, and HCC.

Other Causes of Cirrhosis

Other known causes of HCC include cirrhosis from genetic hemochromatosis, primary biliary cirrhosis (PBC), alpha 1-antitrypsin deficiency, and autoimmune hepatitis. Patients with genetic hemochromatosis and cirrhosis have a relative risk of 20 for HCC [42, 43].

As mentioned above, HCC occurs in patients with PBC. The incidence of HCC in stage 4 PBC is estimated to be between 3% and 5% per year and the frequency between 0.7% and 16% [44–46]. In a study of patients seen at the Mayo Clinic with PBC and HCC, the presence of HCC was predicted in 18 of 19 patients based on a model [44]. Age > 70, male sex, history of blood transfusions, and evidence of portal hypertension were associated with HCC. This study provides evidence that patients with advanced stages of PBC determined by histology or combinations of the above high risk are a target population for HCC surveillance.

Treatment of Early Disease

The purpose of screening and surveillance is to detect a disease early in its course in order to offer a beneficial treatment and ultimately decrease mortality. Once symptoms develop, the disease is often advanced and not amenable to curative therapy via resection, transplantation, or percutaneous ablation [2, 47]. There are no large randomized controlled trials comparing the different modalities of potential curative treatment including resection, transplantation, or radiofrequency ablation for early-stage disease. Surgical resection of HCC is preferred in noncirrhotic patients. Only 5% of the Western population fits this category though up to 40% of Asians do [2]. The 5-year survival after resection is acceptable (>50%). A prospective study conducted between 1989 and 2001 examined the outcome of patients with early HCC treated with partial hepatotectomy who would have also been candidates for transplantation. The median tumor size was 3.5 cm, and the average number of lesions was 1 with a range of 1–3. Approximately 86% of the patients had Child class A cirrhosis. The 1-, 3-, and 5-year survival rates were 85%, 74%, and 69%, respectively, with a median survival of 71 months. The 5-year disease-free survival was 48% with a median of 52 months [48].

In an intention-to-treat analysis comparing orthotopic liver transplant to surgical resection, 164 cirrhotic patients from 1989 to 1997 were evaluated for surgery.

Seventy-seven patients with Child–Pugh class A who were resected and 87 patients with Child–Pugh class B/C were selected for transplantation. The 1-, 3-, and 5-year survival rates for resection were 85%, 62%, and 51% and 84%, 69%, and 69% for transplantation. The overall 5-year survival for resection was 74% for the best candidates who did not have clinically relevant portal hypertension. The results from this study show that surgical resection and OLT provide similar and acceptable survival rates in cirrhotic patients with early HCC [49]. The well-accepted "Milan criteria" highlight the effectiveness of treating early disease. In a prospective cohort study between 1991 and 1994, the efficacy of liver transplant was evaluated in patients who had unresectable HCC. A total of 48 patients underwent transplant; 94% had cirrhosis secondary to HBV, HCV, or both. The criteria used to determine eligibility for transplantation were one nodule less than 5 cm and no more than three tumor nodules each 3 cm in diameter or less (Milan criteria). A total of 36 patients were Child class A of which 28 received anticancer treatment; 15 patients with Child C cirrhosis did not receive any treatment prior to transplant. After transplantation, the patients were followed for a median of 26 months (range 9–54 months). The overall mortality rate was 17%. After 4 years, the actuarial survival rate was 75%, and rate of recurrence-free survival was 83%, comparable to OLT outcomes in patients without HCC. Survival was not affected by patient's age, sex, type of virus, or Child–Pugh stage. The overall and recurrence-free survival rates at 4 years in patients who met predetermined criteria (Milan criteria), which included 35 of the patients, were 85% and 92%, respectively. In patients whose tumors exceed these limits (13 patients), the overall and recurrence-free survival rates were 50% and 59%, respectively. This study shows that early tumor stage was the most important factor affecting overall mortality and recurrence-free survival in patients being considered for transplant and emphasizes the importance of early detection to achieve potential cure [50].

Acceptability of Surveillance

Surveillance programs must be acceptable to health-care providers and individuals at risk. In the USA, it has become standard of care to screen patients with cirrhosis for HCC. In a national survey of 554 members of the AASLD, the majority of responders indicated that they routinely screened patients with cirrhosis using ultrasound and alpha-fetoprotein while 25% also used computed tomography [51]. Additional surveys have shown that gastroenterologists have adequate knowledge of at-risk patients, screening methods and modalities [52]. In Europe and Japan, while screening has become the standard of care for patients at risk of HCC, actual adherence rates are not known [53]. While it appears based on survey data that most hepatologists and gastroenterologists are aware of screening guidelines and abide by them, recent population-based data suggests that actual surveillance rates are much lower. In a study of 1,873 patients with HCC and a prior diagnosis of cirrhosis, only 17% received regular surveillance in the 3 years prior to diagnosis.

Patients seen in an academic center were more likely to have had surveillance. These studies highlight the fact that surveillance strategies are generally accepted but adherence is suboptimal [54, 55].

Effectiveness of Surveillance

The utility of surveillance for HCC in at-risk patients has been debated for some time. Effectiveness and cost effectiveness have been evaluated in various retrospective and prospective studies and models. Unfortunately, there is a paucity of randomized controlled trials in this area, leaving the available data plagued with bias. In this day and age, it is unlikely that additional randomized controlled trials of surveillance vs. no surveillance will be conducted due to ethical concerns. Nevertheless, the body of literature supporting the effectiveness of surveillance is vast. The ultimate objective of HCC surveillance is to decrease mortality from the disease.

Many studies indicate that regular surveillance of patients at risk of HCC increases the chance of detecting potentially curable or treatable tumors attempting to improve patient prognosis [56–59]. This phenomenon is referred to as "stage migration" and does not always correlate with improvements in survival [60].

Screening and surveillance have been recommended for these high-risk subjects; however, there have not been any studies which have shown a reduction in mortality by means of a randomized controlled trial except in HBV carriers in China [57]. Most studies of effectiveness in HCC are nonrandomized and not well controlled. These studies have generally looked favorably on surveillance and its effect on mortality though they generally suffer from significant bias. A retrospective study of 91 patients with HCC in Hawaii showed that patients who were screened had increased median survival when compared to those who were symptomatic (1,399 vs. 234 d, $p = 0.009$) [61]. Another study of patients with chronic viral hepatitis and HCC showed that patients who underwent surveillance were more likely to have smaller and fewer HCC. The adjusted median 2-year survival was also increased in the surveillance group after control for lead and length time bias, assuming tumor doubling time < 90 days [62].

A retrospective study conducted in Japan from 2001 to 2007 evaluated 240 patients who were infected with chronic HCV. These patients were divided into three groups which included patients who received routine surveillance with repeated imaging, another group which received regular doctor visits for chronic liver disease, and the last group which did not undergo any screening or routine medical visits. The prevalence of solitary tumors was significantly higher in the surveillance group, 66%, vs. 24% in the group who received no surveillance or medical visits. The size of the nodules was less than 2 cm in 64% of patients vs. only 5% in the screening and nonscreening groups, respectively. A significantly higher proportion of patients who were diagnosed at stages I and II were candidates for curative procedures [63]. The authors of this study also found that patients who were screened at intervals greater than 12 months presented at later stages of the disease. In addition, HCC-related serological markers including AFP (cutoff at 200 ng/mL) and DCP (cutoff 40 mAU/mL) were negative in 47% of the surveillance group when these patients were diagnosed with HCC. This study showed the poor performance of tumor markers including DCP in detecting early-stage HCC and supported the AASLD guidelines that AFP alone should not be used for HCC screening when ultrasound is not available.

Recently, a retrospective cohort study investigated HCV-infected patients who developed HCC to evaluate the association between HCC surveillance and survival in a large nationwide VA clinical practice setting [64]. This study evaluated the effectiveness of HCC surveillance. Effectiveness takes into account the benefits and harms of an intervention. The study included 1,480 patients who were HCV infected and developed HCC during 1998–2007. Either surveillance with AFP or US was recorded in approximately 78% of the patients within 2 years before they were diagnosed with HCC. Only 2% of patients underwent annual surveillance with both AFP and US during the 2 years prior to HCC diagnosis. 5.7% had an AFP or US every 6 months and 34% had annual surveillance with one modality. In the 2 years before HCC was diagnosed, 57.7% received surveillance with AFP only, 19.4% with both AFP and US, and 0.5% received US only. It appears that most patients received inconsistent surveillance and the use of AFP alone was the most frequent modality. The timing of surveillance was examined in groups of patients based on receiving tests in two consecutive periods, 0–6 months only, 7–24 months only, both periods, and no tests in the two periods. The longest survival was seen in those who received surveillance tests in both time periods, while the shortest survival was observed in patients who received no surveillance in either period. These differences in survival were most pronounced for the 1-year survival rates (50.3% vs. 31.9%), less for the 3 years, and there was no significant difference in survival rates at 5 years. There was a significant 29% reduction in mortality risk among those who received surveillance tests in both time periods and a 20% risk reduction in those who received surveillance in the 0–6-month period only compared with no tests in either period. There was no significant difference in mortality for surveillance recorded only during the 7–24-month period before HCC diagnosis.

A few studies have looked at the effect of Child–Pugh classification score and have shown that surveillance prolongs survival in Child–Pugh class A patients but not in the sicker class C at time of diagnosis [26, 59, 65]. Because most patients with Child C cirrhosis have a severely reduced life expectancy as a result of underlying liver disease, most studies on surveillance have excluded these patients. For Child class B patients, prognostic benefit was seen in an Asian series, while there was borderline advantage seen in Italian Liver Cancer group series. One study has specifically evaluated surveillance for HCC in intermediate/advanced cirrhosis or Child–Pugh classes B and C [66]. In this study, a total of 1,834 HCC patients were seen consecutively from January 1987 to December 2004 at ten medical institutions. A total of 608 patients were selected from the registry, 468 class B and 140 class C cases. The patients were divided into two groups: group 1 included 252 patients in whom HCC was detected using regular surveillance based on liver US and AFP performed every 6 months. Group 2 included 356 cases in whom HCC was detected incidentally, outside any programmed surveillance or during examination for other diseases or because of symptom appearance. The cause of liver disease included HBV, HCV and alcohol, cryptogenic, hereditary hemochromatosis, and PBC. In Child–Pugh class B, the cancer stage and treatment options were better in group 1 than group 2, and the medial survival was 17.1 vs. 12 months, and the 1-, 3-, and 5-year survival rates were 60.4% vs. 49.2%, 26.1% vs. 16.1%, and 10.7% vs. 4.3% in the respective groups. In the Child–Pugh class C patients, cancer stage and treatment distribution were better in group 1 than group 2, but the median survival did not differ, 7.1 months vs. 6.0 months. The authors of this study concluded that in the Italian health-care system, surveillance for early HCC diagnosis increases survival of Child–Pugh class B cirrhotics but not in patients who are Child–Pugh class C.

Liver transplantation is a widely accepted curative treatment for patients with early-stage HCC. Stravitz et al. evaluated the quality of surveillance for HCC and its effect on access to liver transplantation [67]. A total of 269 patients with cirrhosis and HCC were retrospectively categorized into three groups according to the quality of surveillance: standard of care, substandard surveillance, and absence of surveillance in patients who were not recognized to be cirrhotic. Standard-of-care surveillance was defined as performance of liver US or other abdominal imaging (CT or MRI) at least once during the year before cancer diagnosis which included a total of 172 patients. Forty-eight patients were categorized into the substandard surveillance group which was defined as absence of abdominal imaging within the year before cancer diagnosis in a patient with recognized cirrhosis and also included patients who had tumors identified on initial screening examination. The 59 patients underwent abdominal imaging for symptoms or an unrelated indication but were not recognized to have cirrhosis before the time of cancer diagnosis. HCC was diagnosed at stages 1 and 2 in 70% of patients in the surveillance group, 37% of patients in the substandard surveillance group, and 18% of patients in the no surveillance group. Liver transplantation was performed in 32% of patients in surveillance group vs. 13% in substandard surveillance vs. 7% in no surveillance group. The 3-year survival from cancer diagnosis in the no surveillance group was significantly less than the surveillance group (12% vs. 39%). The quality of surveillance had a direct impact on HCC stage at diagnosis, access to liver transplant, and survival.

To date only one randomized controlled trial of surveillance vs. no surveillance has shown a survival benefit to screening with six monthly ultrasound and AFP in a high-risk group in urban Shanghai, China [57]. This randomized controlled trial was conducted on Chinese patients with hepatitis B infection. The study included approximately 18,000 people aged 35–59 years with hepatitis B virus infection or a history of chronic hepatitis. People were randomly divided into two groups, surveillance vs. no surveillance group. The surveillance group was invited to have an AFP (cutoff 20 μg/L) test and undergo ultrasound exam every 6 months. The results showed that in the surveillance group, there were 86 cases of HCC vs. 67 and resection was achieved in 46.5% vs. 7% in the control group; liver transplant was not a treatment option. In addition, there were twice as many stage III cancers in the control

Table 2.2 Stage distribution, treatment, and survival of patients with HCC in the screened and control groups

	Screening group (86)	Control group (67)
Stage[a]		
Stage I	52 (60.5%)	0 (0%)
Stage II	12 (13.9%)	25 (37.2%)
Stage III	22 (25.6%)	42 (62.7%)
Small HCC	39 (45.3%)	0 (0%)
Treatment		
Resection	40 (46.5%)	5 (7.5%)
TACE/PEI	28 (32.6%)	28 (41.8%)
Conservative treatment	18 (20.9%)	34 (50.7%)
Survival (%)[b]		
1-year	65.9	31.2
2-year	59.9	7.2
3-year	52.6	7.2
4-year	52.6	0
5-year	46.4	0

[a]$\chi^2 = 61.41, p < 0.01$
[b]Log-rank $\chi 2 = 35.50, p < 0.01$
Reproduced with permission from Zhang et al. [57]

Table 2.3 Outcome of screening

	Screening group	Control group
Person–years in study	38,444	41,077
HCC occurrence		
No. of cases	86	67
Total incidence (per 100,000)	223.7	163.1
Rate ratio (CI 95%)	1.37 (0.99, 1.89)	
Deaths from HCC		
No. of deaths	32	54
Total mortality (per 100,000)	83.2	131.5
Rate ratio (CI 95%)	0.63 (0.41, 0.98)	

Reproduced with permission from Zhang et al. [57]

group vs. the screening group, 25.6% vs. 62.9%, respectively. The 1-, 3-, and 5-year survival rates were 65.9%, 52.6%, and 46.4% (surveillance) vs. 31.2%, 7.2%, and 0 in the control. There was a 37% reduction in HCC-related mortality in the surveillance group vs. the no surveillance group (Tables 2.2 and 2.3, Fig. 2.1).

Unfortunately, the adherence to surveillance was less than 60%. In addition, the sensitivity of AFP was 69%, and ultrasound was useful for screening. It would be ideal for these tests to be validated in other geographical areas including the West, but it seems unlikely that the West will conduct such randomized clinical trials. In a 16-year population-based study, assessing screening of HBsAg carriers

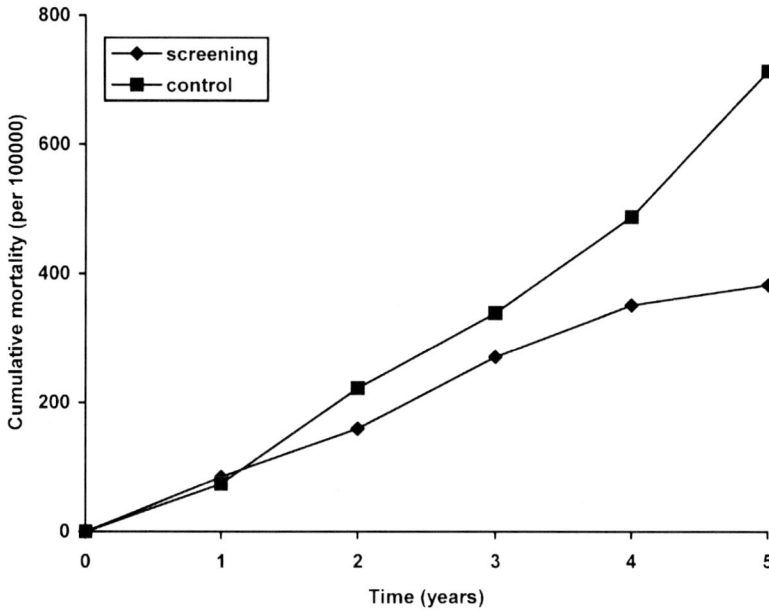

Fig. 2.1 Cumulative mortality in screening group and control group. Modified from Zhang et al. [57]

with semiannual AFP was effective in detecting tumors at a resectable stage and prolonged survival, although this study does suffer from lead-time bias [68]. With a large majority of HCC occurring in Asia in countries like China, many studies indicating effectiveness of screening and surveillance have been conducted in these locations. Another randomized controlled trial from China which included men with chronic HBV between ages 30 and 69 showed that surveillance with ultrasound and AFP resulted in early diagnosis but had no effect on mortality [69]. The screening group included 3,712 men who were screened in six monthly intervals with AFP. Ultrasound was recommended for an abnormal AFP. The population was followed for liver cancer or death. There were 3,712 subjects in the screening group with a mean follow-up of 61.9 months and 1,869 control subjects with a mean follow-up of 62.8 months. The AFP >20 µg/dL in 5.2% of subjects in group A and 5.7% in group B was not statistically significant. A total of 374 cases of liver cancer were diagnosed, with a higher incidence in the screened group vs. the controls although the results were not significant. In addition, the mortality rate among the groups was 1138.1 per 10 [5] in the screened group vs. 1113.9 per 10 [5] in the control group which was not statistically significant. The specificity and sensitivity of AFP in screening were 80.9% and 80.0%, respectively. The study, however, showed that a significantly higher number of cases in the screening group were diagnosed at stage I vs. the control group (27.9% in the screened group vs. 3.7% in the control group). Survival in patients with liver cancer from the screened group was better in the short term, but the advantage disappeared by 5 years. There was no difference in overall mortality, and this is likely attributable to lack of effective treatment. This study, however, is limited because the screening regimen is considered suboptimal by today's guidelines.

Surveillance Tests

Various surveillance tests have been evaluated in the literature. Sensitivity and specificity are inherent to the test being performed. Sensitivity is the probability that a test is positive when true disease exists (true positive). Specificity, on the other hand, refers to the probability that the test is negative when the disease does not exist (true negative). Screening tests must be sensitive and reasonably specific. The accuracy of a test is related to the frequency of the disease in the population and is measured with positive predictive and negative predictive values. Currently, despite new recommendations from AASLD, both serologic and radiologic methods are used in surveillance of HCC. Unfortunately, most studies have evaluated these tests at the time of diagnosis rather than in an at-risk population being screened for disease.

Serologic Markers

The most widely used markers in HCC are alpha-fetoprotein and DCP. There are several reports on the sensitivity and specificity of AFP in surveillance. An AFP value greater than 200 μg/L can be highly specific for hepatocellular cancer, while levels less than 200 would not be informative enough to stop further investigation for HCC [70]. Serum AFP is no longer considered an appropriate surveillance test by AASLD because of the high rates of false-positive and false-negative results in patients with chronic liver disease. AFP level > 20 ng/mL performs poorly as a screening tool because of various reported sensitivities around 60%. Therefore, AFP used alone may miss up to 40% of HCC. Des-gamma-carboxy prothrombin (DCP) or prothrombin induced by vitamin K absence II (PIVKA II) has also been evaluated as a potential serological test. DCP is an abnormal prothrombin molecule generated by malignant cells. Most data regarding DCP comes from Asia, and experience in the West is limited. In a study done by Izuno and colleagues, the usefulness of DCP was evaluated in a group of 137 patients with liver cirrhosis. Patients were followed for an average of 3.4 years, and 35 of the patients developed HCC, with 16 developing a small tumor less than or equal to 2 cm in diameter. Eight patients had a significantly elevated DCP at the time of HCC detection, but these tumors were greater than 2 cm in diameter, and there were multiple or diffuse types. Tumors which were less than 2 cm in diameter were detected by imaging and elevated AFP. The authors concluded that DCP alone is not sensitive enough to detect early small liver cancers [71].

Another prospective surveillance study assessed the optimal test for detection of early HCC in 602 patients with chronic viral hepatitis during a 7-year period [72]. Patients had positive HCV antibodies or HBV surface antigen. Blood samples were obtained at 6- and 12-month intervals for serum AFP, and all patients had abdominal US at least once during each 12-month period. Out of the 602 patients, 426 patients were anti-HCV positive, 163 were hepatitis B surface antigen positive, and 13 were positive for both HCV and HBV. The follow-up range was between 12 and 103 months. A total of 31 cases of HCC were detected. AFP was elevated (range between 8 and 24 ng/mL) in 74% of HCC patients but was also elevated in 10% of non-HCC patients. The maximum sensitivity was 65%, and specificity was 90%. Abdominal US identified all 31 cases. The sensitivity and specificity of US were 100% and 98%, respectively. This study also supports that US was more accurate in detecting HCC, and AFP should not be used as the only test for screening and surveillance for HCC given its low positive predictive value (12%) and sensitivity.

Trevisani et al. studied serum AFP in patients with chronic liver disease. In a case–control study of 170 patients with HCC and 170 controls with chronic liver disease from HBV or HCV, the best discriminating AFP value was 16 ng/mL. A value of 20 ng/mL had a sensitivity of 62.4% and specificity of 89.4%. A 5% prevalence rate of HCC is seen in most liver clinics. In this study, the positive predictive value (PPV) was 84.6% with the 50% tumor prevalence of the study population but decreased to 25.1% at a 5% tumor prevalence. The negative predictive value (NPV) was 69.4% and rose to 97.7% at 5% tumor prevalence. In patients without viral hepatitis, the PPV was 100% at any HCC prevalence, while the NPV ranged from 59.0% to 73%. This study highlights that AFP misses many HCCs and may elevate in the absence of HCC, but elevations may be more indicative of HCC in patients without viral hepatitis [73].

The Hepatitis C Antiviral Long-Term Treatment Against Cirrhosis Trial (HALT-C) study recently supported the efficacy of these serum markers as surveillance tests [74]. The study aim was to compare the accuracy of AFP and DCP in early diagnosis of HCC among patients with chronic HCV who were enrolled into the HALT-C trial. Among the 1,031 patients who were randomized in the study, 39 cases of HCC were detected, 24 of which were in early stage. These patients were compared to 77 controls. The sera were tested 12 months prior to HCC diagnosis. The sensitivity and specificity of DCP at time of diagnosis were 74% and 86% at a cutoff of 40 mAU/mL. On the other hand, the sensitivity and specificity of AFP at the time of diagnosis were 61% and 81% at a cutoff of 20 ng/mL. When the higher values of 150 mAU/mL for DCP and 200 ng/mL for AFP were used, sensitivity dropped to 43% and 22%, respectively. The sensitivity of DCP and AFP 12 months prior to diagnosis was lower still. While lowering cutoff values even further increased sensitivity to around 90%, the loss of specificity would likely lead additional testing in a large number of patients without cancer. While AFP and DCP alone were not very sensitive, the combination of the two was more so. If the markers were combined, the sensitivity increased to 91% at diagnosis and 73% prior to diagnosis with a decrease in specificity 74% and 71%, respectively. While neither marker showed impressive sensitivity, both markers increased significantly in patients with HCC,

Table 2.4 Sensitivity and specificity of DCP alone, AFP alone, and the combination of both markers in differentiating HCC cases from controls at two fixed cutoff values

Months from HCC diagnosis	Sensitivity	Specificity	Sensitivity	Specificity
DCP (mAU/mL)	>=40		>=150	
0	74%	86%	43%	100%
−3	65%	84%	39%	100%
−6	63%	88%	11%	100%
−9	52%	88%	6%	100%
−12	43%	94%	3%	100%
AFP (ng/mL)	>=20		>=200	
0	61%	81%	22%	100%
−3	58%	80%	13%	98%
−6	57%	76%	3%	100%
−9	45%	77%	6%	100%
−12	47%	75%	3%	100%
DCP and/or AFP	DCP>=40 *or* AFP>=20		DCP>=40 *and* AFP>=20	
0	91%	74%	43%	93%
−3	87%	69%	35%	95%
−6	86%	69%	34%	96%
−9	82%	67%	15%	97%
−12	73%	71%	17%	98%

Reproduced with permission from Lok et al. [74]

and tumor diagnosis was triggered by doubling of AFP in 5/39 (12.8%) of cases (Table 2.4).

Lens culinaris agglutinin-reactive AFP or AFP-L3 is an isoform of AFP which has also been studied as a tumor marker for HCC. AFP-L3 is reported as a percentage of AFP-L3 over total AFP level. Prior studies have shown that 10% is a cutoff for the presence of HCC [75]. AFP-L3 has not been well studied for use in surveillance. The clinical utility of AFP, DCP, and AFP-L3 in detecting HCC was assessed in patients with chronic viral disease, with and without HCC. Approximately 230 patients were divided into two groups: group 1 included HCC patients with chronic HCV or HBV, and group 2 included non-HCC patients with HBV or HCV who had chronic hepatitis or cirrhosis. HBV was confirmed with positive HBsAg and HCV with both positive HCV antibody and viral load. A total of 240 were tested for tumor markers. In patients who had HCC and HBV and HCV, the serum levels of DCP, AFP, and AFP-L3 were significantly higher. Using ROC analysis, the cutoff for AFP was 25 ng/mL yielding a sensitivity of 69%, specificity of 87%, and positive predictive value of 69.8% for detecting HCC. Patients with HBV or HCV with cirrhosis and no HCC also had higher AFP levels than in patients with chronic hepatitis. There was no correlation between size of single HCC and AFP, however, showing how it is not a good test for HCC surveillance. The cutoff for AFP-L3 was >10% and demonstrated a sensitivity of 56%, specificity of 90%, and positive predictive value of 56.1% in detecting HCC. However, AFP-L3 also did not correlate with size of single HCC. Finally, for DCP at a cutoff of 84 mAU/mL, the sensitivity, specificity, and positive predictive value were 87%, 85%, and 86.8%, respectively. The DCP level remained below the cutoff value in all patients without HCC. In addition, DCP serum levels correlated with tumor size in single lesion HCC. DCP was not elevated in any patients without HCC [75].

The most recent iteration of the AASLD practice guidelines has recommended against the use of AFP as a surveillance tool in HCC. Despite this, most centers continue to use this tumor marker in combination with radiologic studies to survey for HCC. DCP is less commonly used in the West.

Radiologic Studies

Currently, ultrasound is the method of choice for screening because it appears to have adequate sensitivity, specificity, and accuracy. In addition, it is widely available and relatively inexpensive. Criticisms of ultrasound include that performance of the study can suffer from operator dependence as well as poorer quality images in patients with high body mass index, an increasing problem in the USA. There is a wide variation of sensitivity for ultrasound in published studies, ranging from 23% to 99%. Kim et al. published a study showing that the sensitivity and specificity for HCCs were 38% (6 of 16) and 92% (33 of 36), and those for dysplastic nodules were 0% and 95% (39 of 41), respectively, in a group of 52 patients with liver cirrhosis who were evaluated prior to transplant. Thus, they concluded that ultrasonography is insensitive for detection of HCCs and dysplastic nodules in patients with advanced liver cirrhosis [76].

Alternatively, other studies have shown that ultrasound can have a sensitivity of between 65% and 80% and specificity greater than 90%. A meta-analysis determined the performance characteristics of surveillance with ultrasound for the detection of early HCC defined by the Milan criteria [77]. Surveillance ultrasound detected the majority of tumors before they were clinically symptomatic with a pooled sensitivity of 94%. However, sensitivity was only 63% for detecting early HCC. In this study, AFP did not add additional benefit to ultrasound (Fig. 2.2).

Other imaging modalities are less well evaluated for HCC surveillance. In the USA, contrast enhanced CT or MRI is the modality of choice for diagnosing HCC. These tests are also used with varying frequency to screen for HCC, especially for patients active on the transplant list. According to the AASLD, the performance characteristics of computed tomography (CT) scanning in HCC surveillance are unknown, and thus, no recommendation can be made about CT scanning for individuals in whom US may not allow adequate visibility. In addition, CT exposes the patient to high doses of radiation at frequent intervals. MRI continues to be expensive when compared with ultrasound and is likely not cost effective for surveillance.

A study conducted by Chalasani et al. looked at 285 patients with cirrhosis who were evaluated for liver transplantation between 1994 and 1997. These patients were initially screened for HCC with AFP, US, and CT. One hundred and sixty-six

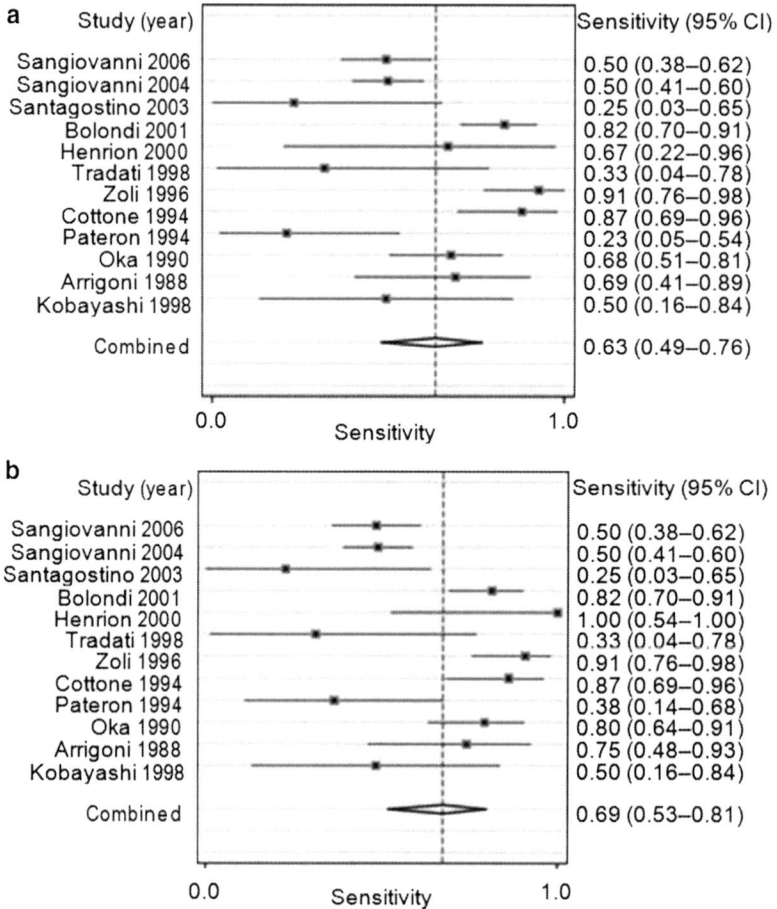

Fig. 2.2 Sensitivity of ultrasound with and without AFP for the detection of early-stage hepatocellular carcinoma (HCC):(**a**) forest plot for the sensitivity of ultrasound to detect early HCC; (**b**) forest plot for the sensitivity of ultrasound with AFP to detect early HCC. Q, chi-squared test of heterogeneity; I^2, inconsistency index. Reproduced with permission from Singal et al

patients who were eligible for liver transplant underwent continued screening with semiannual AFP and ultrasound during a median follow-up of 15 months. There were 27 HCCs found, 22 during initial screening and 5 during extended screening. The sensitivity of CT, AFP at a level of >20 ng/mL, and US were 88%, 62%, and 59%, respectively [78].

According to the AASLD, the performance characteristics of CT scanning in HCC surveillance are unknown, and thus, no recommendation can be made about CT scanning for individuals in whom US may not allow adequate visibility. Such patients tend to be obese with fatty liver disease and cirrhosis.

Timing

Surveillance guidelines by both the European Association for the Study of the Liver (EASL) and AASLD recommend the surveillance interval to be 6 months. This is based on data that the interval from undetectable lesions to those 2-cm diameter is approximately 4–12 months. However, experts in the Far East have adopted a 3-month interval for screening. There is no clear advantage in a 3-month program compared to semiannual surveillance [79]. In addition, a meta-regression analysis showed significantly higher sensitivity for early HCC with ultrasound every 6 months vs. annual surveillance [77].

A surveillance interval of 6–12 months has been proposed based on tumor doubling times in patients with HCV and HBV. In Italy, a study conducted in hemophiliacs with HCV showed similar efficacy between a 6-month and 12-month screening interval to identify potentially curable HCC [80]. Santagostino et al. based their study on prior data that all HCCs detected by yearly ultrasound surveillance of hemophiliacs with HCV and elevated alanine aminotransferase levels were multinodular. Therefore, they designed the study to evaluate if a more intense surveillance with AFP and US improved identification of single nodule tumors. Five hundred and fifty-nine HCV-infected hemophiliacs were divided into two arms: one followed at 6-month intervals and one at 1-year intervals. The overall incidence rate of HCC was 239 per 100,000 per year in the 6-month group and 143 per 100,000 per year in the 12-month group which was not statistically significant. The authors concluded that 6-month surveillance with US did not increase the chances of detection of single nodule tumors [79].

A study by Kim et al. evaluated whether semiannual surveillance affected outcome in patients diagnosed with HCC in Korea. In a total of 400 patients, more were diagnosed with HCC by surveillance with ultrasound and AFP (cutoff 20 ng/mL) every 6 or 12 months. They were divided into two groups: group 1 underwent surveillance every 6 months, while group 2 underwent surveillance annually. Single nodular HCC was more prevalent in group 1 (90.4%) vs. group 2 (72.9%), and curative treatment with resection of ablative therapy was more frequent in group 1 compared to group 2 (18.7% vs. 12.2%). Five-year survival was significantly better in group 1 vs. group 2, supporting that semiannual surveillance allowed for detection of earlier-stage HCC and survival compared to annual surveillance [81].

In a retrospective study comparing Child class A or B patients in Italy, semiannual surveillance was compared to annual surveillance with ultrasound with or without AFP. There were 510 patients in the semiannual surveillance group compared to 139 patients in the annual surveillance group. The cancer stage in the semiannual surveillance group was less severe with more single time <2 cm and less advanced tumors $p < 0.001$. The median observed survival was 45 months vs. 30 months in the semiannual surveillance group compared to the annual surveillance group which shows a significantly increased rate of detection of early HCC decreased advanced tumors in the semiannual group. When the observed survival in the semiannual surveillance group was corrected for lead time bias, the survival advantage remained (40.3 vs. 30 months, $p = 0.028$). These data support the currently recommended semiannual surveillance for high-risk patients to detect early-stage HCC [79].

Cost Effectiveness

Affordability of available testing is a common concern and is especially important if test use will be common as is the case with surveillance. There have been numerous studies assessing the cost effectiveness of surveillance of HCC in patients with cirrhosis. Many factors contribute to treatment outcome like compliance, heterogeneity and etiology of liver disease, and treatment effectiveness.

Patient compliance is a factor that also affects the effectiveness and cost effectiveness of surveillance. In a review by Thompson Coon et al. 1–15% of patients failed to comply with clinic-based surveillance programs in Europe and Japan compared to 42% of the population enrolled in a study in Shanghai [82].

Effectiveness of HCC surveillance is also influenced by the underlying etiology of the liver disease and the annual risk of HCC. There are many published decision analysis/cost-effectiveness models for HCC surveillance which differ in the theoretical population being analyzed and the intervention that is applied. The common theme among these studies is that the efficiency of surveillance is dependent on the incidence of HCC. Unfortunately, there are no experimental data to indicate what level of risk or what incidence of HCC should trigger surveillance. An intervention is considered effective if it provides an increase in longevity of 100 days [83]. In a modeling study of patients with Child class A cirrhosis, researchers found that with an HCC incidence of 1.5% per year, surveillance resulted in an increase in longevity of 3 months. If the incidence was 6%, the survival increase was 9 months [84]. A compilation of other studies has also suggested that in patients with cirrhosis of varying causes, surveillance may be effective when the risk of HCC exceeds 1.5% per year. For this reason, patients with cirrhosis should be offered cirrhosis when the risk of HCC is ≥1.5% per year. The incidence of HCC per 100 person–years in cirrhotic patients with HBV is up to 4.3% vs. 5–8% in HCV patients. In alcohol-related cirrhosis and PBC, the annual risk is up to 1.8% [34]. Patients who suffer from these diseases meet this incidence threshold and should undergo surveillance. However, this cutoff of 1.5% per year cannot be applied to HBV carriers without cirrhosis. In these patients, surveillance should be started once the incidence of HCC exceeds 0.2% per year according to AASLD guidelines [2].

Surveillance programs in which cost–utility ratios are measured at < $50,000 per quality-adjusted life year saved are thought to be cost effective [85]. In a Markov model study of patients with chronic HCV cirrhosis, screening with AFP and either ultrasound or CT was associated with incremental cost–utility ratios of 26,689 and 25,232 US dollars per quality-adjusted life year, respectively. Use of MRI increased this number to $118,000 [15]. Another study found that biannual AFP with annual US provided the most quality-adjusted life year increase while maintaining the cost-effective ratio below the $50,000/QALY threshold. Increasing the frequency of ultrasound to biannual resulted in an increase in cost to $73,789 per QALY [14]. Another recent study from England was conducted in cirrhotic patients using a decision analytic model [86]. Comparisons were made between various surveillance algorithms using AFP with or without ultrasound at semiannual and annual intervals. The model estimated that compared with no surveillance, 6-month AFP and US tripled the number of people with operable tumors at diagnosis and halved the number of people who would die from HCC. At a willingness to pay threshold of 30,000 pounds per quality-adjusted life year (QALY), the most intensive surveillance protocol simulated with 6 monthly AFP and US was most cost effective in individuals with HBV-related cirrhosis.

Other studies have suggested that surveillance for HCC in patients with cirrhosis is not cost effective. In a study conducted by Bolondi et al., the cost effectiveness of surveillance in patients with cirrhosis was evaluated during 1989–1991 in Italy. The control group included 104 patients who had incidentally detected HCC vs. 313 patients with liver cirrhosis. Surveillance was conducted in 6-month intervals with US and AFP. Sixty-one cases of HCC were detected with an incidence of 4.1% per year of follow-up. Only 42 out of 61 patients were able to undergo curative treatment with surgical resection, liver transplantation, or local therapy. The survival rate of the 61 patients with the liver tumors was significantly longer than the controls. The overall cost of the surveillance program was $753,226, the cost per treatable HCC was $17,934, and the cost per year of life saved was $112,993 [58]. As these data show, the cost effectiveness of surveillance for HCC remains controversial, and the decision to proceed must weigh available resources and treatments.

Recall Policies

According to the WHO criteria for a surveillance or screening program, there must be policies set up to address abnormalities seen or identified on a screening test. This policy is termed a recall policy. Recall policies are the policies instituted to deal with an abnormal screening test result. The tests and interval follow-up are different. Recall policies cover investigations and follow-up that determine whether an initial abnormality identified on surveillance is an HCC or not. The process starts with an abnormal result, i.e., any nodule not seen on a prior study should be considered abnormal. Often, abnormalities such as a lesion seen on US are followed up by a CT scan or MRI, and if the results are still equivocal, biopsy is pursued. The AASLD has presented well-accepted guidelines for recall after an abnormal screening ultrasound (Fig. 2.3).

```
                              ┌─────────────┐
                              │ Liver nodule│
                              └─────────────┘
              ┌──────────────────────┴──────────────────────┐
          ┌───────┐                                     ┌───────┐
          │ < 1 cm│                                     │ > 1 cm│
          └───────┘                                     └───────┘
              │                                             │
     ┌─────────────────┐                      ┌──────────────────────────┐
     │ Repeat US at 3  │◄─────────────┐       │ 4-phase MDCT/ dynamic    │
     │ months          │              │       │ contrast enhanced MRI    │
     └─────────────────┘              │       └──────────────────────────┘
              │                       │                    │
      ┌───────┴───────┐               │       ┌──────────────────────────┐
      │               │               │       │ Arterial hypervascularity│
┌──────────────┐ ┌────────┐           │       │ AND venous or delayed    │
│Growing/changing││ Stable │──────────┘       │ phase washout            │
│character     │ └────────┘                   └──────────────────────────┘
└──────────────┘
      │                    ┌───────┐   ┌──────────────────┐        ┌────┐
      │                    │  Yes  │   │ Other contrast   │        │ No │
      │                    └───────┘   │ enhanced study (CT│◄──────│    │
┌──────────────┐                       │ or MRI)          │        └────┘
│ Investigate  │           ┌───────┐   └──────────────────┘
│ according to │           │  HCC  │   ┌──────────────────────────┐ ┌────────┐
│ size         │           └───────┘   │ Arterial hypervascularity│ │ Biopsy │
└──────────────┘                       │ AND venous or delayed    │ └────────┘
                                       │ phase washout            │
                                       └──────────────────────────┘
                              ┌───────┐          ┌────┐
                              │  Yes  │          │ No │
                              └───────┘          └────┘
```

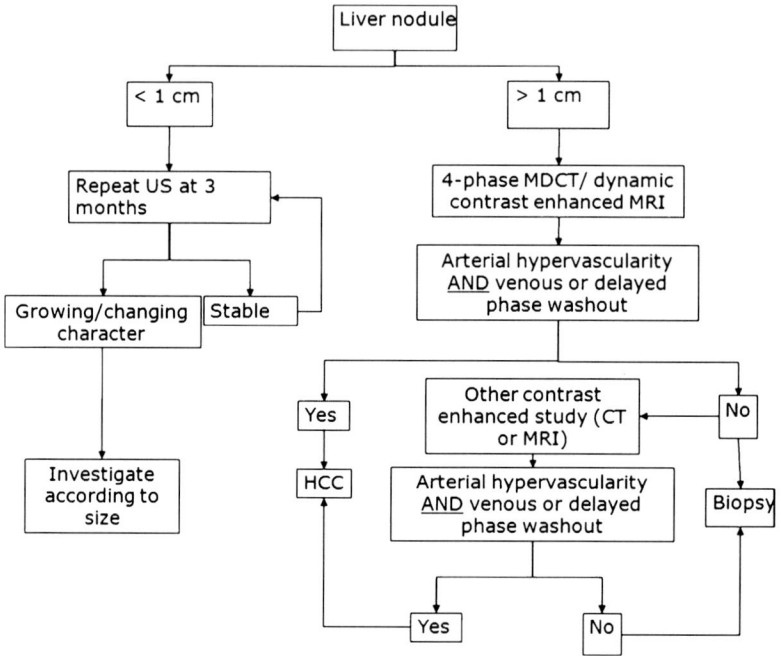

Fig. 2.3 Diagnostic algorithm for suspected HCC. Reproduced with permission from Bruix et al. [2]

Conclusion

HCC is one of the fastest growing cancers worldwide and is associated with a high mortality rate when detected after the appearance of symptoms. Much like other malignancies such as breast cancer, cervical cancer, and even colon cancer, early detection can allow for therapeutic benefit and appears to be cost effective in high-risk populations. High-risk populations for HCC differ geographically, as the etiology of HCC is different in developing vs. developed countries. HBV still accounts for the majority of HCC cases in Asia and the Eastern world, while HCV and NAFLD are currently on the rise in the Western world and account for a large proportion of cases of HCC. Therefore, surveillance for HCC is currently recommended by EASL and AASLD using ultrasound for identifying early stages of HCC, and this has become current standard of care in cirrhotics. Detecting HCC early allows for curative treatments such as resection, liver transplant, and RFA and may be associated with better survival. Thus far, however, only one randomized controlled trial has shown a mortality benefit in screening for HCC in HBV patients [57]. However, the remainder of the studies which are often retrospective reviews or cohort studies has shown a benefit in early diagnosis of HCC. Current guidelines recommend at-risk patients be screened by US at 6–12-month intervals, ideally

6-month intervals. The sensitivity of US is variable ranging from 65% to 80%, and specificity has shown to be greater than 90% [58]. AFP is no longer included in the surveillance guidelines given its poor sensitivity and specificity, as indicated by various studies. Other modalities such as CT and MRI have not been well investigated for screening for HCC, but are in place to further evaluate abnormalities detected on US. It appears that the majority of gastroenterologists and hepatologists provide some sort of HCC screening for their patients [78], though there have been several studies that have shown that surveillance is underutilized in the USA [55, 87]. About 28% of patients diagnosed with HCC underwent regular surveillance, and the patients who underwent surveillance were ten times more likely to be offered curative therapy [87].

Regular surveillance should play a role in reducing mortality from HCC, and it should be widely instituted [88].

References

1. Meissner HI, Smith RA, Rimer BK, et al. Promoting cancer screening: Learning from experience. Cancer. 2004;101(5 Suppl):1107–17.
2. Bruix J, Sherman M. Management of hepatocellular carcinoma: an update. Hepatology. 2011;53(3):1020–2.
3. Omata M, Lesmana LA, Tateishi R, et al. Asian Pacific Association for the Study of the Liver consensus recommendations on hepatocellular carcinoma. Hepatol Int. 2010;4(2):439–74.
4. Bruix J, Sherman M, Llovet JM, et al. Clinical management of hepatocellular carcinoma. Conclusions of the Barcelona-2000 EASL conference. European Association for the Study of the Liver. J Hepatol. 2001;35(3):421–30.
5. National Comprehensive Cancer Network, Inc. The NCCN Clinical Practice Guidelines in Oncology. Hepatobiliary Cancers (Version 1.2011). http://www.NCCN.org. Accessed June 28, 2011.
6. Sherman M. Hepatocellular carcinoma: epidemiology, surveillance, and diagnosis. Semin Liver Dis. 2010;30(1):3–16.
7. American Cancer Society. Cancer Facts and Figures 2010. http://www.cancer.org/acs/groups/content/@nho/documents/document/acpsc-024113.pdf. Accessed February 1, 2011.
8. Liver Cancer Incidence and Mortality Worldwide in 2008. http://globocan.iarc.fr/factsheets/cancers/liver.asp. Accessed January 10, 2011.
9. McGlynn KA, Tsao L, Hsing AW, Devesa SS, Fraumeni Jr JF. International trends and patterns of primary liver cancer. Int J Cancer. 2001;94(2):290–6.
10. El-Serag HB. Hepatocellular carcinoma: an epidemiologic view. J Clin Gastroenterol. 2002;35(5 Suppl 2):S72–8.
11. El-Serag HB, Davila JA, Petersen NJ, McGlynn KA. The continuing increase in the incidence of hepatocellular carcinoma in the United States: an update. Ann Intern Med. 2003;139(10):817–23.
12. El-Serag HB, Mason AC. Rising incidence of hepatocellular carcinoma in the United States. N Engl J Med. 1999;340(10):745–50.
13. Kuo YH, Lu SN, Chen CL, et al. Hepatocellular carcinoma surveillance and appropriate treatment options improve survival for patients with liver cirrhosis. Eur J Cancer. 2010;46(4):744–51.
14. Lin OS, Keeffe EB, Sanders GD, Owens DK. Cost-effectiveness of screening for hepatocellular carcinoma in patients with cirrhosis due to chronic hepatitis C. Aliment Pharmacol Ther. 2004;19(11):1159–72.
15. Arguedas MR, Chen VK, Eloubeidi MA, Fallon MB. Screening for hepatocellular carcinoma in patients with hepatitis C cirrhosis: a cost-utility analysis. Am J Gastroenterol. 2003;98(3):679–90.

16. Beasley RP, Hwang LY, Lin CC, Chien CS. Hepatocellular carcinoma and hepatitis B virus. A prospective study of 22 707 men in Taiwan. Lancet. 1981;2(8256):1129–33.
17. Beasley RP. Hepatitis B virus. The major etiology of hepatocellular carcinoma. Cancer. 1988;61(10):1942–56.
18. Liaw YF, Lin DY, Chen TJ, Chu CM. Natural course after the development of cirrhosis in patients with chronic type B hepatitis: a prospective study. Liver. 1989;9(4):235–41.
19. Chen CJ, Yang HI, Su J, et al. Risk of hepatocellular carcinoma across a biological gradient of serum hepatitis B virus DNA level. J Am Med Assoc. 2006;295(1):65–73.
20. Yang HI, Lu SN, Liaw YF, et al. Hepatitis B e antigen and the risk of hepatocellular carcinoma. N Engl J Med. 2002;347(3):168–74.
21. Yang HI, Yeh SH, Chen PJ, et al. Associations between hepatitis B virus genotype and mutants and the risk of hepatocellular carcinoma. J Natl Cancer Inst. 2008;100(16):1134–43.
22. Evans AA, O'Connell AP, Pugh JC, et al. Geographic variation in viral load among hepatitis B carriers with differing risks of hepatocellular carcinoma. Cancer Epidemiol Biomarkers Prev. 1998;7(7):559–65.
23. Kew MC, Macerollo P. Effect of age on the etiologic role of the hepatitis B virus in hepatocellular carcinoma in blacks. Gastroenterology. 1988;94(2):439–42.
24. Chen JD, Yang HI, Iloeje UH, et al. Carriers of inactive hepatitis B virus are still at risk for hepatocellular carcinoma and liver-related death. Gastroenterology. 2010;138(5):1747–54.
25. Yang HI, Sherman M, Su J, et al. Nomograms for risk of hepatocellular carcinoma in patients with chronic hepatitis B virus infection. J Clin Oncol. 2010;28(14):2437–44.
26. Yuen MF, Tanaka Y, Fong DY, et al. Independent risk factors and predictive score for the development of hepatocellular carcinoma in chronic hepatitis B. J Hepatol. 2009;50(1):80–8.
27. El-Serag HB. Hepatocellular carcinoma: recent trends in the United States. Gastroenterology. 2004;127(5 Suppl 1):S27–34.
28. Goodgame B, Shaheen NJ, Galanko J, El-Serag HB. The risk of end stage liver disease and hepatocellular carcinoma among persons infected with hepatitis C virus: publication bias? Am J Gastroenterol. 2003;98(11):2535–42.
29. Lok AS, Seeff LB, Morgan TR, et al. Incidence of hepatocellular carcinoma and associated risk factors in hepatitis C-related advanced liver disease. Gastroenterology. 2009;136(1):138–48.
30. Sun CA, Wu DM, Lin CC, et al. Incidence and cofactors of hepatitis C virus-related hepatocellular carcinoma: a prospective study of 12,008 men in Taiwan. Am J Epidemiol. 2003;157(8):674–82.
31. Singal AK, Singh A, Jaganmohan S, et al. Antiviral therapy reduces risk of hepatocellular carcinoma in patients with hepatitis C virus-related cirrhosis. Clin Gastroenterol Hepatol. 2010;8(2):192–9.
32. Giordano TP, Kramer JR, Souchek J, Richardson P, El-Serag HB. Cirrhosis and hepatocellular carcinoma in HIV-infected veterans with and without the hepatitis C virus: a cohort study, 1992–2001. Arch Intern Med. 2004;164(21):2349–54.
33. Di Bisceglie AM. Hepatitis C and hepatocellular carcinoma. Hepatology. 1997;26(3 Suppl 1):34S–8.
34. Fattovich G, Stroffolini T, Zagni I, Donato F. Hepatocellular carcinoma in cirrhosis: incidence and risk factors. Gastroenterology. 2004;127(5 Suppl 1):S35–50.
35. Donato F, Tagger A, Gelatti U, et al. Alcohol and hepatocellular carcinoma: the effect of lifetime intake and hepatitis virus infections in men and women. Am J Epidemiol. 2002;155(4):323–31.
36. Hassan MM, Hwang LY, Hatten CJ, et al. Risk factors for hepatocellular carcinoma: synergism of alcohol with viral hepatitis and diabetes mellitus. Hepatology. 2002;36(5):1206–13.
37. Ratziu V, Giral P, Charlotte F, et al. Liver fibrosis in overweight patients. Gastroenterology. 2000;118(6):1117–23.
38. Ratziu V, Bonyhay L, Di Martino V, et al. Survival, liver failure, and hepatocellular carcinoma in obesity-related cryptogenic cirrhosis. Hepatology. 2002;35(6):1485–93.

39. Calle EE, Rodriguez C, Walker-Thurmond K, Thun MJ. Overweight, obesity, and mortality from cancer in a prospectively studied cohort of U.S. adults. N Engl J Med. 2003;348(17): 1625–38.
40. Marrero JA, Fontana RJ, Su GL, Conjeevaram HS, Emick DM, Lok AS. NAFLD may be a common underlying liver disease in patients with hepatocellular carcinoma in the United States. Hepatology. 2002;36(6):1349–54.
41. El-Serag HB, Tran T, Everhart JE. Diabetes increases the risk of chronic liver disease and hepatocellular carcinoma. Gastroenterology. 2004;126(2):460–8.
42. Elmberg M, Hultcrantz R, Ekbom A, et al. Cancer risk in patients with hereditary hemochromatosis and in their first-degree relatives. Gastroenterology. 2003;125(6):1733–41.
43. Fracanzani AL, Conte D, Fraquelli M, et al. Increased cancer risk in a cohort of 230 patients with hereditary hemochromatosis in comparison to matched control patients with non-iron-related chronic liver disease. Hepatology. 2001;33(3):647–51.
44. Silveira MG, Suzuki A, Lindor KD. Surveillance for hepatocellular carcinoma in patients with primary biliary cirrhosis. Hepatology. 2008;48(4):1149–56.
45. Deutsch M, Papatheodoridis GV, Tzakou A, Hadziyannis SJ. Risk of hepatocellular carcinoma and extrahepatic malignancies in primary biliary cirrhosis. Eur J Gastroenterol Hepatol. 2008;20(1):5–9.
46. Turissini SB, Kaplan MM. Hepatocellular carcinoma in primary biliary cirrhosis. Am J Gastroenterol. 1997;92(4):676–8.
47. Llovet JM, Burroughs A, Bruix J. Hepatocellular carcinoma. Lancet. 2003;362(9399): 1907–17.
48. Cha CH, Ruo L, Fong Y, et al. Resection of hepatocellular carcinoma in patients otherwise eligible for transplantation. Ann Surg. 2003;238(3):315–21. discussion 321–313.
49. Llovet JM, Fuster J, Bruix J. Intention-to-treat analysis of surgical treatment for early hepatocellular carcinoma: resection versus transplantation. Hepatology. 1999;30(6):1434–40.
50. Mazzaferro V, Regalia E, Doci R, et al. Liver transplantation for the treatment of small hepatocellular carcinomas in patients with cirrhosis. N Engl J Med. 1996;334(11):693–9.
51. Chalasani N, Said A, Ness R, Hoen H, Lumeng L. Screening for hepatocellular carcinoma in patients with cirrhosis in the United States: results of a national survey. Am J Gastroenterol. 1999;94(8):2224–9.
52. Sharma P, Saini SD, Kuhn LB, et al. Knowledge of hepatocellular carcinoma screening guidelines and clinical practices among gastroenterologists. Dig Dis Sci. 2011;56(2):569–77.
53. Colombo M. Screening and diagnosis of hepatocellular carcinoma. Liver Int. 2009;29 Suppl 1:143–7.
54. Davila JA, Morgan RO, Richardson PA, Du XL, McGlynn KA, El-Serag HB. Use of surveillance for hepatocellular carcinoma among patients with cirrhosis in the United States. Hepatology. 2010;52(1):132–41.
55. Davila JA, Weston A, Smalley W, El-Serag HB. Utilization of screening for hepatocellular carcinoma in the United States. J Clin Gastroenterol. 2007;41(8):777–82.
56. Sangiovanni A, Del Ninno E, Fasani P, et al. Increased survival of cirrhotic patients with a hepatocellular carcinoma detected during surveillance. Gastroenterology. 2004;126(4):1005–14.
57. Zhang BH, Yang BH, Tang ZY. Randomized controlled trial of screening for hepatocellular carcinoma. J Cancer Res Clin Oncol. 2004;130(7):417–22.
58. Bolondi L, Sofia S, Siringo S, et al. Surveillance programme of cirrhotic patients for early diagnosis and treatment of hepatocellular carcinoma: a cost effectiveness analysis. Gut. 2001;48(2):251–9.
59. Trevisani F, De NS, Rapaccini G, et al. Semiannual and annual surveillance of cirrhotic patients for hepatocellular carcinoma: effects on cancer stage and patient survival (Italian experience). Am J Gastroenterol. 2002;97(3):734–44.
60. Feinstein AR, Sosin DM, Wells CK. The Will Rogers phenomenon. Stage migration and new diagnostic techniques as a source of misleading statistics for survival in cancer. N Engl J Med. 1985;312(25):1604–8.

61. Wong LL, Limm WM, Severino R, Wong LM. Improved survival with screening for hepato-cellular carcinoma. Liver Transplant. 2000;6(3):320–5.
62. Wong GL, Wong VW, Tan GM, et al. Surveillance programme for hepatocellular carcinoma improves the survival of patients with chronic viral hepatitis. Liver Int. 2008;28(1):79–87.
63. Noda I, Kitamoto M, Nakahara H, et al. Regular surveillance by imaging for early detection and better prognosis of hepatocellular carcinoma in patients infected with hepatitis C virus. J Gastroenterol. 2010;45(1):105–12.
64. El-Serag HB, Kramer JR, Chen GJ, Duan Z, Richardson PA, Davila JA. Effectiveness of AFP and ultrasound tests on hepatocellular carcinoma mortality in HCV-infected patients in the USA. Gut. 2011;60(7):992–7.
65. Yuen MF, Cheng CC, Lauder IJ, Lam SK, Ooi CG, Lai CL. Early detection of hepatocellular carcinoma increases the chance of treatment: Hong Kong experience. Hepatology. 2000;31(2):330–5.
66. Trevisani F, Santi V, Gramenzi A, et al. Surveillance for early diagnosis of hepatocellular car-cinoma: is it effective in intermediate/advanced cirrhosis? Am J Gastroenterol. 2007;102(11): 2448–57. quiz 2458.
67. Stravitz RT, Heuman DM, Chand N, et al. Surveillance for hepatocellular carcinoma in patients with cirrhosis improves outcome. Am J Med. 2008;121(2):119–26.
68. McMahon BJ, Bulkow L, Harpster A, et al. Screening for hepatocellular carcinoma in Alaska natives infected with chronic hepatitis B: a 16-year population-based study. Hepatology. 2000;32(4 Pt 1):842–6.
69. Chen JG, Parkin DM, Chen QG, et al. Screening for liver cancer: results of a randomised con-trolled trial in Qidong, China. J Med Screen. 2003;10(4):204–9.
70. Gupta S, Bent S, Kohlwes J. Test characteristics of alpha-fetoprotein for detecting hepatocel-lular carcinoma in patients with hepatitis C. A systematic review and critical analysis. Ann Intern Med. 2003;139(1):46–50.
71. Izuno K, Fujiyama S, Yamasaki K, Sato M, Sato T. Early detection of hepatocellular carci-noma associated with cirrhosis by combined assay of des-gamma-carboxy prothrombin and alpha-fetoprotein: a prospective study. Hepatogastroenterology. 1995;42(4):387–93.
72. Tong MJ, Blatt LM, Kao VW. Surveillance for hepatocellular carcinoma in patients with chronic viral hepatitis in the United States of America. J Gastroenterol Hepatol. 2001;16(5): 553–9.
73. Trevisani F, D'Intino PE, Morselli-Labate AM, et al. Serum alpha-fetoprotein for diagnosis of hepatocellular carcinoma in patients with chronic liver disease: influence of HBsAg and anti-HCV status. J Hepatol. 2001;34(4):570–5.
74. Lok AS, Sterling RK, Everhart JE, et al. Des-gamma-carboxy prothrombin and alpha-fetopro-tein as biomarkers for the early detection of hepatocellular carcinoma. Gastroenterology. 2010;138(2):493–502.
75. Durazo FA, Blatt LM, Corey WG, et al. Des-gamma-carboxyprothrombin, alpha-fetoprotein and AFP-L3 in patients with chronic hepatitis, cirrhosis and hepatocellular carcinoma. J Gastroenterol Hepatol. 2008;23(10):1541–8.
76. Kim CK, Lim JH, Lee WJ. Detection of hepatocellular carcinomas and dysplastic nodules in cirrhotic liver: accuracy of ultrasonography in transplant patients. J Ultrasound Med. 2001;20(2):99–104.
77. Singal A, Volk ML, Waljee A, et al. Meta-analysis: surveillance with ultrasound for early-stage hepatocellular carcinoma in patients with cirrhosis. Aliment Pharmacol Ther. 2009;30(1): 37–47.
78. Chalasani N, Horlander Sr JC, Said A, et al. Screening for hepatocellular carcinoma in patients with advanced cirrhosis. Am J Gastroenterol. 1999;94(10):2988–93.
79. Santi V, Trevisani F, Gramenzi A, et al. Semiannual surveillance is superior to annual surveil-lance for the detection of early hepatocellular carcinoma and patient survival. J Hepatol. 2010;53(2):291–7.
80. Santagostino E, Colombo M, Rivi M, et al. A 6-month versus a 12-month surveillance for hepatocellular carcinoma in 559 hemophiliacs infected with the hepatitis C virus. Blood. 2003;102(1):78–82.

81. Kim DY, Han KH, Ahn SH, et al. Semiannual surveillance for hepatocellular carcinoma improved patient survival compared to annual surveillance (Korean experience). Hepatology. 2007;46(S1):403A.
82. Thompson Coon J, Rogers G, Hewson P, et al. Surveillance of cirrhosis for hepatocellular carcinoma: systematic review and economic analysis. Health Technol Assess. 2007;11(34): 1–206.
83. Naimark D, Naglie G, Detsky AS. The meaning of life expectancy: what is a clinically significant gain? J Gen Intern Med. 1994;9(12):702–7.
84. Sarasin FP, Giostra E, Hadengue A. Cost-effectiveness of screening for detection of small hepatocellular carcinoma in western patients with Child-Pugh class A cirrhosis. Am J Med. 1996;101(4):422–34.
85. Andersson KL, Salomon JA, Goldie SJ, Chung RT. Cost effectiveness of alternative surveillance strategies for hepatocellular carcinoma in patients with cirrhosis. Clin Gastroenterol Hepatol. 2008;6(12):1418–24.
86. Thompson Coon J, Rogers G, Hewson P, et al. Surveillance of cirrhosis for hepatocellular carcinoma: a cost-utility analysis. Br J Cancer. 2008;98(7):1166–75.
87. Leykum LK, El-Serag HB, Cornell J, Papadopoulos KP. Screening for hepatocellular carcinoma among veterans with hepatitis C on disease stage, treatment received, and survival. Clin Gastroenterol Hepatol. 2007;5(4):508–12.
88. Sherman M. Surveillance of hepatocellular carcinoma: we must do better. Am J Med. 2008;121(2):89–90.

Chapter 3
Radiologic Diagnosis of Hepatocellular Carcinoma

Stephen Thomas and Aytekin Oto

Introduction

Hepatocellular carcinoma (HCC) is the most common primary malignancy of the liver accounting for one million deaths annually worldwide. The incidence of HCC in North America has almost doubled during the past 20 years, more significantly among younger people aged 40–60 years [1]. Cirrhosis carries an increased risk of developing HCC with the greatest risk in patients with hepatitis B and C. Of the patients chronically infected with hepatitis C, 25% are expected to progress to cirrhosis [2]. In the setting of cirrhosis, HCC develops at an annual rate of 1%–4% with 25%–30% of patients with hepatitis C and cirrhosis developing HCC. Patients with hepatitis B and hepatitis C coinfection have the highest risk of developing HCC [3]. HCC is mostly asymptomatic and is often detected at a late stage. HCC growth can be sporadic, and screening must be performed at appropriate intervals to detect lesions early [4].

Currently, many treatment options exist for HCC including surgical resection, radiofrequency ablation, percutaneous ethanol ablation, transcatheter chemoembolization, Yttrium-90 radioembolization, and liver transplantation. Some focused minimally invasive therapies can be curative, and others offer a bridge to transplantation. However, improved long-term outcomes depend on successful HCC surveillance for early detection and intervention [5]. Thus, the challenge of screening is early and cost-effective tumor detection in the setting of hepatic cirrhosis.

Screening for HCC is done noninvasively using ultrasound, computed tomography, and magnetic resonance imaging. Each diagnostic modality employs a different technique to examine the hepatic parenchyma with differing levels of accuracy for lesion detection. Often multiple modalities are needed to detect and subsequently

S. Thomas, MD (✉) • A. Oto, MD
Department of Radiology, University of Chicago, Chicago, IL, USA
e-mail: sthomas@radiology.bsd.uchicago.edu

N. Reau and F.F. Poordad (eds.), *Primary Liver Cancer: Surveillance, Diagnosis and Treatment*, Clinical Gastroenterology, DOI 10.1007/978-1-61779-863-4_3,
© Springer Science+Business Media New York 2012

characterize focal hepatic lesions. A working knowledge of the types of lesions that occur in hepatic cirrhosis is necessary as some of the lesions can have overlapping imaging characteristics.

Nodular Hepatocellular Lesions

The 1995 International Working Party panel published a set of guidelines for classifying and describing nodular hepatocellular lesions. The panel created two broad categories of hepatocellular nodules: (a) regenerative lesions and (b) dysplastic or neoplastic lesions [6]. Regenerative lesions include regenerative nodules, lobar or segmental hyperplasia, and focal nodular hyperplasia. Regenerative nodules that occur in the cirrhotic liver are referred to as cirrhotic nodules and are surrounded by fibrous septa while those that arise in an otherwise normal liver are surrounded by normal liver parenchyma. Lobar or segmental hyperplasia and focal nodular hyperplasia usually occur in a noncirrhotic liver. When regenerative nodules contain iron, they are referred to as siderotic or iron containing. Dysplastic and neoplastic cirrhotic lesions include dysplastic foci and nodules, hepatocellular carcinomas, and some hepatocellular adenomas, although the latter typically occur in the noncirrhotic liver.

This framework provides us with four classes of lesions that are typically found in the cirrhotic liver: regenerative nodules, dysplastic foci, dysplastic nodules, and hepatocellular carcinomas. This scheme also provides a basic framework for the carcinogenesis of HCC (Fig. 3.1) with a stepwise sequence of events as follows: regenerative nodule, dysplastic nodule, small HCC, and large HCC [7]. During the process of carcinogenesis for HCC, tumor angiogenesis takes place, which is important in the transformation of regenerative nodules into dysplastic nodules and small

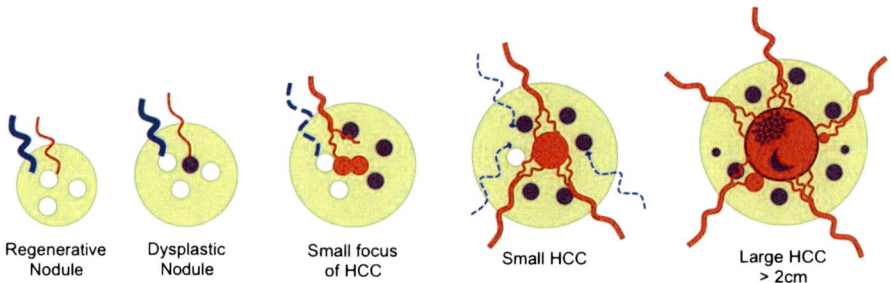

| Regenerative Nodule | Dysplastic Nodule | Small focus of HCC | Small HCC | Large HCC > 2cm |

Fig. 3.1 Concept of stepwise sequence of carcinogenesis in HCC where a regenerative nodule grows and undergoes cellular atypia to form a dysplastic nodule. The dysplastic nodule undergoes malignant transformation forming a small focus of HCC that eventually grows to occupy the entire nodule. A key change in the pathway is an increase in neovascularity with a shift from portal venous to hepatic arterial blood supply

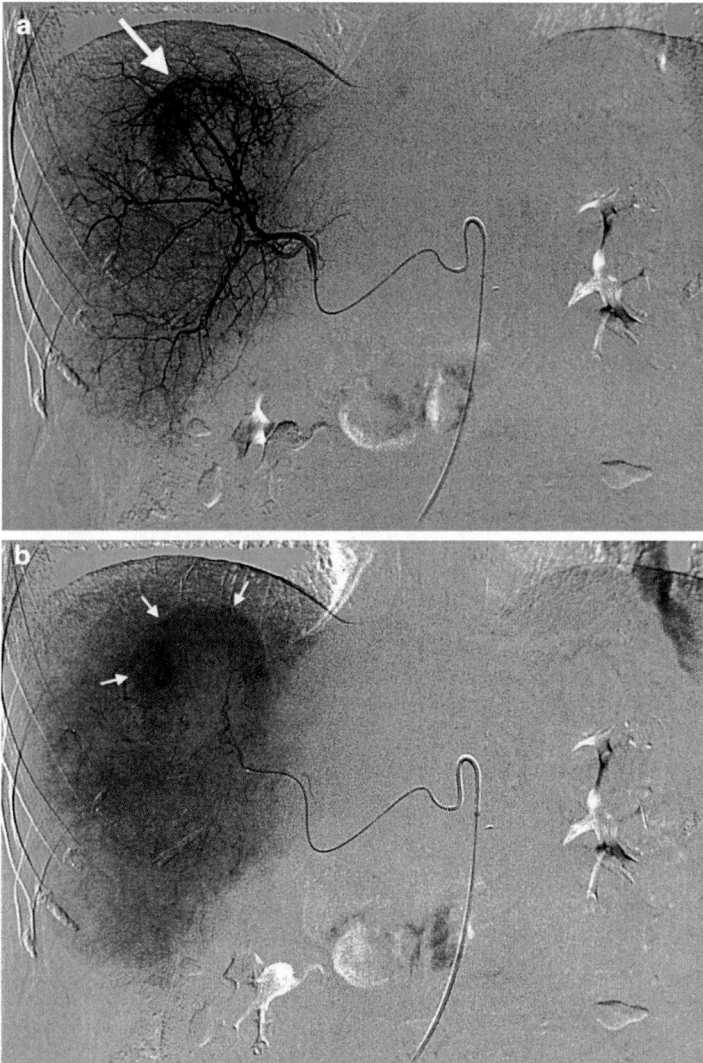

Fig. 3.2 Conventional catheter angiography of the hepatic artery in a patient with known HCC demonstrating neovascularization. (**a**) Arterial phase of the exam shows the neovascularization and proliferation of arterial vessels around the mass (*arrow*). (**b**) Parenchymal phase of the injection shows the tumor blush and which outlines it from surrounding liver (*arrows*)

HCC. The tumor angiogenesis plays an important role in the imaging of a cirrhotic liver. As nodules progress to HCC, they tend to have a greater arterial vascular supply compared to regenerative and dysplastic nodules, which have a primary portal venous supply (Fig. 3.2) [8].

Ultrasound in the Diagnosis of Hepatocellular Carcinoma

Ultrasound (US) is the most widely used tool to screen for HCC. US has added benefits as it is noninvasive and widely available, lacks ionizing radiation, and has been shown to be cost-effective with annual or semiannual screening [9]. However, US requires highly skilled operators to produce diagnostic images and detect and characterize hepatic lesions [10]. The quality of the study also heavily depends on the patient's physical condition and body habitus.

Ultrasound is a useful tool in evaluating hepatic cirrhosis. Cirrhotic livers have a nodular surface contour due to macronodular (>3 mm) regenerative nodules and intervening fibrous septa. The nodular surface contour of the liver is best evaluated with a high-frequency probe [11]. Evaluation of the hepatic parenchyma is performed with a lower-frequency probe as the coarsened, echogenic cirrhotic echotexture limits beam penetration [12].

On gray-scale ultrasound, HCCs have a varied appearance with lesions appearing hypo-, iso-, or hyperechoic to background liver with the hypoechoic pattern being the most common (approximately 76%) (Fig. 3.3a) [13–15]. Small (<2 cm)

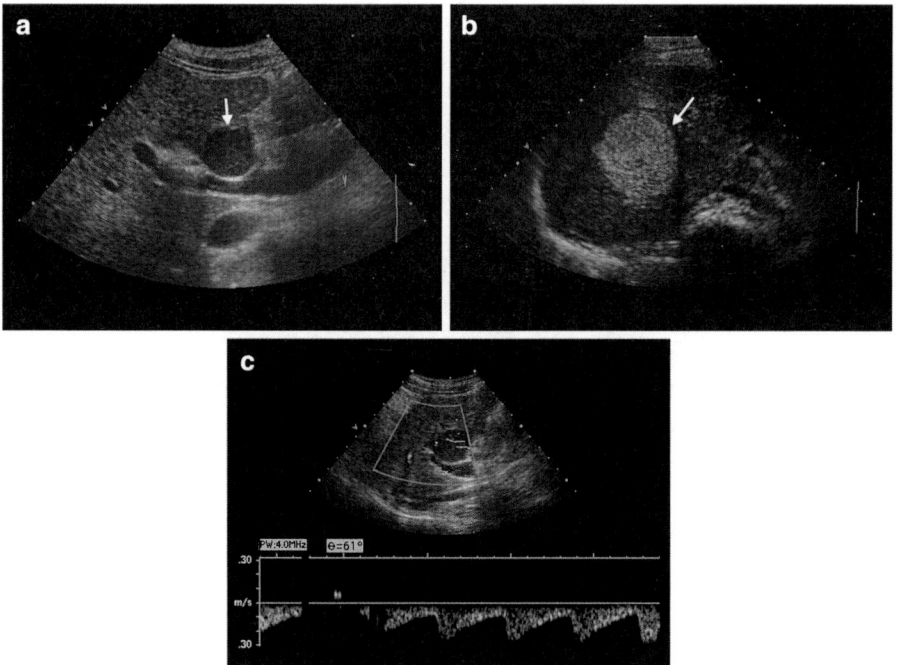

Fig. 3.3 Ultrasound images from patients with cirrhosis undergoing screening showing the different appearances of HCC. (**a**) Small exophytic rounded lesion that is hypoechoic to the liver parenchyma (*arrow*). (**b**) US images from another patient showing a large hyperechoic mass in the liver (*arrow*). (**c**) Color and spectral Doppler ultrasound showing color flow with an arterialized waveform within the lesion

lesions detected at US are mostly hypoechoic with respect to the adjacent liver parenchyma and may require further characterization to rule out the presence of malignancy. Approximately 17% of HCCs show a hyperechoic pattern, which have been reportedly found in patients with lower AFP levels and higher prevalence of hepatitis C [16] (Fig. 3.3b). HCCs that are isoechoic or have a nodule within a nodule pattern tend to occur less frequently with a reported frequency of approximately 3% each [16]. The sonographic appearance of the lesion has not shown to correlate with tumor differentiation [16]. The overall sensitivity of US for detection of HCC ranges between 40% and 81% and a specificity of 80%–100% [17–20]. US has a lower sensitivity for detecting early HCC with sensitivities as low as 25% [21]. The use of ultrasound to image diffuse infiltrative tumors, intrahepatic venous invasion, and displacement or compression of vessels or bile ducts remains a limitation of the modality.

Ultrasound has a unique ability to noninvasively image blood flow with color Doppler and spectral Doppler techniques. Doppler techniques can easily detect blood flow, can characterize the waveform patterns, and can be performed with almost all-standard ultrasound probes [22]. Standard ultrasound liver protocol includes imaging of the portal vein allowing detection of portal hypertension and portosystemic shunts. In the evaluation of focal hepatic lesions, Doppler ultrasound can be used to image the vascularity of hepatic lesions with the majority (approximately 75%) of HCCs showing internal vascularity (Fig. 3.3c) [23]. Doppler US can help in the staging of HCC, especially to evaluate tumor extension into the portal vein. The presence of intrathrombus pulsatile spectral Doppler flow has a reported sensitivity of 62% and specificity of 95% for the detection of malignant tumor thrombus in the portal vein [24].

The real-time imaging ability of ultrasound makes it an excellent modality to guide percutaneous procedures. Percutaneous US-guided fine-needle aspiration biopsy (FNAB) and core needle biopsy are performed for definitive tissue diagnosis. The diagnostic accuracy of US-guided fine-needle biopsies is very high with a reported accuracy of greater than 90% for focal liver lesions [25]. When portal venous invasion is suspected, US-guided fine-needle aspiration of portal venous thrombus can be performed to confirm portal extension (Fig. 3.4) [26]. Percutaneous US-guided radiofrequency or ethanol ablation of HCCs has been effectively used to treat lesions and can be used as a bridge to liver translation [27, 28].

Contrast-enhanced ultrasound (CEUS) with microbubble ultrasound contrast agents (UCAs) offers ultrasound the ability to characterize focal liver lesions based on vascularity [29]. UCAs are gas bubbles stabilized by a membrane. The microbubble sizes vary from 3 to 5 μm, which allow them to escape filtration in the pulmonary circuit, and they are too large to enter the interstitium. The covering layer is based on perfluorocarbons with a phospholipid membrane, providing low solubility and favorable resonance behavior at low acoustic pressures. UCAs, when injected intravenously, demonstrate strong nonlinear harmonic responses when insonated with low acoustic pressure and generate specific signals without being destroyed when insonated at low mechanical index allowing continuous real-time imaging [30]. UCAs have been used in guiding and monitoring therapy with percutaneous

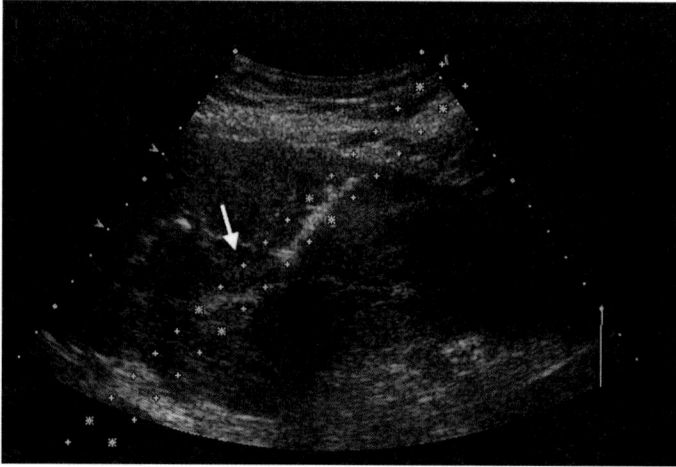

Fig. 3.4 Patient with known HCC with suspected portal venous extension. Percutaneous core needle biopsy of portal venous thrombus (*arrow*) to confirm venous invasion. *Dotted lines* represent the needle guide with the echogenic needle track

ablation. Intraoperative use of UCAs has helped decrease the need of re-treatment by detecting partially unablated tumors [31].

Computed Tomography in the Diagnosis of Hepatocellular Carcinoma

Multidetector CT (MDCT) plays a vital role in the imaging of cirrhosis and detection and characterization of focal hepatic lesions. The introduction of multidetector row CT scanners in the 1990s allowed for faster imaging times as rotational speed increased and improved temporal resolution. The shorter imaging times allowed imaging during the critical arterial phase and coverage of the entire liver in 10 s or less [32]. Multiple detector row CT allowed for improved spatial resolution, and thinner sections allowed better resolution in the z-axis [33]. The sensitivity for detection of HCC increases with smaller slice thickness with a mean reported sensitivity of 76% on 2.5-mm images, 73% on 5-mm images, and 67% on 7.5-mm images. However, a thinner slice thickness has the potential to detect intrahepatic vascular shunts and other benign vascular lesions and thus increase false-positive results [34].

A standard liver CT protocol consists of an unenhanced and a dynamic contrast-enhanced study including hepatic arterial (25–35 s), portal venous (70–80 s), and delayed phases (3 min after contrast administration). The hepatic arterial phase added to the unenhanced and portal venous phase will allow the detection of approximately 30% more tumor lesions and in approximately 10% of HCC patients will be the only phase to show the lesions [35–37]. Arterial phase imaging is performed with a nonionic iodine containing contrast medium (iodine content 300–350 mg/ml) injected at 3–5 ml/s intravenously by a power injector. No significant differences have been found between injection rates of 3 ml or 5 ml/s, and higher injection rates (5 ml/s) show an increase in the false-positive lesions such as intrahepatic shunts [32].

Evaluation of the cirrhotic liver by CT is complicated by replacement of the normal-homogenous parenchyma by areas of fibrosis, scarring, and nodular regeneration. Fibrosis manifests as areas of low attenuation on unenhanced CT and can be nearly isoattenuating to hepatic parenchyma on contrast-enhanced sequences. Fibrosis may be diffuse or focal. Four patterns of diffuse fibrosis have been described and include patchy, poorly defined regions, thin perilobular bands, thick bridging bands that surround regenerative nodules, and diffuse fibrosis that causes perilobular (bull's eye) cuffing [38]. Confluent hepatic fibrosis appears as mass-like areas of signal or attenuation difference that extends from the hilum to the capsule. Confluent fibrosis is associated with capsular retraction and volume loss, which is useful sign in differentiating it from HCC; the latter tends to show mass effect or an exophytic border [39].

CT easily detects macronodular changes as they distort the hepatic surface contour. Micronodular changes are rarely seen on CT, as the parenchyma appears homogenous after contrast administration. On CT, regenerative nodules are isoattenuating on an unenhanced exam. Iron deposits in regenerating nodules can make them slightly hyperattenuating (Fig. 3.5a) as they are surrounded by lower attenuation fibrosis [40]. Regenerative nodules typically do not enhance on the arterial phase as their blood supply is almost exclusively from portal vein (Fig. 3.5b) [41].

Dysplastic nodules have cellular atypia without frank malignant changes and are considered precursors to HCC. Small dysplastic nodules (<5 mm) are difficult to detect at imaging; however, they are commonly found in the explant specimens. Larger nodules may be higher in attenuation on unenhanced imaging and become isoattenuating after contrast administration [40].

The main CT finding of HCC in the cirrhotic liver is the depiction of changes in the vascular supply of liver nodules due to neoangiogenesis, as described during hepatic angiography [42]. The imaging features of HCC at CT vary depending on the size of the lesion. Smaller lesions are homogeneously enhancing, whereas larger lesions (>5 cm) tend to show mosaic enhancement pattern and some show delayed capsular enhancement [43]. The presence of arterial enhancement followed by washout on portal venous or delayed phases of imaging yields a sensitivity and specificity of 90% and 95%, respectively (Fig. 3.6) [44]. The enhancement patterns are crucial for the characterization of HCC. According to the AASLD practice guidelines, in patients with cirrhosis, liver lesions measuring larger than 1 cm can be noninvasively diagnosed as HCC, if they demonstrate enhancement at the arterial phase and washout on delayed phase on CT. If the classic pattern is not present, a subsequent study either CT or MR can be performed to detect enhancement characteristics. If the lesion is less than 1 cm, diagnosis can be made if similar enhancement characteristics are noted on both CT and MRI [45, 46].

However, some HCCs only demonstrate enhancement at the arterial phase without washout, and some only demonstrate washout without arterial phase enhancement.

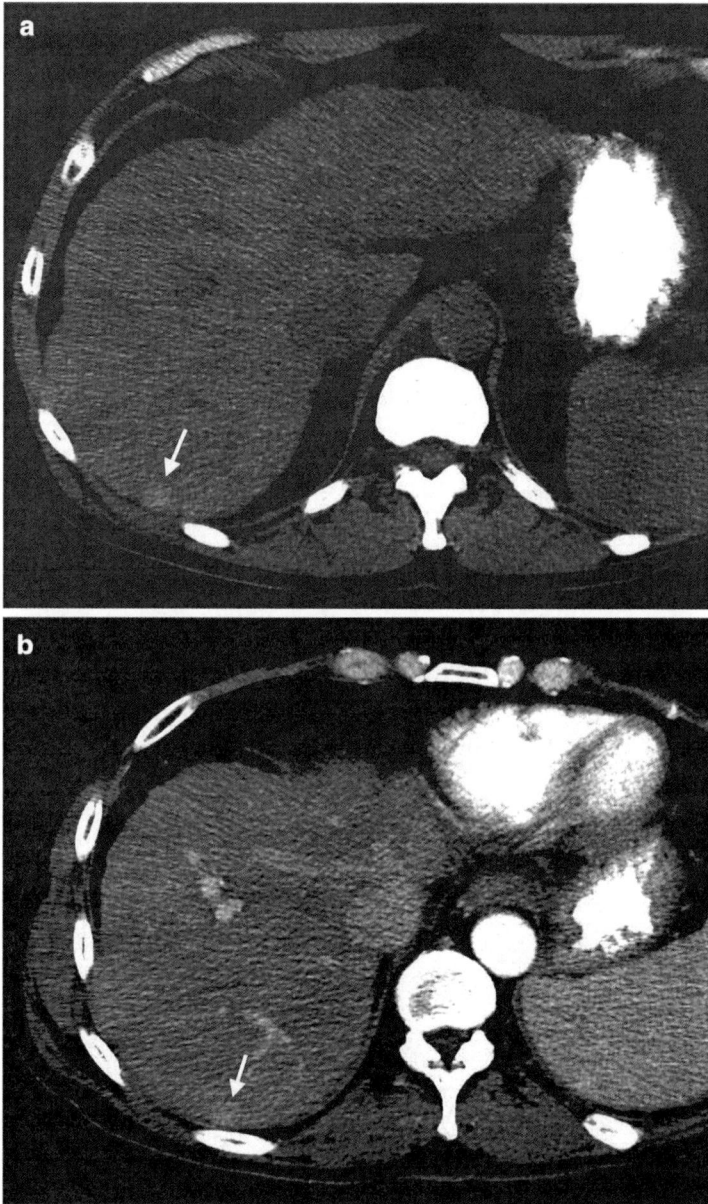

Fig. 3.5 Axial noncontrast CT of the liver showing iron-containing regenerative nodule in a screening CT. (**a**) The nodule is hyperattenuating (*arrow*) compared to background liver on unenhanced CT. (**b**) Arterial phase of the same patient showing no appreciable enhancement of the nodule (*arrow*)

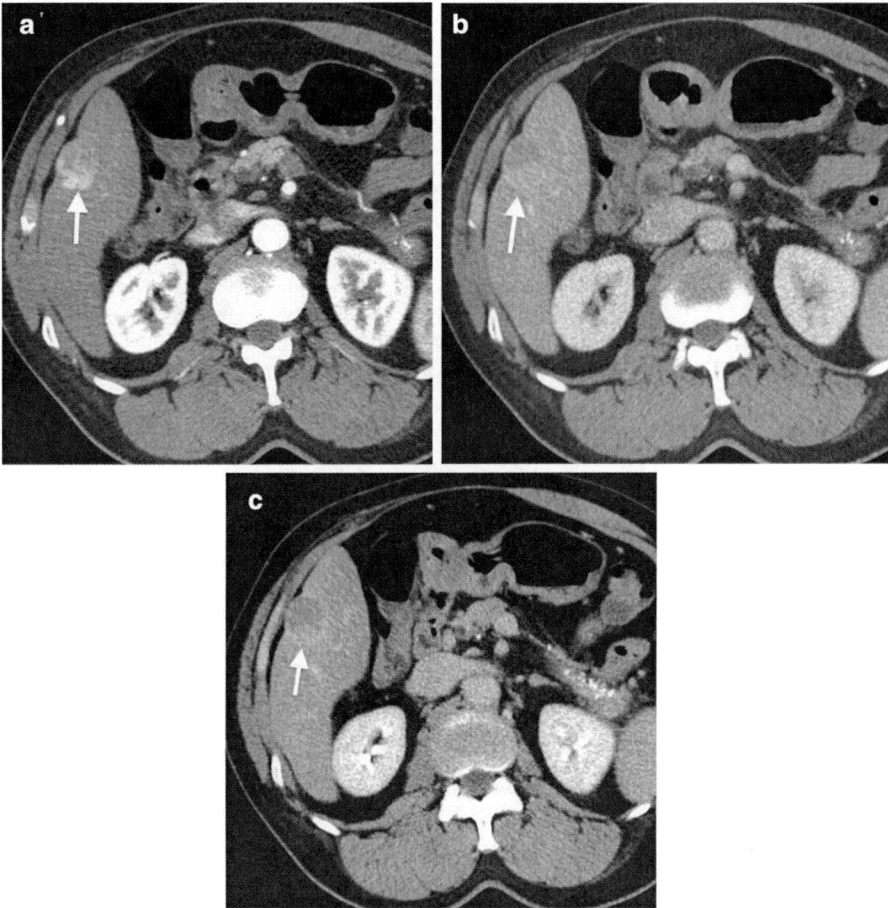

Fig. 3.6 Screening multiphase contrast-enhanced CT of the liver in a hepatitis C patient demonstrating the classic enhancement pattern of HCC. (**a**) Peripherally located arterial enhancing lesion (*arrow*) that bulges the hepatic contour. (**b**) Portal venous phase shows part of the lesion is isoattenuating to liver (*arrow*) and portion of the lesion has washed out. (**c**) Delayed phase shows progressive washout of the lesion with a subtle capsule (*arrow*)

Some HCCs may remain isointense/dense to the liver on all phases. Lack of reliable criteria to detect or characterize HCC other than vascular changes is the main reason for false-positive findings (e.g., arteriovenous shunts, dysplastic nodules with pathological vascularization) or false-negative findings (e.g., well-differentiated HCC without arterial hyperenhancement, hypovascular HCC).

The overall range sensitivity for detecting HCC using triple-phase CT is 50–94% and specificity of 80–96% [17, 18, 20, 47–50]. Despite technological advances, CT remains insensitive to detect subcentimeter HCC (33–45%) [51]. Several lesions including hemangiomas, focal confluent fibrosis, peliosis, benign regenerative nodules, and transient hepatic attenuation difference can simulate small HCC lesions on

CT [52]. Since CT depicts the vascularity of lesions, it is difficult to distinguish between simple regenerative nodules, high-grade dysplastic nodules, and early HCC in the cirrhotic liver, as there can be overlap in imaging findings.

Magnetic Resonance Imaging in the Diagnosis of Hepatocellular Carcinoma

Magnetic resonance imaging (MRI) is useful in the detection and characterization of focal hepatic lesions. The development of fast gradients, parallel imaging, and employment of higher field strengths allow for breath-hold imaging and dynamic contrast exams. Newer imaging techniques such as diffusion-weighted imaging (DWI) have shown utility in imaging HCC. MRI, unlike CT, does not expose the patients to ionizing radiation and is a more appropriate screening tool in the high-risk patient population for radiation who may otherwise undergo regular screening by CT.

A standard MR screening liver protocol includes axial and coronal single-shot T2-weighted imaging (WI), axial fast spin echo T2 with fat saturation (FS), axial gradient-recalled echo (GRE) in and opposed phase imaging, and pre- and dynamic postgadolinium-enhanced three-dimensional gradient-echo FS. The sequences are typically performed with breath-hold technique to reduce motion artifacts. The post-contrast sequences can be used to evaluate vascular anatomy and vascular invasion.

Similar to CT, the cirrhotic liver poses problems in detection and characterization of hepatic lesions due to distortion of the parenchyma. Unlike CT, MR inherently has better soft tissue discrimination aiding in nodule detection and characterization. Fibrosis is usually iso- to hypointense on T1-weighted imaging (WI) and hyperintense to liver parenchyma on T2-WI. Areas of fibrosis may show mild enhancement after the administration of gadolinium-based contrast agents [53, 54].

On MR, iron-free regenerative nodules are usually isointense on T1- and T2-WI, while iron-containing nodules are hypointense on T1- and T2-WI (Fig. 3.7) and do not show arterial enhancement [41, 55, 56]. Regenerative nodules are not hyperintense on T2-WI except in the setting of chronic Budd–Chiari syndrome [57]. Rarely, large regenerative nodules may undergo ischemic coagulative necrosis and appear hyperintense on T2-WI [58].

MR imaging shows dysplastic nodules as usually hyperintense to surrounding liver on T1-WI and hypointense on T2-WI [3]. Dysplastic nodules may show arterial enhancement, which likely reflects early neoplastic angiogenesis. Subtraction imaging can help detection of enhancement of nodules that are hyperintense on precontrast T1-weighted imaging (Fig. 3.8) [41, 59]. It is difficult to distinguish between iron-containing regenerative and dysplastic nodules, as both appear hypointense in T1- and T2-WI. Despite its better tissue discrimination, MR imaging has poor sensitivity for detecting dysplastic nodules [60].

Small HCCs have variable patterns of signal intensity on T1- and T2-WI and may appear similar to dysplastic nodules [3]. HCCs smaller than 1.5 cm are often isointense on T1-WI, and larger lesions can be T1 hyperintense. Signal intensity of

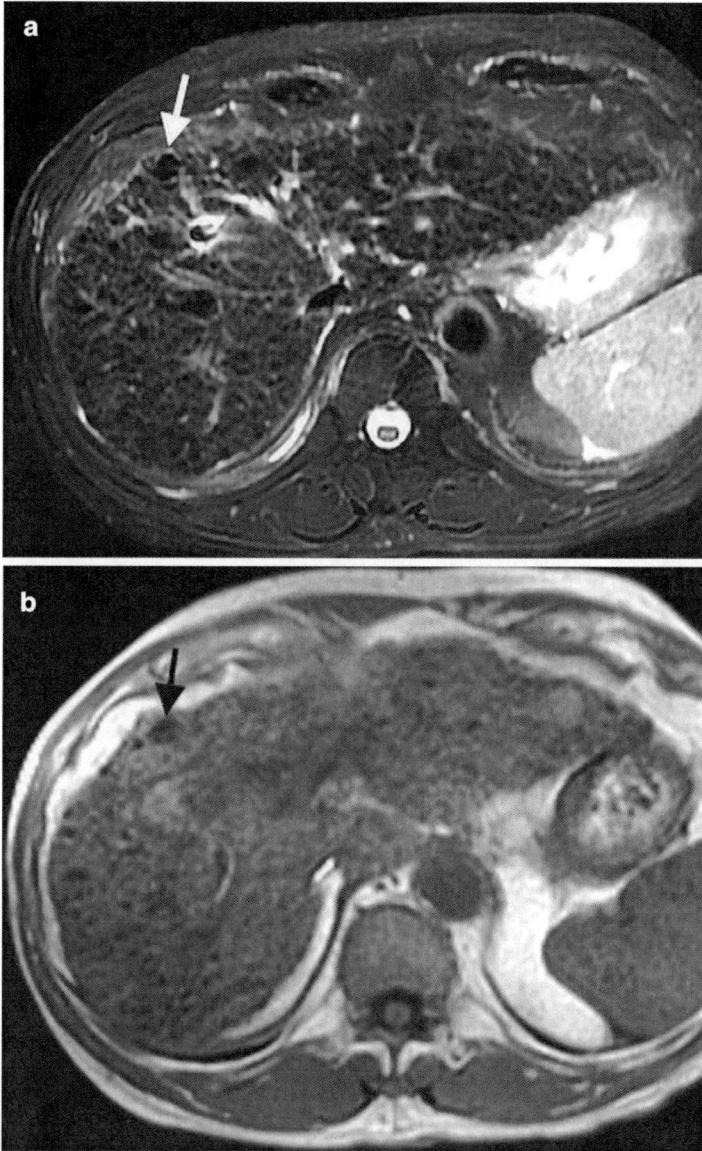

Fig. 3.7 Screening MRI in a patient with cirrhosis showing a typical siderotic nodule. (**a**) Axial T2 fat-suppressed image showing a T2 hypointense nodule (*arrow*). (**b**) Axial T1 SPGR image showing the nodule is T1 hypointense

lesions is related to tumoral differentiation and the presence of iron, lipid, copper, and glycogen [61–63]. HCCs can have variable signal intensity on T2-WI with most lesions either hyper- or isointense to liver. T2 hypointensity and isointensity are correlated with better-differentiated lesions [61].

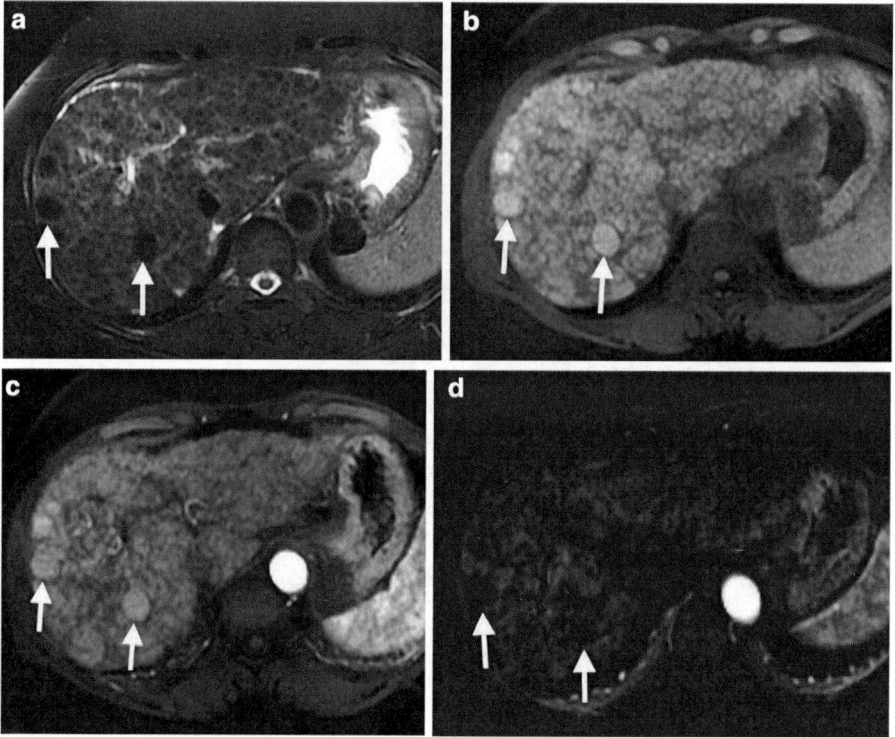

Fig. 3.8 Screening MRI in a cirrhotic liver with multiple dysplastic nodules. (**a**) Axial T2 fat-suppressed image showing multiple hypointense modules (*arrows*). (**b**) Axial T1 FSPGR FS pre-contrast images showing multiple T1 hyperintense nodules (*arrows*). (**c**) Postcontrast axial T1 FSPGR FS sequence showing the nodules are hyperintense making determining arterial enhancement difficult (*arrows*). (**d**) Subtraction image created from the postcontrast and precontrast sequences confirms the lack of enhancement as the nodules appear as areas of signal void (*arrows*)

Early HCCs may show a rare "nodule within a nodule" pattern where a small focus of T2 hypointensity is present in a hypo- or isointense nodule (Fig. 3.9) [64]. Well-differentiated HCCs may have microscopic lipid, which can be detected using in- and opposed-phase techniques (Fig. 3.10). The technique uses the phase shift between fat and water to produce images and is useful in detecting cellular lipids. Lesions that contain fat show signal loss on out-of-phase images. Lipid distribution in the nodule is dependent on nodule size and tends to be evenly distributed throughout smaller lesions, whereas in larger lesions, the fat tends to be focal [65].

Since HCCs demonstrate variable signal intensities on T1- and T2-WI, dynamic contrast-enhanced MR plays an important role in detecting and characterizing lesions. Gadolinium chelate-based contrast agents produce T1 shortening that can be detected on T1-WI. The pattern of enhancement is dependent on lesion size and tumoral differentiation. Small HCCs (<2 cm) show uniform intense arterial enhancement, while larger lesions have a heterogeneous enhancement pattern with

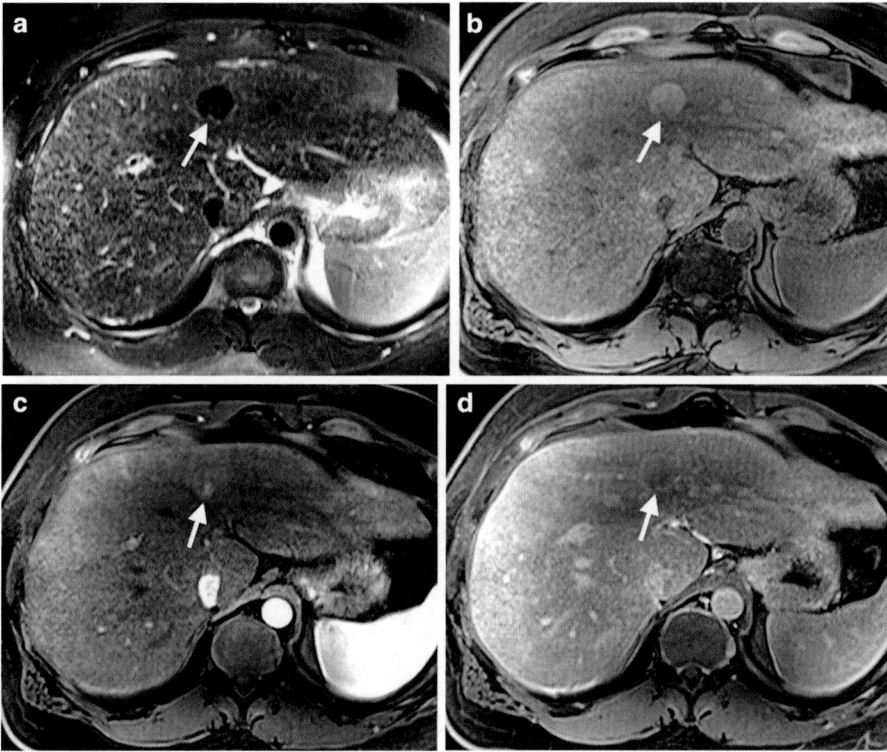

Fig. 3.9 MRI of a cirrhotic liver showing development of a focus of HCC within a dysplastic nodule referred to as a nodule in a nodule pattern. (**a**) Axial T2 fat-suppressed image showing a T2 hypointense nodule (*arrow*). (**b**) Precontrast T1 FSPGR FS image showing a distinct hypointense nodule within a larger hyperintense nodule (*arrow*). (**c**) Postcontrast T1 FSPGR FS image demonstrates enhancement of the nodule (*arrow*). (**d**) Delayed-phase imaging shows washout of the lesion with a developing capsular rim (*arrow*)

10%–15% of small lesions only identified on arterial phase [66, 67].The mosaic pattern of enhancement of larger lesions is a configuration of confluent small nodules separated by thin septa and necrotic areas within the tumor. The degree of enhancement is partly due to the larger sinusoidal spaces in moderately and poorly differentiated tumors [68]. HCCs can show venous "washout" and appear hypointense to liver on venous phase of imaging and are an important predictor of malignancy [69, 70]. The combination of arterial enhancement and venous washout is very specific of HCC with the probability of malignancy less than 10% if both arterial phase enhancement and venous phase washout are absent [70].

The presence of a fibrous capsule (FC) is a characteristic finding in hepatocellular carcinoma. The capsule consists of an inner layer rich in fibrous component and an outer layer containing various numbers of small vessels, newly formed bile duct, and prominent sinusoids [71–73]. The tumor capsule becomes thicker with

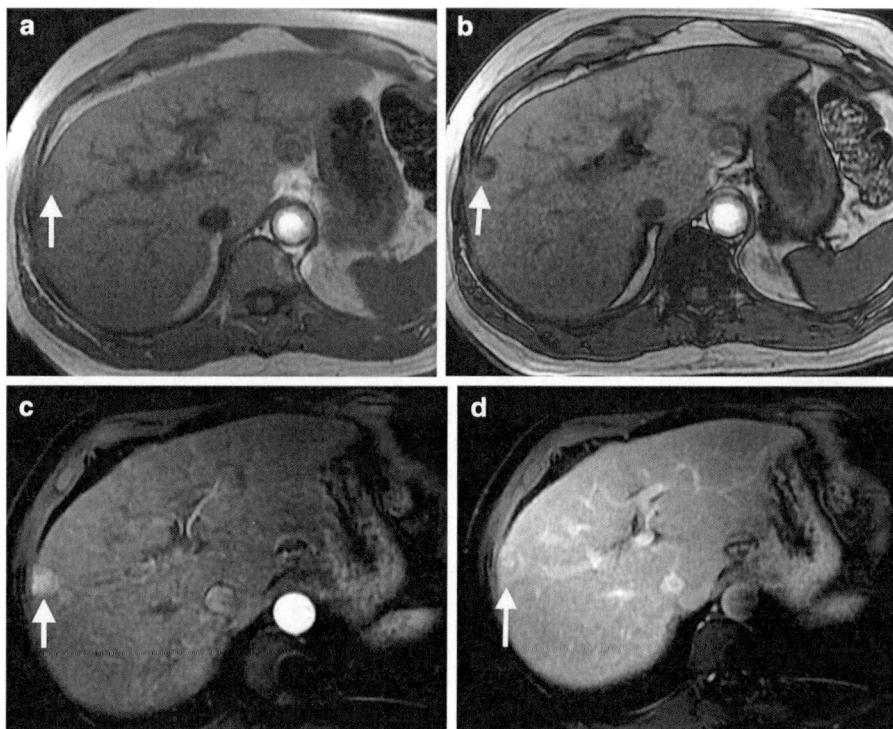

Fig. 3.10 Screening MRI shows a peripheral lesion containing lipid. (**a**) In-phase T1 SPGR shows a nodule (*arrow*) that is nearly isointense to liver. (**b**) Opposed-phase T1 SPGR shows signal loss in the nodule (*arrow*) indicating the nodule contains lipids. (**c**) Postcontrast T1 FSPGR FS shows brisk arterial enhancement of the lesion (*arrow*). (**d**) Postcontrast T1 FSPGR delayed phase shows washout and a subtle capsule around the lesion

increasing tumor size. In contrast, the term "pseudocapsule" is used for nonspecific tissue changes that may be present surrounding the lesion. HCCs with an FC tend to be larger, moderately to poorly differentiated, and have portal venous invasion and intrahepatic metastasis. They are associated with a significantly poorer clinical outcome [74].

The capsule is usually a hypointense thin rim on T1- and T2-WI with enhancement on portal venous phase of contrast enhancement. The presence of the capsule correlates with tumoral differentiation with the majority of the lesions found to be moderately to poorly differentiated [75].

Vascular invasion occurs frequently in HCC and with more frequent invasion of the portal than the hepatic veins. Microscopic invasion (59%) is more common than macroscopic invasion (16%) (Fig. 3.11). Lesions with vascular invasion tend to be larger, have a higher serum α-fetoprotein level, and show less frequent encapsulation [76].

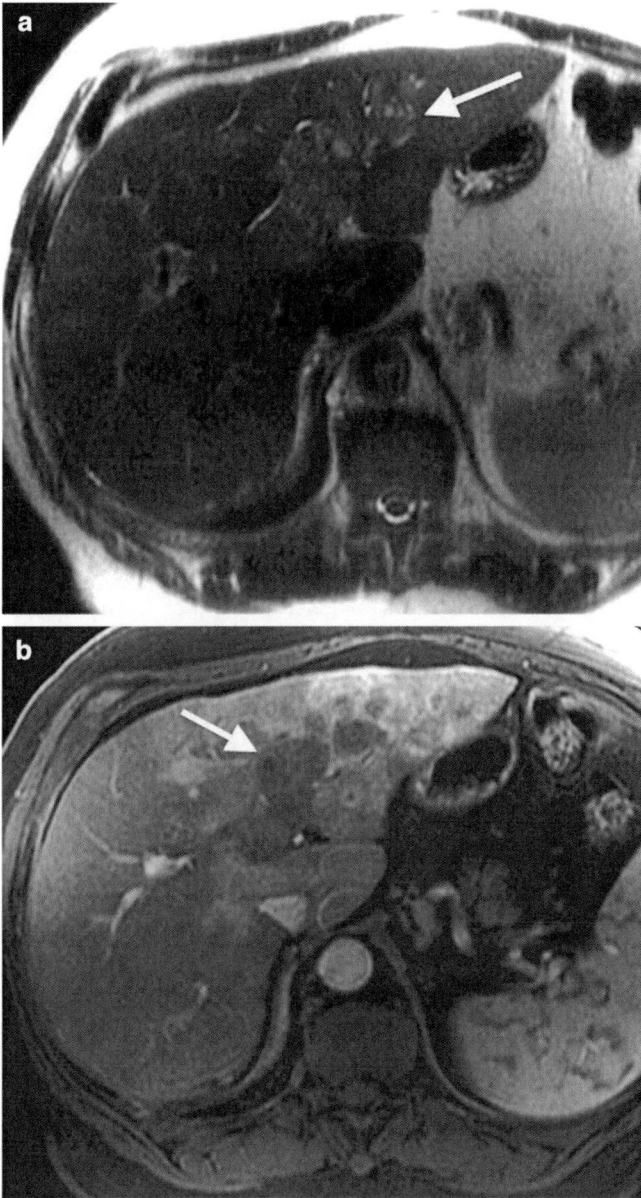

Fig. 3.11 Screening MRI in a patient with suspected HCC shows extensive disease in the left lobe of the liver with portal venous extension. (**a**) T2-WI shows expansion of the left portal vein with thrombus that is T2 hyperintense to liver (*arrow*). (**b**) Postcontrast T1 FSPGR shows expansion of the portal vein with heterogeneously enhancing tumor thrombus (*arrow*) and arterially enhancing tumor in the left lobe

On T1- and T2-WI imaging, vascular invasion can be as a signal flow void. With gadolinium-enhanced MR imaging, the tumor thrombus typically shows arterial enhancement and a filling defect on portal venous phases [66, 77].

Extrahepatic metastasis occurs in patients with advanced intrahepatic tumor (stage IVA). Common sites of metastasis include lungs, regional nodes, adrenal, bone, peritoneum, and omentum [78, 79]. Upper abdominal lymphadenopathy is a common finding in chronic liver disease, and metastatic involvement cannot be excluded based on size. Features such as arterial enhancement and interval growth can predict malignant lymph node involvement [78].

Diffusion-Weighted MRI: DW imaging is a new tool, which has shown utility to detect and characterize HCC. The sequence exploits the random motion of water molecules and produces signal in areas where there is decreased motion of water molecules. The degree of restriction to water diffusion in biologic tissue is inversely correlated to the tissue cellularity and the integrity of cell membranes [80]. DWI is noninvasive and does not require contrast agents, and with new scanner generations, faster gradient coils, parallel imaging, and processing power, breath-hold DW imaging with echoplanar imaging is feasible with a high image quality and robustness [81].

DW imaging can help increase the detection rate of focal liver lesions, especially due to the black-blood effect, which helps to perceive even very small lesions or lesions directly adjacent to vessels [82]. DW imaging has shown benefit in improved detection of HCC compared to conventional MRI, due to better characterization of lesions smaller than 2 cm (Fig. 3.12) [83]. DW imaging has shown utility in discriminating between bland and neoplastic portal vein thrombus, which can help in disease staging [84].

Hepatocyte-Specific Contrast Agent (HSCA): Most MR gadolinium-based contrast agents are extracellular and are distributed in the vascular and interstitial spaces. Hepatocyte-specific gadolinium-based contrast agents are taken up by the hepatocytes and are considered combined extracellular and hepatocyte-specific agents. Some of the currently available agents include gadobenate dimeglumine (Gd-BOPTA, MultiHance®: Bracco Imaging SpA, Milan, Italy) and gadoxetic acid (Gd-EOB-DTPA Primovist, Bayer Schering Pharma; Eovist, Bayer HealthCare, in the United States) with reported biliary excretion of 5% and 50%, respectively [85].

HSCAs are administered as a bolus infusion and allow for imaging arterial, portal venous, and the hepatobiliary phase, which is at 40 and 20 min for Gd-BOPTA and Gd-EOB-DTPA, respectively [85]. The utility of HSCAs has been shown in detecting additional small metastasis, which appears hypointense to bright background liver increasing lesion conspicuity. Low-grade dysplastic nodules can take up contrast, while high-grade dysplastic nodules do not take up contrast as the number of expressed organic ion transporters in dysplastic nodules decreases [86]. However, HSCAs do not necessary improve HCC lesion conspicuity as well-differentiated HCCs can take up these agents. Poorly differentiated HCCs do not take up hepatocyte-specific agents [87].

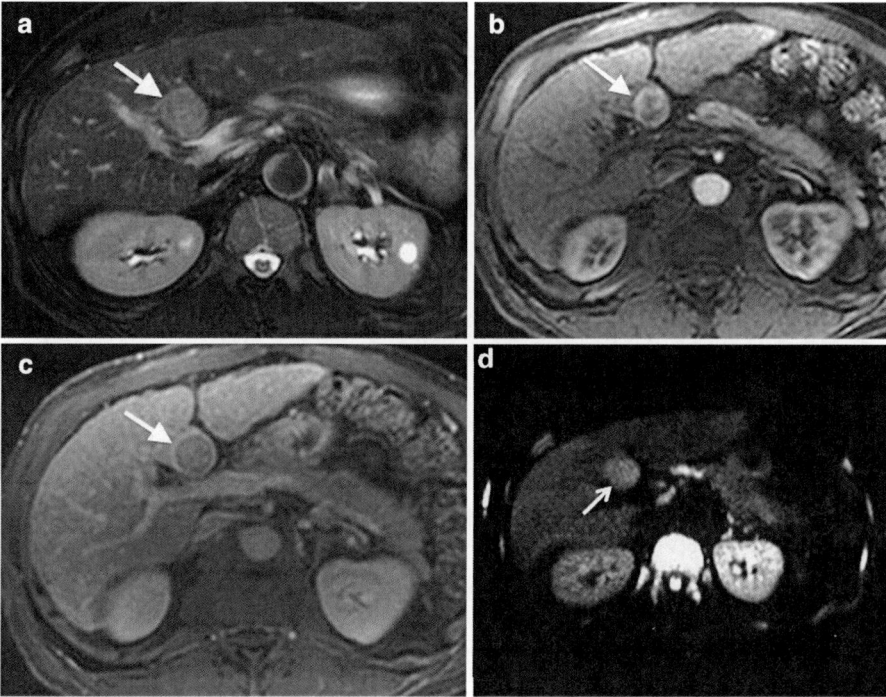

Fig. 3.12 Screening MRI in a hepatitis C patient showing the utility of diffusion-weighted imaging. (**a**) Axial T2-WI fat-suppressed image showing a mildly T2 hyperintense lesion (*arrow*). (**b**) Postcontrast T1 FSPGR FS arterial phase sequence shows brisk enhancement of the lesion (*arrow*). (**c**) Postcontrast T1 FSPGR fat-suppressed delayed phase shows washout of the lesion with a peripheral capsule typical for HCC (*arrow*). (**d**) Axial (noncontrast) DWI image of the lesion clearly depicts the lesion as a hyperintense lesion (*arrow*) compared to background liver

Positron Emission Tomography-Computed Tomography in the Diagnosis of Hepatocellular Carcinoma

Positron emission tomography-computed tomography (PET-CT) with fluorine-18-labeled 2-fluoro-2-deoxy-D-glucose (FDG) has not shown promise in the detection of HCC with reported sensitivities between 50% and 55% with lower sensitivities for well-differentiated and moderately differentiated lesions [88, 89]. PET has shown an 83% detection rate for extrahepatic metastases larger than 1 cm in greatest diameter and is used in staging advanced disease [90].

Summary

Detecting and characterizing lesions in a cirrhotic liver is a challenging task. The early detection of HCC is important to guide curative therapies focused on small lesions. Advances in technology have helped in detecting smaller lesions and characterizing them. Regular screening with an accepted modality offers the best chance at detection HCC at an early stage.

Ultrasound plays an important role in screening for HCC. The use of Doppler imaging and contrast-enhanced ultrasound has shown benefit in the detection and characterization of hepatic lesions over gray-scale imaging alone. In addition to screening, US plays an important role in percutaneous image-guided therapeutics and postintervention monitoring. However, US is limited by the operator, technique, patient's condition, and tissue acoustics. CT and MR are the mainstay for the detection and characterization of hepatic lesions. MR with its superior tissue discrimination and newer pulse sequences such as diffusion-weighted imaging and hepatocyte-specific contrast agents can help better characterize lesions. MR is limited as it is more time-consuming, has increased cost, and requires patient cooperation for breath holding. CT is widely available, but when used as a screening tool every 6–12 months over many years, there is significant radiation exposure.

Each of the screening modalities has benefits and drawbacks, and no consensus currently exists on which modality is best for screening. Ultrasound is currently widely used for screening as it is widely available and has a demonstrable cost benefit over other modalities.

References

1. El-Serag HB. Hepatocellular carcinoma: recent trends in the United States. Gastroenterology. 2004;127(5 Suppl 1):S27–34.
2. Flamm SL. Chronic hepatitis C virus infection. J Am Med Assoc. 2003;289(18):2413–7.
3. Earls JP, et al. Dysplastic nodules and hepatocellular carcinoma: thin-section MR imaging of explanted cirrhotic livers with pathologic correlation. Radiology. 1996;201(1):207–14.
4. Cottone M, et al. Asymptomatic hepatocellular carcinoma in child's A cirrhosis. A comparison of natural history and surgical treatment. Gastroenterology. 1989;96(6):1566–71.
5. Kuo YH, et al. Hepatocellular carcinoma surveillance and appropriate treatment options improve survival for patients with liver cirrhosis. Eur J Cancer. 2010;46(4):744–51.
6. International Working Party. Terminology of nodular hepatocellular lesions. Hepatology. 1995;22(3):983–93.
7. Sakamoto M, Hirohashi S, Shimosato Y. Early stages of multistep hepatocarcinogenesis: adenomatous hyperplasia and early hepatocellular carcinoma. Hum Pathol. 1991;22(2):172–8.
8. van den Bos IC, et al. Stepwise carcinogenesis of hepatocellular carcinoma in the cirrhotic liver: demonstration on serial MR imaging. J Magn Res Imag. 2006;24(5):1071–80.
9. Andersson KL, et al. Cost effectiveness of alternative surveillance strategies for hepatocellular carcinoma in patients with cirrhosis. Clin Gastroenterol Hepatol. 2008;6(12):1418–24.
10. Ando E, et al. Surveillance program for early detection of hepatocellular carcinoma in Japan: results of specialized department of liver disease. J Clin Gastroenterol. 2006;40(10):942–8.

11. Ferral H, et al. Cirrhosis: diagnosis by liver surface analysis with high-frequency ultrasound. Gastrointestinal Radiol. 1992;17(1):74–8.
12. Aube C, et al. Ultrasonographic diagnosis of hepatic fibrosis or cirrhosis. J Hepatol. 1999;30(3):472–8.
13. Li D, Hann LE. A practical approach to analyzing focal lesions in the liver. Ultrasound Quarter. 2005;21(3):187–200.
14. Sheu JC, et al. Hepatocellular carcinoma: US evolution in the early stage. Radiology. 1985;155(2):463–7.
15. Choi BI, Takayasu K, Han MC. Small hepatocellular carcinomas and associated nodular lesions of the liver: pathology, pathogenesis, and imaging findings. Am J Roentgenol. 1993;160(6):1177–87.
16. Rapaccini GL, et al. Hepatocellular carcinomas <2 cm in diameter complicating cirrhosis: ultrasound and clinical features in 153 consecutive patients. Liver Int. 2004;24(2):124–30.
17. Rizzi PM, et al. Accuracy of radiology in detection of hepatocellular carcinoma before liver transplantation. Gastroenterology. 1994;107(5):1425–9.
18. Miller WJ, Federle MP, Campbell WL. Diagnosis and staging of hepatocellular carcinoma: comparison of CT and sonography in 36 liver transplantation patients. Am J Roentgenol. 1991;157(2):303–6.
19. Bennett GL, et al. Sonographic detection of hepatocellular carcinoma and dysplastic nodules in cirrhosis: correlation of pretransplantation sonography and liver explant pathology in 200 patients. Am J Roentgenol. 2002;179(1):75–80.
20. Libbrecht L, et al. Focal lesions in cirrhotic explant livers: pathological evaluation and accuracy of pretransplantation imaging examinations. Liver Transplant. 2002;8(9):749–61.
21. Singal A, et al. Meta-analysis: surveillance with ultrasound for early-stage hepatocellular carcinoma in patients with cirrhosis. Aliment Pharmacol Ther. 2009;30(1):37–47.
22. McNaughton DA, Abu-Yousef MM. Doppler US of the liver made simple. Radiographics. 2011;31(1):161–88.
23. Nino-Murcia M, et al. Color flow Doppler characterization of focal hepatic lesions. Am J Roentgenol. 1992;159(6):1195–7.
24. Dodd 3rd GD, et al. Portal vein thrombosis in patients with cirrhosis: does sonographic detection of intrathrombus flow allow differentiation of benign and malignant thrombus? Am J Roentgenol. 1995;165(3):573–7.
25. Buscarini L, et al. Ultrasound-guided fine-needle biopsy of focal liver lesions: techniques, diagnostic accuracy and complications. A retrospective study on 2091 biopsies. J Hepatol. 1990;11(3):344–8.
26. Cedrone A, et al. Portal vein thrombosis complicating hepatocellular carcinoma. Value of ultrasound-guided fine-needle biopsy of the thrombus in the therapeutic management. Liver. 1996;16(2):94–8.
27. McGhana JP, Dodd 3rd GD. Radiofrequency ablation of the liver: current status. Am J Roentgenol. 2001;176(1):3–16.
28. Fontana RJ, et al. Percutaneous radiofrequency thermal ablation of hepatocellular carcinoma: a safe and effective bridge to liver transplantation. Liver Transplant. 2002;8(12):1165–74.
29. Nicolau C, Vilana R, Bru C. The use of contrast-enhanced ultrasound in the management of the cirrhotic patient and for detection of HCC. Eur Radiol. 2004;14 Suppl 8:P63–71.
30. Wilson SR, Burns PN. Microbubble-enhanced US in body imaging: what role? Radiology. 2010;257(1):24–39.
31. Solbiati L, et al. Guidance and monitoring of radiofrequency liver tumor ablation with contrast-enhanced ultrasound. Eur J Radiol. 2004;51(Suppl):S19–23.
32. Ichikawa T, et al. Hypervascular hepatocellular carcinoma: can double arterial phase imaging with multidetector CT improve tumor depiction in the cirrhotic liver? Am J Roentgenol. 2002;179(3):751–8.
33. Atasoy C, Akyar S. Multidetector CT: contributions in liver imaging. Eur J Radiol. 2004;52(1): 2–17.

34. Kawata S, et al. Multidetector CT: diagnostic impact of slice thickness on detection of hypervascular hepatocellular carcinoma. Am J Roentgenol. 2002;179(1):61–6.
35. Baron RL, et al. Hepatocellular carcinoma: evaluation with biphasic, contrast-enhanced, helical CT. Radiology. 1996;199(2):505–11.
36. Oliver 3rd JH, et al. Detecting hepatocellular carcinoma: value of unenhanced or arterial phase CT imaging or both used in conjunction with conventional portal venous phase contrast-enhanced CT imaging. Am J Roentgenol. 1996;167(1):71–7.
37. Oliver 3rd JH, Baron RL. Helical biphasic contrast-enhanced CT of the liver: technique, indications, interpretation, and pitfalls. Radiology. 1996;201(1):1–14.
38. Dodd 3rd GD, et al. Spectrum of imaging findings of the liver in end-stage cirrhosis: part I, gross morphology and diffuse abnormalities. Am J Roentgenol. 1999;173(4):1031–6.
39. Ohtomo K, et al. Confluent hepatic fibrosis in advanced cirrhosis: evaluation with MR imaging. Radiology. 1993;189(3):871–4.
40. Dodd 3rd GD, et al. Spectrum of imaging findings of the liver in end-stage cirrhosis: Part II, focal abnormalities. Am J Roentgenol. 1999;173(5):1185–92.
41. Krinsky GA, Lee VS. MR imaging of cirrhotic nodules. Abdominal Imag. 2000;25(5):471–82.
42. Matsui O. Imaging of multistep human hepatocarcinogenesis by CT during intra-arterial contrast injection. Intervirology. 2004;47(3–5):271–6.
43. Lalonde L, et al. Capsule and mosaic pattern of hepatocellular carcinoma: correlation between CT and MR imaging. Gastrointestinal Radiol. 1992;17(3):241–4.
44. Quaglia A, et al. Classification tool for the systematic histological assessment of hepatocellular carcinoma, macroregenerative nodules, and dysplastic nodules in cirrhotic liver. World J Gastroenterol. 2005;11(40):6262–8.
45. Sherman M. The radiological diagnosis of hepatocellular carcinoma. Am J Gastroenterol. 2010;105(3):610–2.
46. Bruix J, Sherman M. Management of hepatocellular carcinoma: an update. Hepatology. 2011;53(3):1020–2.
47. Miller WJ, et al. Malignancies in patients with cirrhosis: CT sensitivity and specificity in 200 consecutive transplant patients. Radiology. 1994;193(3):645–50.
48. Kim CK, Lim JH, Lee WJ. Detection of hepatocellular carcinomas and dysplastic nodules in cirrhotic liver: accuracy of ultrasonography in transplant patients. J Ultrasound Med. 2001;20(2):99–104.
49. Peterson MS, et al. Pretransplantation surveillance for possible hepatocellular carcinoma in patients with cirrhosis: epidemiology and CT-based tumor detection rate in 430 cases with surgical pathologic correlation. Radiology. 2000;217(3):743–9.
50. Brancatelli G, et al. Helical CT screening for hepatocellular carcinoma in patients with cirrhosis: frequency and causes of false-positive interpretation. Am J Roentgenol. 2003;180(4):1007–14.
51. Kim SH, et al. Diagnostic accuracy of multi-/single-detector row CT and contrast-enhanced MRI in the detection of hepatocellular carcinomas meeting the milan criteria before liver transplantation. Intervirology. 2008;51 Suppl 1:52–60.
52. Ariff B, et al. Imaging of liver cancer. World J Gastroenterol. 2009;15(11):1289–300.
53. Hayashida M, et al. Small hepatocellular carcinomas in cirrhosis: differences in contrast enhancement effects between helical CT and MR imaging during multiphasic dynamic imaging. Magn Reson Imag. 2008;26(1):65–71.
54. Faria SC, et al. MR imaging of liver fibrosis: current state of the art. Radiographics. 2009;29(6):1615–35.
55. Krinsky GA, et al. Siderotic nodules in the cirrhotic liver at MR imaging with explant correlation: no increased frequency of dysplastic nodules and hepatocellular carcinoma. Radiology. 2001;218(1):47–53.
56. Krinsky GA, Israel G. Nondysplastic nodules that are hyperintense on T1-weighted gradient-echo MR imaging: frequency in cirrhotic patients undergoing transplantation. Am J Roentgenol. 2003;180(4):1023–7.

57. Ohtomo K, et al. Confluent hepatic fibrosis in advanced cirrhosis: appearance at CT. Radiology. 1993;188(1):31–5.
58. Kim T, Baron RL, Nalesnik MA. Infarcted regenerative nodules in cirrhosis: CT and MR imaging findings with pathologic correlation. Am J Roentgenol. 2000;175(4):1121–5.
59. Krinsky GA, et al. Dysplastic nodules in cirrhotic liver: arterial phase enhancement at CT and MR imaging—a case report. Radiology. 1998;209(2):461–4.
60. Krinsky GA, et al. Hepatocellular carcinoma and dysplastic nodules in patients with cirrhosis: prospective diagnosis with MR imaging and explantation correlation. Radiology. 2001;219(2): 445–54.
61. Ebara M, et al. Small hepatocellular carcinoma: relationship of signal intensity to histopathologic findings and metal content of the tumor and surrounding hepatic parenchyma. Radiology. 1999;210(1):81–8.
62. Kelekis NL, et al. Hepatocellular carcinoma in North America: a multiinstitutional study of appearance on T1-weighted, T2-weighted, and serial gadolinium-enhanced gradient-echo images. Am J Roentgenol. 1998;170(4):1005–13.
63. Koushima Y, et al. Small hepatocellular carcinoma: assessment with T1-weighted spin-echo magnetic resonance imaging with and without fat suppression. Eur J Radiol. 2002;41(1):34–41.
64. Muramatsu Y, et al. Early hepatocellular carcinoma: MR imaging. Radiology. 1991;181(1): 209–13.
65. Yoshikawa J, et al. Fatty metamorphosis in hepatocellular carcinoma: radiologic features in 10 cases. Am J Roentgenol. 1988;151(4):717–20.
66. Hussain SM, Semelka RC, Mitchell DG. MR imaging of hepatocellular carcinoma. Magn Res Imag Clin North Am. 2002;10(1):31–52.
67. Baron, R.L. and M.S. Peterson, From the RSNA refresher courses: screening the cirrhotic liver for hepatocellular carcinoma with CT and MR imaging: opportunities and pitfalls. Radiographics : a review publication of the Radiological Society of North America, Inc, 2001. 21 Spec No: pp. S117–32.
68. Yamashita Y, et al. Spin-echo and dynamic gadolinium-enhanced FLASH MR imaging of hepatocellular carcinoma: correlation with histopathologic findings. J Magn Reson Imag. 1994;4(1):83–90.
69. Marrero JA, et al. Improving the prediction of hepatocellular carcinoma in cirrhotic patients with an arterially-enhancing liver mass. Liver Transplant. 2005;11(3):281–9.
70. Carlos RC, et al. Developing a prediction rule to assess hepatic malignancy in patients with cirrhosis. Am J Roentgenol. 2003;180(4):893–900.
71. Kadoya M, et al. Hepatocellular carcinoma: correlation of MR imaging and histopathologic findings. Radiology. 1992;183(3):819–25.
72. Okuda K, et al. Clinicopathologic features of encapsulated hepatocellular carcinoma: a study of 26 cases. Cancer. 1977;40(3):1240–5.
73. Ng IO, et al. Tumor encapsulation in hepatocellular carcinoma. A pathologic study of 189 cases. Cancer. 1992;70(1):45–9.
74. Iguchi T, et al. Both fibrous capsule formation and extracapsular penetration are powerful predictors of poor survival in human hepatocellular carcinoma: a histological assessment of 365 patients in Japan. Anna Surg Oncol. 2009;16(9):2539–46.
75. Ishigami K, et al. Hepatocellular carcinoma with a pseudocapsule on gadolinium-enhanced MR images: correlation with histopathologic findings. Radiology. 2009;250(2):435–43.
76. Tsai TJ, et al. Clinical significance of microscopic tumor venous invasion in patients with resectable hepatocellular carcinoma. Surgery. 2000;127(6):603–8.
77. Low RN. MR imaging of the liver using gadolinium chelates. Magn Reson Imag Clin North Am. 2001;9(4):717–43. vi.
78. Katyal S, et al. Extrahepatic metastases of hepatocellular carcinoma. Radiology. 2000;216(3): 698–703.
79. Lee YT, Geer DA. Primary liver cancer: pattern of metastasis. J Surg Oncol. 1987;36(1):26–31.
80. Koh DM, Collins DJ. Diffusion-weighted MRI in the body: applications and challenges in oncology. Am J Roentgenol. 2007;188(6):1622–35.

81. Taouli B, et al. Evaluation of liver diffusion isotropy and characterization of focal hepatic lesions with two single-shot echo-planar MR imaging sequences: prospective study in 66 patients. Radiology. 2003;226(1):71–8.
82. Zech CJ, et al. Black-blood diffusion-weighted EPI acquisition of the liver with parallel imaging: comparison with a standard T2-weighted sequence for detection of focal liver lesions. Investig Radiol. 2008;43(4):261–6.
83. Vandecaveye V, et al. Diffusion-weighted MRI provides additional value to conventional dynamic contrast-enhanced MRI for detection of hepatocellular carcinoma. Eur Radiol. 2009;19(10):2456–66.
84. Catalano OA, et al. Differentiation of malignant thrombus from bland thrombus of the portal vein in patients with hepatocellular carcinoma: application of diffusion-weighted MR imaging. Radiology. 2010;254(1):154–62.
85. Fidler J, Hough D. Hepatocyte-specific magnetic resonance imaging contrast agents. Hepatology. 2011;53(2):678–82.
86. Cruite I, et al. Gadoxetate disodium-enhanced MRI of the liver: part 2, protocol optimization and lesion appearance in the cirrhotic liver. Am J Roentgenol. 2010;195(1):29–41.
87. Manfredi R, et al. Delayed MR imaging of hepatocellular carcinoma enhanced by gadobenate dimeglumine (Gd-BOPTA). J Magn Reson Imag. 1999;9(5):704–10.
88. Trojan J, et al. Fluorine-18 FDG positron emission tomography for imaging of hepatocellular carcinoma. Am J Gastroenterol. 1999;94(11):3314–9.
89. Khan MA, et al. Positron emission tomography scanning in the evaluation of hepatocellular carcinoma. J Hepatol. 2000;32(5):792–7.
90. Sugiyama M, et al. 18 F-FDG PET in the detection of extrahepatic metastases from hepatocellular carcinoma. J Gastroenterol. 2004;39(10):961–8.

Chapter 4
Pathology of Hepatocellular Carcinoma

Shriram Jakate and Deborah Giusto

Hepatocellular carcinoma (HCC) is the most common primary malignant neoplasm of the liver. HCC is intriguing at multiple levels including its remarkable geographic variation, strong etiological association with hepatitis viral infections, certain carcinogens and metabolic diseases, preference for males, and predisposition to develop in cirrhosis or chronic liver injury from any cause [1]. HCC developing in the setting of cirrhosis is far more common in low incidence regions such as North America (as many as 90% of patients may be cirrhotic) than in high incidence regions such as Eastern Asia and Africa (only about 50% of patients may be cirrhotic), where hepatitis B virus is the most common cause of chronic liver disease [2]. Differences in geographical and age incidences are linked to variations in associated risk factors: HCV, HBV (+/− HDV), EtOH, aflatoxin B1, tobacco, NAFLD, hemochromatosis, tyrosinemia, alpha-1-antitrypsin deficiency, etc. These varied etiological factors also contribute toward complex and heterogeneous molecular genetic cellular changes and pathways during hepatocarcinogenesis. It is quite rare for HCC, except the fibrolamellar variant, to occur in patients who have no underlying liver disease at all.

HCC is usually detected after clinical suspicion with signs and symptoms such as right upper quadrant abdominal pain, hepatomegaly, palpable mass, weight loss, or rapid hepatic decompensation. Unusual presentations include identification of HCC after metastasis or with various rare paraneoplastic syndromes. Presymptomatic HCC may be identified through active surveillance screening of high-risk patients for serum tumor marker such as alpha-fetoprotein (AFP) and imaging studies.

S. Jakate, MD, FRCPath (✉)
Department of Pathology, Rush University Medical Center,
1750 West Harrison Street, Chicago, IL 60612, USA
e-mail: sjakate@rush.edu

D. Giusto, MD
4Path Pathology Services, 9050 West 81st Street, Justice, IL 60458, USA
e-mail: DGiusto@4path.com

N. Reau and F.F. Poordad (eds.), *Primary Liver Cancer: Surveillance, Diagnosis and Treatment*, Clinical Gastroenterology, DOI 10.1007/978-1-61779-863-4_4,
© Springer Science+Business Media New York 2012

Previously undetected and unknown HCC may be incidentally found at autopsy or during evaluation of explanted native liver after orthotopic liver transplantation. When HCC occurs in the prototypical clinical setting and shows striking elevation in serum marker and demonstrates characteristic imaging on dynamic computed tomography (CT) or magnetic resonance (MR), pathological tissue confirmation of HCC may sometimes not be considered necessary before therapy. In such cases, ablation and/or other therapeutic options are executed with the presumed diagnosis of HCC. However, in the majority of cases, tumor tissue is procured to microscopically verify that the mass is HCC.

Tissue Procurement for Pathological Diagnosis of HCC

The most common method of obtaining tissue to diagnose HCC is image-guided fine-needle aspiration or biopsy. For accurate and complete cytological and/or histological assessment of the tumor, it is crucial that the needle is well targeted into the mass and sufficient sample is obtained to not only carry out routine stains but also perform the necessary immunohistochemical markers. Seeding of tumor along the needle tract remains a potential risk, but it may be minimized under optimal circumstances [3]. If needle core biopsies are planned, it is beneficial to procure two separate samples: one, targeted from the mass, and the, second randomly away from the mass to assess the native liver disease in the background. The tumor biopsy itself may have attached adjacent liver available for review, but the random "away" sample is more useful in assessing the diffuseness and cause of chronic liver injury. When a tumor mass develops in a cirrhotic liver, not only the likelihood of HCC is greatly increased but also the possibility of metastatic tumor is markedly reduced [4], possibly owing to the remarkable portacaval circulatory shunting that occurs in cirrhosis. Occasionally, a resectable tumor is surgically excised with presumptive diagnosis of HCC and no preoperative biopsy confirmation.

Gross or Macroscopic Features of HCC

HCC is often a spherical nodule which is larger than the surrounding cirrhotic nodules and stands out with a contrasting appearance—pale (Fig. 4.1), cholestatic or dark, or variegated with variable mixtures of these depending upon the cellular contents (fat, bile, glycogen, etc.). Post-ablated tumors tend to be highly necrotic but continue to retain their spherical form. Most HCCs are soft since these are predominantly comprised of cells without desmoplastic stroma (exceptions are variants such as fibrolamellar HCC and scirrhous HCC). HCCs may be single or multiple and may form a large expansile mass with or without smaller nodules. Gross HCC classifications have been documented in multiple large series of cases [5]. Overall, most HCCs display the following patterns in decreasing order of frequency: expanding solitary nodule with apparent encapsulation and discrete margins ("massive" type),

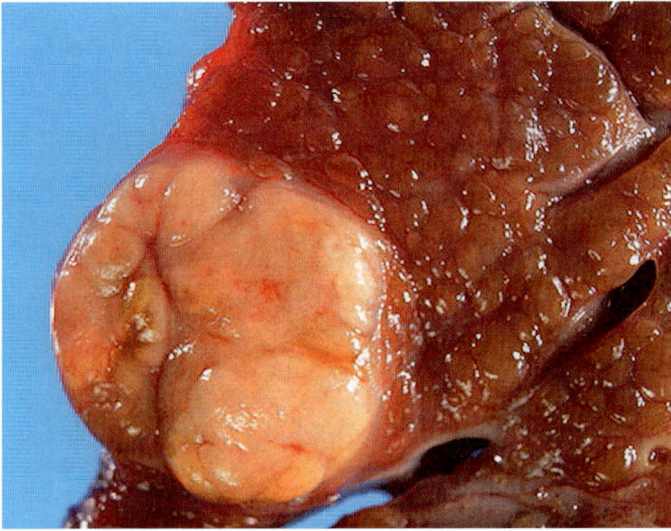

Fig. 4.1 Cut surface of an explanted liver showing an encapsulated pale HCC tumor mass arising in a cirrhotic liver

multiple discrete nodules with apparent encapsulation which may or may not be satellites of a solitary large nodule ("nodular" type), and several small nodules with replacing rather than expanding growth pattern and without encapsulation ("infiltrative," "diffuse," "cirrhotomimetic" or "spreading" types). Tumor embolization may also be visible in larger blood vessels on gross examination.

Microscopic Features of HCC

Tumor cells in HCC tend to simulate non-neoplastic hepatocytes. At the well-differentiated end of the HCC spectrum, this similarity is the most striking. Diagnosis of HCC thus requires demonstration of hepatocellular differentiation by tumor cells which may be based on growth pattern, cytological features, immunohistochemical staining, or combination of any of these. There are several different architectural growth patterns. The trabecular pattern is most commonly observed in well-differentiated and moderately differentiated HCCs and is also referred to as the "plate-like" pattern. With this pattern, the tumor cells grow in cords of variable thickness, separated by sinusoids which are lined by endothelial cells. Unlike normal hepatocytes which have a single layer of trabeculae, HCC cells tend to have thicker cell plates with two or more cell thickness (Fig. 4.2). The more well differentiated the tumor, the thinner the trabeculae. Sometimes the trabeculae contain a dilated bile canaliculus or may centrally degenerate which creates a pseudoglandular or acinar pattern. Poorly differentiated or undifferentiated HCCs may entirely lack trabecular or acinar patterns. The stroma between the tumor cell plates consists of sinusoid-like blood spaces lined by a single layer of

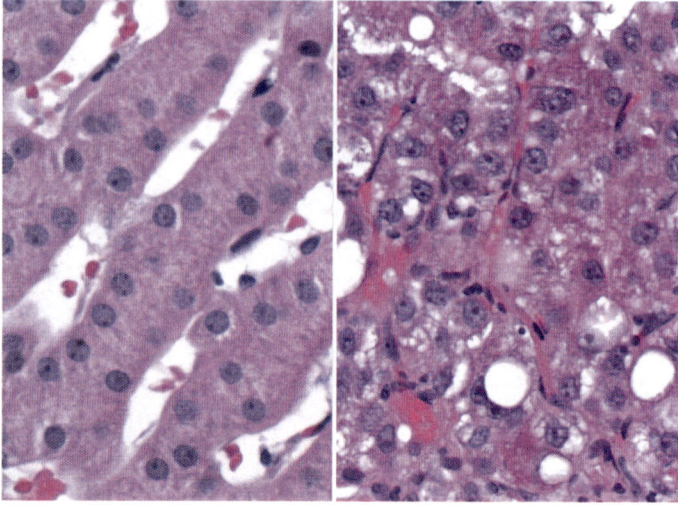

Fig. 4.2 Histological contrast between normal hepatocytes (*left*) and HCC cells (*right*). HCC cells show thickened cell plates, irregular nuclear margins, prominent nucleoli, and high nuclear-to-cytoplasmic ratios. Routine hematoxylin and eosin stain (magnification ×600)

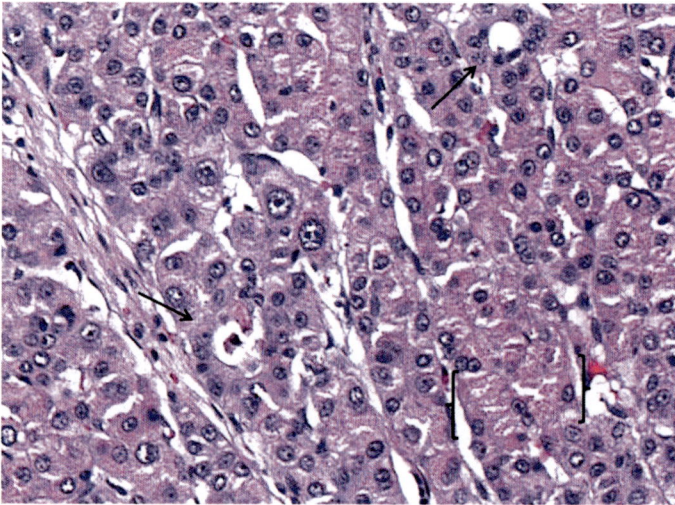

Fig. 4.3 Microphotograph of moderately differentiated HCC showing high nuclear-to-cytoplasmic ratios, trabeculae with stratified cell plates (*braces*), and focal pseudogland formation (*arrows*). Routine hematoxylin and eosin stain (magnification ×400)

endothelial cells. Cytologically, HCC cells are polyhedral-like epithelial cells that have distinct cell membranes, moderate amount of eosinophilic finely granular cytoplasm, and vesicular nuclei with prominent nucleoli. In comparison with non-neoplastic hepatocytes, the HCC cells have a high nuclear-to-cytoplasmic ratios, nuclear irregularity, hyperchromasia, and variable enlargement of nucleoli

(Fig. 4.3). Bile canaliculi may be visible between tumor cells and retention of bile may be seen intracellularly and in the canaliculi. Any of a wide variety of cytoplasmic contents may be encountered within HCC cells that include aggregated proteins, lipids, and trace elements. These are generally epiphenomena of injury and bear no relevance to the etiology of the underlying liver disease or the tumor differentiation. The cytoplasmic contents include fat, glycogen, Mallory bodies, hyaline bodies, pale bodies, fibrinogen, alpha-1-antitrypsin, iron (iron content is generally lower in HCC compared to the surrounding liver), and copper.

Immunohistochemical Features of HCC

Immunohistochemical studies can be utilized to determine the hepatocytic origin of malignant tumor cells (thus distinguishing HCC for metastatic tumors), assess the effect of HCC on sinusoidal endothelial cells (as a surrogate marker for HCC), and differentiate malignant (HCC) cells from reactive hepatocytes [6].

Hepatocytic origin is strongly favored with granular cytoplasmic positivity for HepPar1 (Fig. 4.4), also known as hepatocyte-specific antigen. This marker may be falsely negative in poorly differentiated HCC and rarely falsely positive in carcinomas from other organs. Carcinoembryonic antigen—polyclonal (CEAp) and CD10—may highlight the bile canaliculi specifically creating a distinctive pericanalicular staining pattern (Fig. 4.5). Since the bile canaliculus is a unique structure exclusive to a hepatocyte, a hepatocellular origin may be presumed with such pericanalicular staining. Hepatocytic origin is not established by cytokeratin staining but use of a panel of cytokeratins is helpful while differentiating HCC from cholangiocarcinoma and most metastatic carcinomas; HCC is positive for cytokeratin 8/18

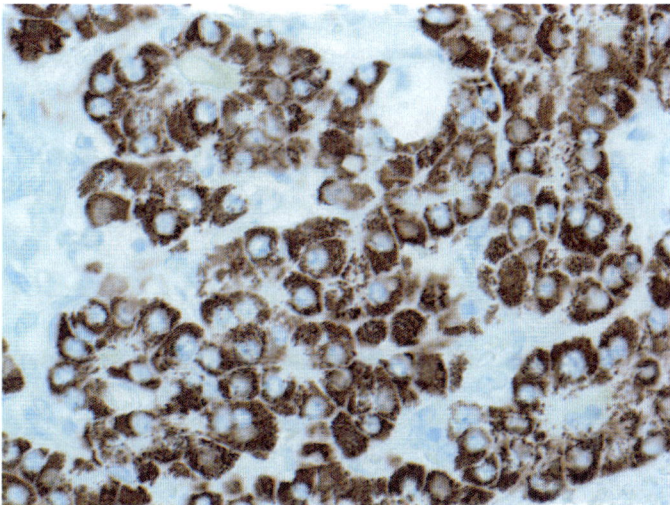

Fig. 4.4 Strongly positive granular cytoplasmic immunoreactivity for HepPar1 in HCC (magnification ×400)

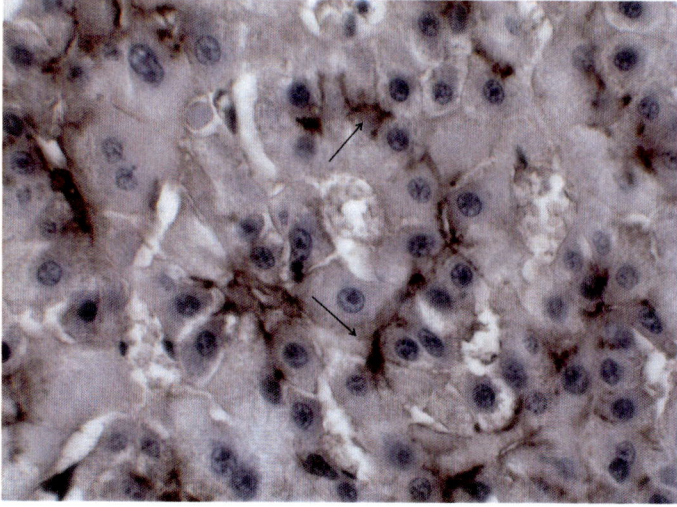

Fig. 4.5 HCC showing pericanalicular reactivity (*arrows*) for CEAp, characteristic of hepatocellular origin (magnification ×400)

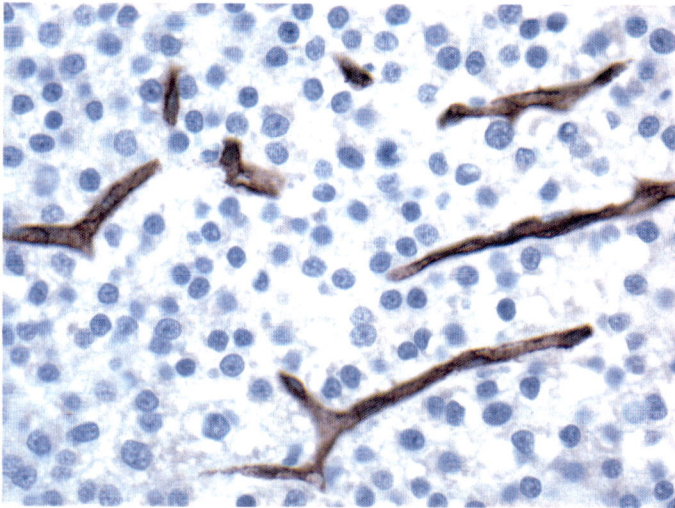

Fig. 4.6 Strong over-expression of CD34 positive sinusoidal endothelial cells ("capillarization" of sinusoids) in HCC (magnification ×200)

and generally negative for cytokeratin 7 (while cholangiocarcinoma and the majority of metastatic carcinomas are positive) and negative for cytokeratin 20 (positive in metastatic colon carcinoma).

Sinusoidal endothelial cells normally do not overexpress CD34. In HCC, however, there is overexpression of CD34 attributed to capillarization of the sinusoids

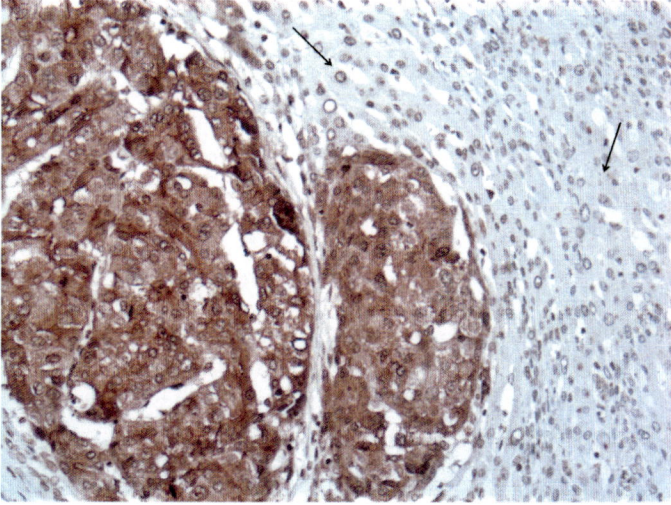

Fig. 4.7 Strongly positive cytoplasmic glypican 3 immunoreactivity exclusively for HCC tumor nodules. Adjacent non-neoplastic hepatocytes (*arrows*) are negative (magnification×200)

(Fig. 4.6). CD34 staining pattern also helps in highlighting the multilayered cell plates of HCC. Similar sinusoidal staining pattern may be seen with vimentin.

Some immunomarkers are helpful in discriminating reactive or dysplastic hepatocytes from HCC cells. Glypican 3 (GPC3) (Fig. 4.7) is a highly sensitive marker for hepatocellular malignancy. Positivity for other markers such as heat shock protein 70 (HSP70) or glutamine synthetase (GS) also favors HCC [7]. While high *serum* level of AFP is found in HCC and it is helpful in screening and post-therapeutic monitoring, positive AFP immunostaining on HCC tumor tissue is found in only a small minority of cases.

Molecular Changes in HCC

Most HCCs arise in the setting of chronic liver disease. Considering the wide spectrum of underlying etiological conditions, it is not surprising that molecular alterations in HCC are similarly varied and inconsistent and include both genetic (point mutations, deletions) and epigenetic (methylations, amplifications, micro-satellite instability) phenomena. These result in dysregulation of normal cellular functions such as controlled growth, differentiation, and apoptosis. Regardless of their diversity and complexity, molecular changes help in understanding the processes of hepatocarcinogenesis, potential preventive measures, and targeting of therapy. Molecular studies also help in differentiating between intrahepatic metastasis of a single original tumor mass versus separate multiclonal tumor nodules in multifocal HCC.

Variants of HCC

One variant, fibrolamellar HCC, is distinctly different from HCC in multiple crucial ways as follows: (1) No association exists with underlying liver disease or cirrhosis. (2) Unlike male predominance in HCC, there is nearly equal gender distribution. (3) Mean age of presentation is much younger at about 26 years. (4) Serum AFP levels are usually normal. (5) Prognosis is better for equivalent size of HCC likely due to fibrolamellar HCC being generally slow-growing and resectable, patients almost always symptomatic with earlier detection and the adjacent liver having no underlying disease. (6) The majority occur in the left lobe of liver, contributing to the resectability. Grossly, this variant may have a central scar and nodular appearance (Fig. 4.8) mimicking focal nodular hyperplasia (FNH). Microscopically, it derives its name from the presence of dense hyalinized collagen in a linear lamellar pattern. Trapped in this collagen are single and small groups of hepatocytic-appearing tumor cells that are distinctly large with large vesicular and hyperchromatic nuclei and prominent nucleoli.

Several other variants are described [8] that are largely prognostically similar to typical HCC, but may present diagnostic difficulties due to variations as follows: (1) glandular rather than trabecular architecture (pseudoglandular HCC), (2) dense fibrous stroma rather than intervening sinusoids (scirrhous HCC), (3) clear rather than granular eosinophilic cytoplasm (clear cell HCC), (4) mixed conventional HCC and cholangiocarcinoma (combined hepatocellular-cholangiocarcinoma), (5) spindled

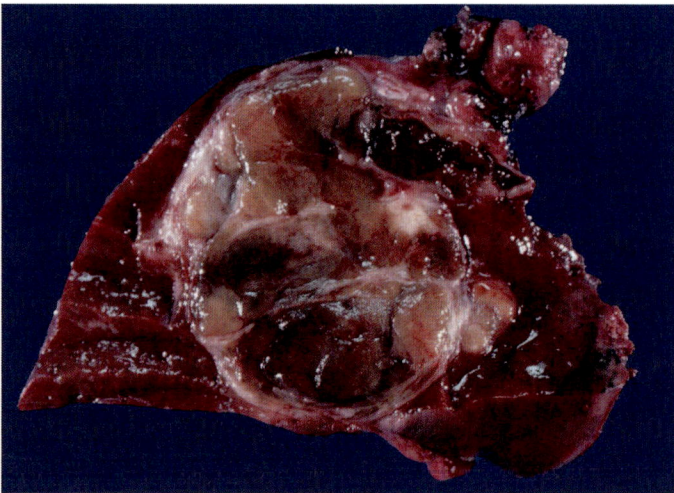

Fig. 4.8 Cut surface of resected fibrolamellar HCC variant showing nodular mass with central stellate scar and non-cirrhotic surrounding liver

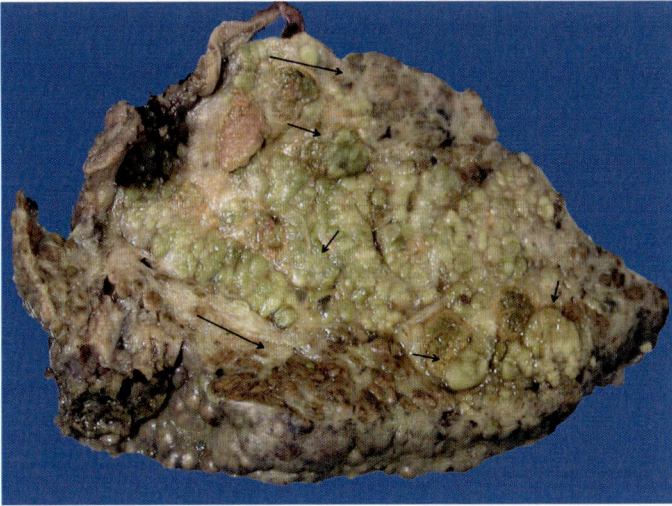

Fig. 4.9   Cut surface of diffuse cirrhosis-like HCC where almost the entire liver is replaced by small cholestatic or pale nodules of HCC (*short arrows*). Non-neoplastic cirrhotic brown nodules are seen at the periphery (*long arrows*)

rather than hepatocytic-appearing cells (sarcomatoid HCC), (6) clinically and radiographically undetected HCC diffusely spread throughout the liver as small cirrhotic-like nodules [9] (diffuse cirrhosis-like HCC, Fig. 4.9), and (7) HCC not present intrahepatically within the liver, but a mass projecting out, generally from the inferior or posterior surface of the right lobe (pedunculated HCC).

Differential Diagnosis

A moderately differentiated HCC occurring in a cirrhotic liver with characteristic microscopic features is relatively easy to diagnose and generally not confused with any other primary or metastatic neoplasm. A small (<2 cm), well-differentiated HCC may be quite difficult to differentiate from dysplastic nodule with high-grade dysplasia (HGDN—itself a precancerous entity). Potential distinctions between the two include diffuse and not focal cellular changes (particularly small cell change) in HCC, stromal or portal tumor infiltration in HCC, exclusively unpaired arteries in HCC and minimal cell plate stratification (<3-cell thick) in HGDN. Positivity for markers such as glypican 3, heat shock protein 70 or glutamine synthetase favors HCC over HGDN [7]. When distinction between HGDN and HCC remains unsettled, the mass may be described as "Early HCC."

Pseudoglandular pattern may create likeness to adenocarcinoma (metastatic or primary cholangiocarcinoma). This can usually be resolved with the use of immunomarkers: a panel of cytokeratins (8/18, 7, 19, and 20—HCC is positive for 8/18

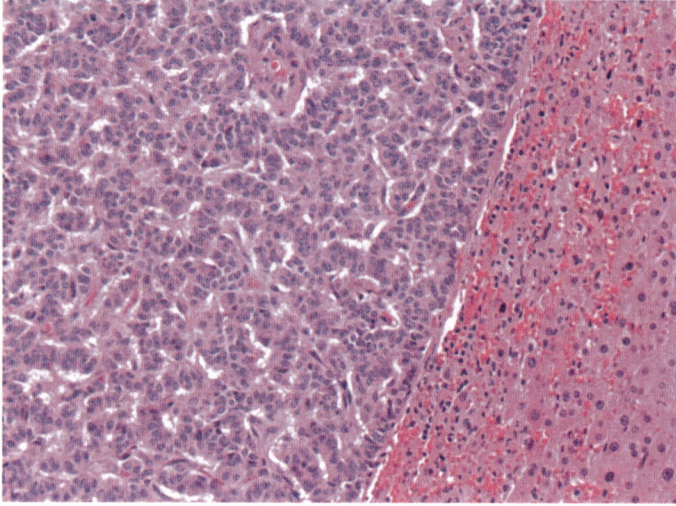

Fig. 4.10 Trabecular pattern of tumor (*left*) mimics HCC, but coarse nuclear chromatin pattern suggests (metastatic) neuroendocrine carcinoma. Subsequent work-up confirmed a pancreatic primary (pancreatic neuroendocrine or islet cell tumor). Routine hematoxylin and eosin stain (magnification ×200)

and generally negative for others); markers for hepatocytic differentiation such as HepPar1, pericanalicular CEAp, and pericanalicular CD10; and markers indicative of (hepatocytic) malignancy including GPC3, HSP70, or GS.

Metastatic well-differentiated neuroendocrine carcinomas (NEC) bear striking resemblance to HCC with their trabecular and pseudoglandular patterns and monomorphic cells. Coarse clumped nuclear chromatin in NEC versus vesicular nucleus in HCC is a subtle distinction (Fig. 4.10). NEC is positive for pan-neuroendocrine markers synaptophysin and chromogranin and negative for markers of hepatocytic differentiation. Further studies may identify the potential primaries such as ileum (CDX-2 positive), pancreas (imaging showing a mass), lung (TTF1 positive), and breast (ER positive).

Sometimes abundance of clear cells in HCC creates mimicry to renal cell or adrenal cortical carcinoma. Additionally, cytokeratin staining pattern is similar in all of these three carcinomas. Immunostains for hepatocytic differentiation and markers favoring renal (RCC, PAX2) or adrenal (inhibin) carcinomas are helpful in resolving the diagnoses.

Rare cases of undifferentiated HCC may need to be differentiated from melanoma, sarcoma, and lymphoma. Specific immunohistochemical markers for these can be utilized to arrive at the diagnoses.

Grading and Staging

Histological grade of HCC is a reflection of differentiation and only indistinctly relates to tumor behavior and size. Most larger (>3 cm) HCCs are not uniform in their grade and display better differentiation toward the periphery and poorer differentiation near the center. At one end of the spectrum, at the lowest grade, the tumor is well differentiated, easily histologically recognizable as hepatocytic, challenging in terms of distinguishing from reactive benign or dysplastic hepatocytes and generally small (<2 cm). At the other end of the spectrum, the undifferentiated or poorly differentiated HCCs are larger and barely recognizable as of hepatocytic origin. These may be hard to differentiate from metastatic or other primary malignant tumors. The majority of HCCs are mid-grade and moderately differentiated and histologically reasonably identifiable as of hepatocellular origin.

The WHO HCC grading is as follows: (1) Well-differentiated HCC—cells with mild atypia and increased nuclear-to-cytoplasmic ratio in a thin trabecular pattern and often with pseudo-glandular structures. (2) Moderately differentiated HCC—cells have abundant eosinophilic cytoplasm and round nuclei with distinct nucleoli. A pseudoglandular pattern is also frequent, and pseudoglands often contain bile or proteinaceous fluid. Trabecular growth is three or more cells in thickness. (3) Poorly differentiated HCC—cells show an increased nuclear-to-cytoplasmic ratio and frequently moderate-to-marked pleomorphism. The growth pattern is solid without distinct sinusoid-like blood spaces. (4) Undifferentiated HCC—cells contain little cytoplasm and are spindle or round-shaped. The growth pattern is solid.

The WHO HCC staging is as follows: T1—solitary tumor without vascular invasion. T2—solitary tumor with vascular invasion or multiple tumors, not >5 cm. T3—any multiple tumors >5 cm (T3a) or tumor involving a major branch of portal or hepatic veins (T3b); and T4—tumor with direct invasion of adjacent organs other than the gallbladder or with perforation of visceral peritoneum.

Components of staging such as tumor size and number along with distribution (right, left, or both lobes) are crucial for qualification for orthotopic liver transplant (OLT) [10].

References

1. Theise ND, Curado MP, Franceschi S, et al. Hepatocellular carcinoma. In: Bosman FT, Carneiro F, Hruban RH, et al., editors. WHO classification of tumors of the digestive system. Lyon: IARC; 2010. pp. 205–16.
2. Goodman ZD, Terracciano LM. Tumors and tumor-like lesions of the liver. In: Burt AD, Portman BC, Ferrell LD, editors. MacSween's pathology of the liver. Churchill Livingstone: Elsevier; 2007. pp. 771–88.
3. Rowe LR, Mulvihill SJ, Emerson L, et al. Subcutaneous tumor seeding following needle core biopsy of hepatocellular carcinoma. Diagn Cytopathol. 2007;35:717–21.
4. Pereira-Lima JE, Lichtenfels E, Barbosa FS, et al. Prevalence study of metastases in cirrhotic livers. Hepatogastroenterology. 2003;53:1490–5.

5. Ishak KG, Goodman ZD, Stocker JT. Hepatocellular carcinoma. In: Rosai J, Sobin L, editors. Tumors of the liver and intrahepatic bile ducts. Washington, DC: Armed Forces Institute of Pathology; 2001. pp. 203–5.
6. Kakar S, Gown AM, Goodman ZD, et al. Best practices in diagnostic immunohistochemistry: hepatocellular carcinoma versus metastatic neoplasms. Arch Pathol Lab Med. 2007;131: 1648–54.
7. Tommaso LD, Franchi G, Park YN, et al. Diagnostic value of HSP70, glypican 3, and glutamine synthetase in hepatocellular nodules in cirrhosis. Hepatology. 2007;45:725–34.
8. Jakate S, Giusto D. Hepatocellular carcinoma variants. In: Ferrell LD, Kakar S, editors. Liver pathology. New York: demosMEDICAL; 2011. pp. 407–29 (Consultant pathology, vol. 4).
9. Jakate S, Yabes A, Giusto D, et al. Diffuse cirrhosis-like hepatocellular carcinoma: a clinically and radiographically undetected variant mimicking cirrhosis. Am J Surg Pathol. 2010;34: 935–41.
10. Duffy JP, Vardanian A, Benjamin E, et al. Liver transplantation criteria for hepatocellular carcinoma should be expanded: a 22-year experience with 467 patients at UCLA. Ann Surg. 2007;246:502–9.

Chapter 5
Differential Diagnosis of Focal Hepatic Lesions

Russell N. Wesson and Andrew M. Cameron

Abbreviations

AASLD	American association for the study of liver diseases
AFP	Alpha fetoprotein
AJCC	American Joint Committee on Cancer
BilIN	Biliary intraepithelial neoplasia
CA	Cancer antigen
CEA	Carcinoembyonic antigen
CT	Computerized tomography
FDG-PET	Fluorodeoxyglucose positron emission tomography
FNH	Focal nodular hyperplasia
HCC	Hepatocellular carcinoma
ICC	Intrahepatic cholangiocarcinoma
IPNB	Intraductal papillary neoplasm of the bile duct
MRI	Magnetic resonance imaging
US	Ultrasound

R.N. Wesson, MD • A.M. Cameron, MD, PhD (✉)
Department of Surgery, The Johns Hopkins Hospital, Baltimore, MD, USA
e-mail: acamero5@jhmi.edu

N. Reau and F.F. Poordad (eds.), *Primary Liver Cancer: Surveillance, Diagnosis
and Treatment*, Clinical Gastroenterology, DOI 10.1007/978-1-61779-863-4_5,
© Springer Science+Business Media New York 2012

Introduction

Liver lesions are an increasingly common finding. The broad variety of lesions that exist (Figs. 5.1 and 5.2) necessitates a thorough understanding of the nuances in differential diagnosis prior to approaching management decisions. Lesions are not only found in patients with symptomatic complaints, but are increasingly being detected incidentally at imaging. Lesions of the liver will be discovered in patients with extrahepatic disease where their presence has the potential to alter management. In each case, knowledge of the differential diagnosis aids the construction of a plan of management. Where treatment decisions hinge on subtle findings, consequences of interpretation are great and can mean the difference between reassurance and observation or pursuit of one of a wide variety of interventions. The purpose of this chapter is to illustrate the more common liver tumors with which clinicians may be presented and provide insight into diagnostic nuances as they currently exist.

Liver lesions may be categorized in several ways. Since presentation involves imaging, classification (Table 5.1) into solid or cystic tumors is useful, while a benign or malignant description of behavior informs management.

Hemangioma

Estimates of the prevalence of hepatic hemangiomas range from 0.4% to 7% [1, 2], placing hemangiomas as the most common benign liver lesion. Hemangiomas are approximately three times more common in women than men [2, 3] and are considered congenital vascular malformations thought to enlarge by ectasia rather than hyperplasia [4, 5]. Estrogen receptors are found in some tumors and blood vessels, and these vascular malformations have been associated with endogenous and exogenous estrogen with relationships to puberty, pregnancy, oral contraceptives, and androgen use reported in prospective series and case reports [6–10].

Pathology

Grossly, these compressible hypervascular lesions are well circumscribed, reddish purple in appearance, and are often surrounded by a thin capsule. Their size may vary from a few millimeters to many centimeters. Through common acceptance, lesions greater than 4 cm have been termed giant hemangiomas [11, 12]. More often, hemangiomas occur in the right liver due to its increased volume.

Microscopically, histologic analysis reveals large cavernous blood-filled spaces of varying sizes lined by a single layer of flat endothelial cells and separated by thin fibrous septae [13]. Areas of thrombosis may lead to collagenous scarring and rare calcification.

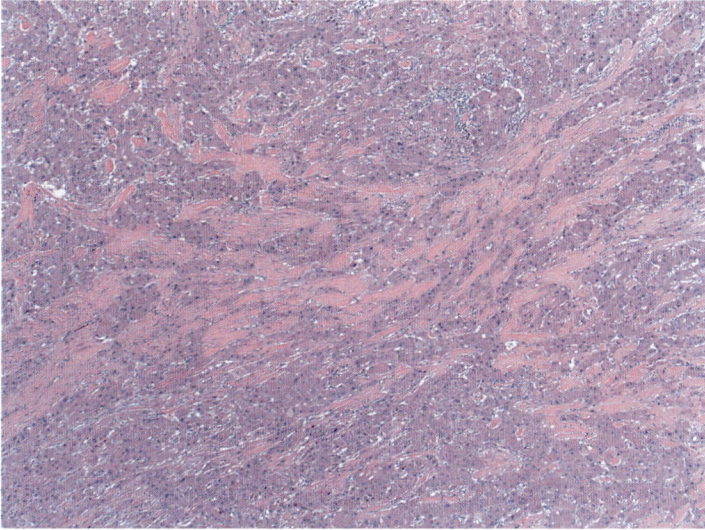

Fig. 5.1 Normal liver architecture (×20)

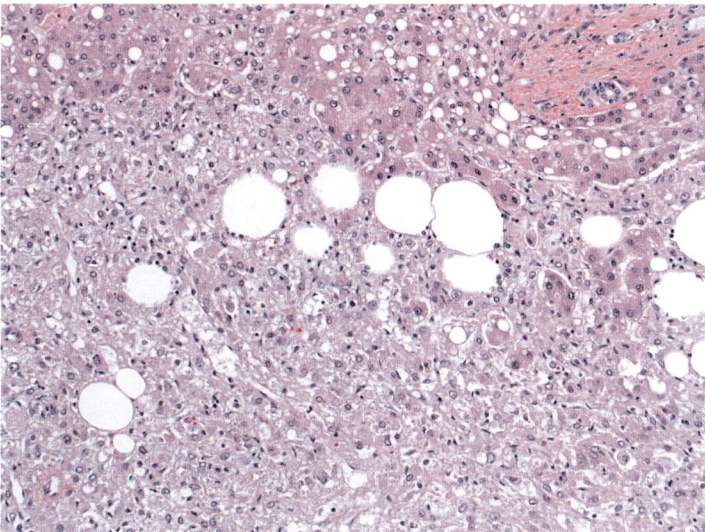

Fig. 5.2 Angiomyolipoma of the liver (×64)

Presentation

Hemangiomas occur across all age groups and may be solitary or multiple, with nearly half of individuals having more than one lesion. Most hemangiomas are small (<4 cm), and the majority of patients are asymptomatic, even with larger

Table 5.1 Abbreviated classification of neoplasms and tumorlike lesions of the liver

	Cystic lesions	Solid lesions					
	Biliary	Infectious	Mesenchymal	Hepatocellular	Focal Nodular Hyperplasia	Nodular Regenerative Hyperplasia	Biliary
Benign	Simple cyst Multiple cysts associated with polycystic liver disease Biliary cystadenoma	Pyogenic, amebic Hydatid	Hemangioma Infantile Hemangioendothelioma Angiomyolipoma Leiomyoma Lymphangioma Inflammatory pseudotumor	Hepatic adenoma Focal fatty change, focal fatty sparing			Bile duct adenoma Bile duct Hamartoma Biliary papilloma
Malignant	Biliary cystadenocarcinoma		Angiosarcoma Epithelioid hemangioendothelioma Lymphoma	Hepatocellular carcinoma	Carcinosarcoma	Hepato-blastoma	Intrahepatic Cholangiocarcinoma
Metastatic disease							

tumors. Larger lesions may produce a variety of symptoms and signs related to compression of adjacent structures or distension of Glisson's capsule. Presentation may consequently be with pain or discomfort. Other symptoms related to compression of adjacent structures are nonspecific and can include nausea, vomiting, early satiety, weight loss, dyspepsia, and dysphagia. However, pain and discomfort have been found to be due to other causes in about half of patients with symptoms [3, 5]. Pain occurring acutely has been described with acute thrombosis or bleeding within the hemangioma and consequent distension of the capsule although this is uncommon [14]. As with other liver lesions, abnormal liver function tests may be present but are nonspecific. Spontaneous intraperitoneal bleeding of hemangiomas has been reported to occur in 1–4% of lesions, with roughly 40 reports of spontaneous rupture of massive hemangiomas present in the literature. Rupture can be life-threatening [15].

Rare presentations include the syndrome of Kasabach–Merritt. This has been reported to occur in very large hemangiomas and presents with thrombocytopenia and consumptive coagulopathy including hypofibrinogenemia and elevated fibrin degradation products. Fragmentation of red blood cells is present and is secondary to platelet trapping within the hemangioma [16]. Other rare presentations of hemangiomas include reports of hepatic hemangiomatosis with innumerable hemangiomas found diffusely throughout the liver [17, 18].

Natural History

The majority of hemangiomas remain unchanged over time with several longitudinal clinical and radiological studies demonstrating stability [2, 3, 19–21]. Farges and colleagues [3] reported their series of 163 hepatic hemangiomas with a mean follow-up of 92 months. Only nine hemangiomas increased in size, while seven decreased in size.

Radiologic Appearance

The appearance of hemangiomas is characteristic on cross-sectional imaging and usually sufficient for diagnosis. Initially, a well-defined hypodense mass will be found within the liver, sometimes with evidence of calcification, scarring, and fibrosis. In practice, multiple imaging techniques are often used. In one series [5], the mean number of imaging studies performed prior to definitive diagnosis was 2.9. Ultrasound typically reveals a well-demarcated homogenous hyperechoic mass in the setting of normal surrounding liver. Color Doppler has been used but does not improve the diagnostic accuracy of ultrasound with blood flow demonstrated within hemangiomas in only 10–50% [22, 23]. Contrast-enhanced ultrasound using microbubbles may enhance the specificity of diagnosis [24]. In patients with underlying liver disease or a history of malignancy, confirmatory studies should be obtained as ultrasound features of hemangiomas may have similar acoustic patterns similar to hepatocellular carcinoma and hepatic metastases.

In one series, CT established or confirmed the diagnosis of hemangioma in 73% of scans [5]. A well-demarcated hypodense mass is usually seen on noncontrast CT scan. Calcification is present in 10% of cases. The classic progressive centripetal enhancement with areas of pooling at the periphery is seen on contrast CT images, although this enhancement pattern is related to size of the lesion [25]. Peripheral nodular enhancement occurs in the early phase on contrast CT of larger lesions. After a delay, larger lesions typically opacify and remain isodense or hyperdense on delayed scans. This characteristic finding has a positive predictive value greater than 80% for hemangioma [26]. Areas without enhancement may be due to thrombosis, fibrosis, or scarring. Small lesions may have an atypical enhancement pattern and appearance [27, 28].

CT may also be useful in the unusual circumstance where therapy is considered. CT angiography may assist in the identification of feeding vessels which may arise from the either or both hepatic arteries. Accessory feeding vessels may be present and arise from the intercostal, phrenic, epigastric, gastric, or superior mesenteric arteries [5].

It is generally believed that MRI is superior to CT for hepatic lesion characterization [29]. MRI (Fig. 5.3) has been assessed by multiple investigators who report a greater than 90% sensitivity and specificity [30–32]. Consistent with their aqueous constituent, T1-weighted images are hypointense with high signal intensity demonstrated on T2-weighted images. Gadolinium results in early peripheral nodular or globular enhancement with progressive centripetal filling as seen on CT scan. This pattern may be absent on smaller lesions <2 cm due to rapid filling. Small hemangiomas which demonstrate this rapid uniform enhancement may therefore be indistinguishable from hypervascular metastases of hepatocellular carcinoma [27]. Where doubt persists, a Tc99-labeled red cell scan can be performed to assist in making a definitive diagnosis. Series have shown this modality to have a specificity approximating 100%, with false positives due to rare hypervascular malignancies and angiosarcomas [33]. Angiography is reserved for atypical cases that cannot be diagnosed definitively after multiple imaging tests [34]. The characteristic "cotton wool" appearance and demonstration of a large feeding vessel are classic features.

Role of Percutaneous Biopsy

Biopsy has been associated with significant hemorrhage and fatality [35, 36]. Additionally, in some series, diagnostic material was only obtained in two thirds of cases. Hence, needle aspiration or biopsy in the evaluation of a possible hemangioma cannot be recommended. Biopsy may be useful intraoperatively where frozen section may facilitate confirmation of diagnosis in select cases where a definitive diagnosis has not been made prior to surgery [5].

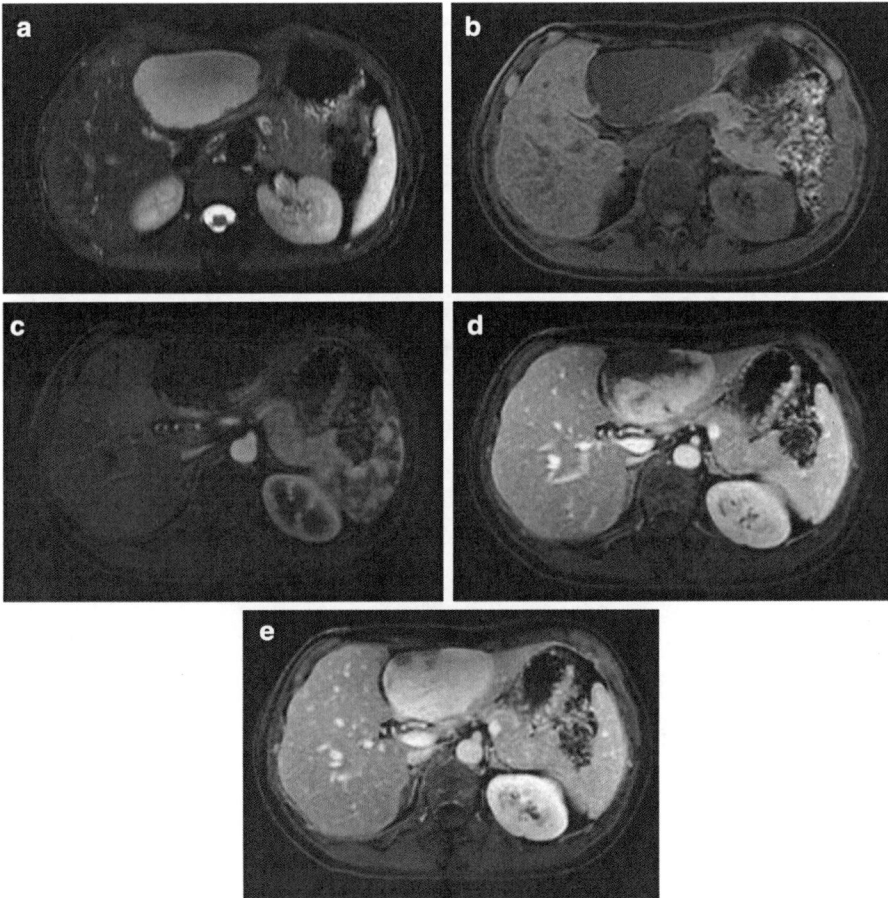

Fig. 5.3 MRI—hemangioma of the liver. (**a**) T2-weighted image—well-defined hyperintense mass with smooth margins within the left liver lobe, (**b**) pre-gadolinium, (**c**) postcontrast at 20 s showing hypointense lesion with peripheral nodular enhancement, (**d**) postcontrast at 70 s, (**e**) postcontrast at 3 min showing progressive centripetal enhancement to complete filling

Hepatocellular Adenoma

These benign tumors of the liver are of epithelial origin and are relatively uncommon. They are usually solitary and occur in women four times as often as men, usually within the age range of 20–40 years. Their increased occurrence in women appears to be due to their association with estrogen use, particularly as found in oral contraceptives. Multiple adenomas have been described, occurring with prolonged oral contraceptive and androgen use, in patients with glycogen storage disease and in the entity of hepatic adenomatosis.

Considered extremely rare prior to the 1960s [37], the increasing incidence of hepatic adenoma with oral contraceptive use was first described in 1973 by Janet

Baum at Michigan [38]. Over the last few decades, the incidence has increased in parallel with the increased use of the oral contraceptives [37–40], with current estimates of the incidence around 1 per 100,000 in women who have never used oral contraceptives as compared to 3–4 per 100,000 in long-term users [41]. Case–control studies suggest exposure to estrogen is an important etiological factor with both duration [40, 41] and dose implicated [42, 43]. Reports of remission and recurrence exist while levels of estrogen fluctuate with both contraceptive use and pregnancy. Several cases of adenoma rupture during pregnancy have been reported. These are associated with a high maternal and fetal mortality.

Anabolic steroid use (C17 alkylating steroids) has also associated with the development and enlargement of hepatic adenomas.

Finally, patients with type I and type III glycogen storage disease appear to be susceptible to the development of hepatic adenomas. The incidence in type I glycogen storage disease has been reported to be as high as 50–75% with up to 25% of patients with type III disease developing adenoma in some series [44, 45].

Pathology

These tumors range in size from 1 to 30 cm and are usually solitary. Similar to other liver lesions and likely due to the increased mass of a normal right lobe, they are more often in the right hemiliver. Occasionally, they may be pedicled. In gross appearance, they are smooth and tan, and have a soft consistency occasionally with areas of hemorrhage and necrosis which is responsible for a heterogenous appearance on imaging. There are usually prominent blood vessels on the surface as well as within the tumor, and due to the absence of a fibrous capsule, hemorrhage into the liver or peritoneum may occur.

Microscopically (Fig. 5.4), hepatocellular adenomas are composed of benign hepatocytes arranged in sheets and cords without the acinar architecture of normal liver. Cells are usually larger and paler than surrounding nontumor hepatocytes due to increased cytoplasmic glycogen and fat. The nuclei of the tumor cells are typically uniform and regular, the nuclear-to-cytoplasmic ratio is low, and mitoses are almost never seen. A well-developed reticulin framework is usually present in the tumor. The sinusoids, with flattened endothelial lining cells, are usually compressed, contributing to the sheetlike appearance. Bile ducts are not found in HCA, but ductules and progenitor cells may be present [46]. A feature is the lack of a significant number of Kupffer cells, which leads to the cold appearance of hepatic adenomas on Tc99m-labeled sulfur colloid scan. Importantly, the distinction from well-differentiated hepatocellular carcinoma is sometimes difficult [47].

From a molecular standpoint, recent discoveries have led to the suggestion of a division of hepatic adenomas into three groups after a multicenter series of adenomas were analyzed according to genotype [48]. Hepatic adenomas with inactivating mutations in hepatocyte nuclear factor 1 alpha were phenotypically characterized by marked steatosis, lack of cytological abnormalities, and no inflammatory

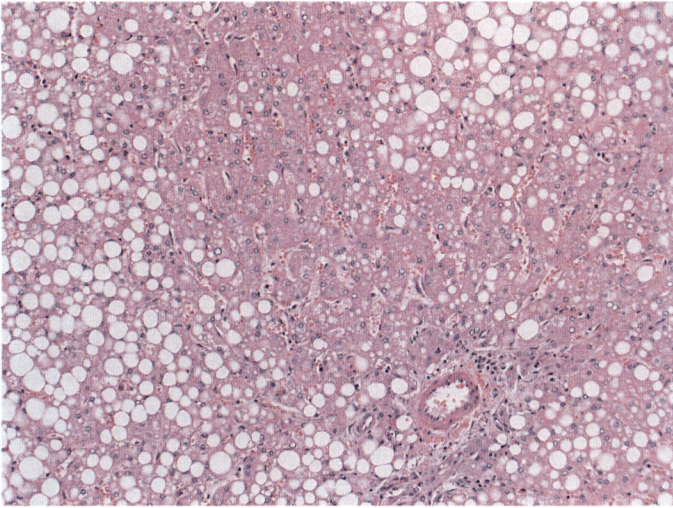

Fig. 5.4 Hepatocellular adenoma (×64)

infiltrates; these were contrasted by tumors with activating mutations in beta-catenin also characterized by steatosis but with frequent cytologic atypia. The third group of tumors without mutation was divided into two subgroups based on the presence or absence of an inflammatory infiltrate. The subgroup described with an inflammatory infiltrate resembled telangiectatic focal nodular hyperplasias, with frequent cytological abnormalities, ductular reaction, and dystrophic vessels. In this series, hepatocellular carcinoma associated with adenoma or borderline lesions between carcinoma and adenoma was found in 46% of the beta-catenin-mutated tumors, whereas they were never observed in inflammatory lesions and were rarely found in HNF1-mutated tumors. Furthermore, radiologic features on MRI have been found to correlate with the different subtypes [49]. The telangiectatic variant of FNH has now been recognized as a variant of hepatic adenoma and is now designated as inflammatory adenoma or telangiectatic adenoma (Fig. 5.5) [50, 51].

Presentation

Clinical presentation [39, 52–55] is often related to pain and discomfort. Jaundice has been described, and a mass may be palpable on examination. Occasionally, rupture and hemorrhage into the peritoneum occurs and presents with hypotension and pain which may be severe and result in mortality. Associations with bleeding include a long history of contraceptive use, the presence of abdominal pain, and subcapsular location of the adenoma. Other lesions present incidentally at imaging for unrelated reasons. Elevation of gamma-glutamyl transpeptidase and alkaline phosphatase may be present. Due to their nonspecificity, however, liver function tests do not usually

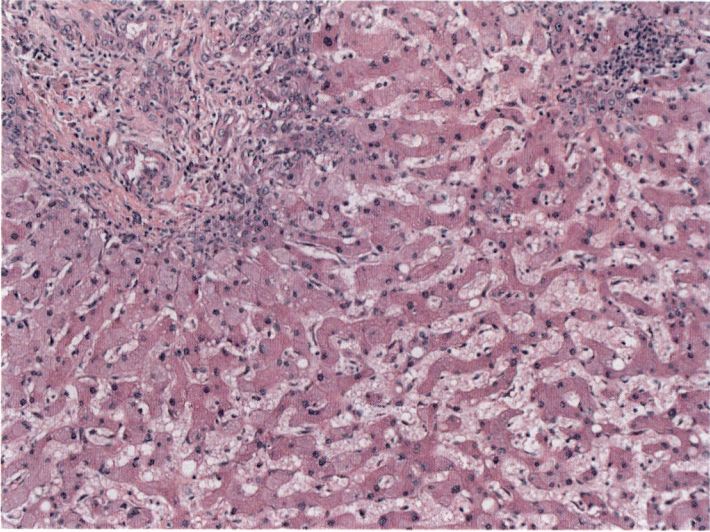

Fig. 5.5 Hepatocellular adenoma—telangiectatic variant (×64)

contribute to the diagnosis. Information on the risk of malignancy developing within the hepatic adenoma is limited. Small series suggest that it may be between 8% and 13% [55, 56] with common associations being an increase in size and an elevation in serum AFP. These features would not be expected in adenoma alone. Where more than ten adenomas exist in the absence of an association with steroid use and glycogen storage disease, the rare entity of adenomatosis is described and definition fulfilled. It is radiologically and histologically similar to hepatic adenoma. This entity may have a higher rate of bleeding than hepatic adenomas [57].

Radiologic Appearance

Imaging characteristics are critical to the diagnosis of adenoma, with different modalities having different levels of diagnostic utility. On ultrasound, characteristics are nonspecific: Adenomas are single, well-demarcated lesions with a hyperechoic appearance due to the presence of high lipid content within the lesion. The presence of intratumoral hemorrhage may lead to heterogeneity with areas of calcification and necrosis also apparent. Blood vessels may be seen within and around the tumor differentiating it from focal nodular hyperplasia [58].

CT imaging shows a well-demarcated isodense to hypodense lesion. However, because adenomas consist almost entirely of uniform hepatocytes and a variable number of Kupffer cells, most adenomas are nearly isoattenuating relative to normal liver on unenhanced, portal venous phase, and delayed-phase images [59]. In patients with fatty liver, adenomas are hyperattenuating during all phases of contrast enhancement as well as on unenhanced images. Adenomas sometimes have an

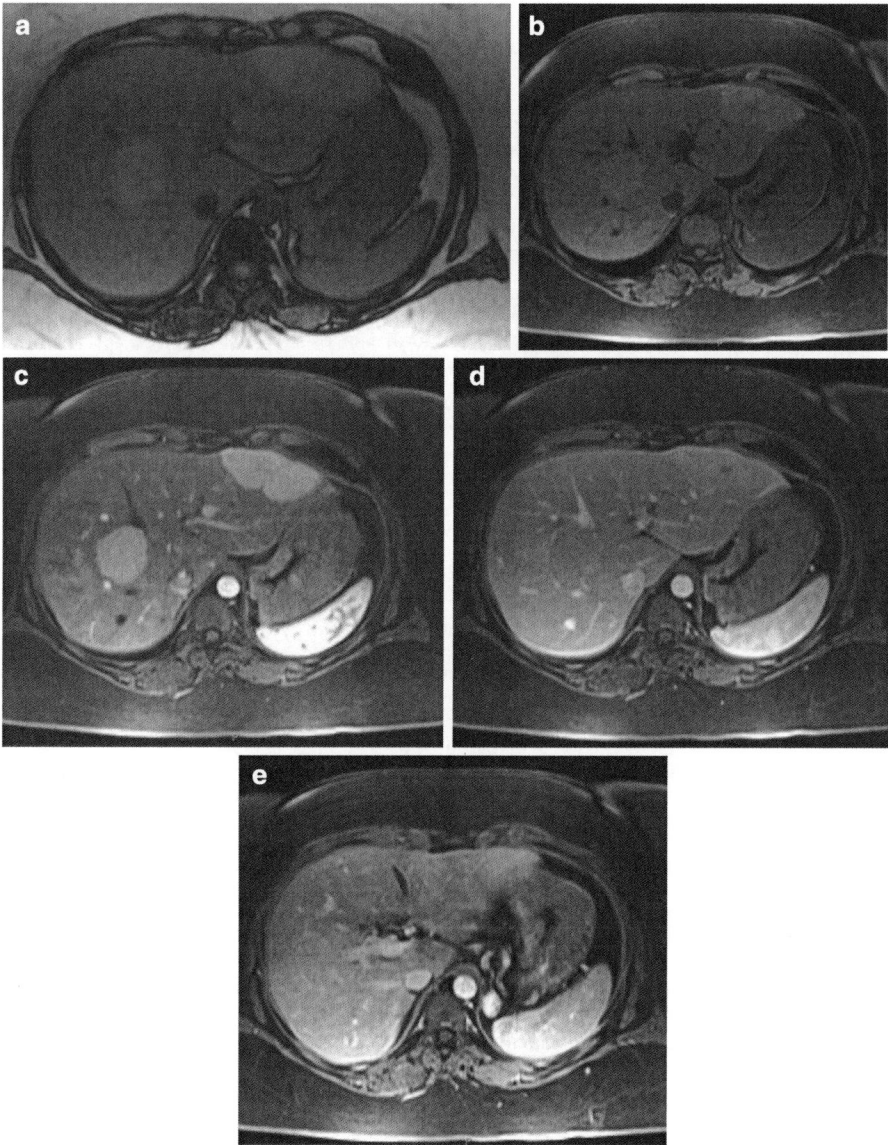

Fig. 5.6 MRI—hepatocellular adenoma. (**a**) Out-of-phase image, (**b**) T2-weighted image, (**c**) arterial phase, (**d**) venous phase, (**e**) delayed phase

encapsulated appearance (30%) and are occasionally calcified (10%). Contrast scans demonstrate peripheral enhancement with subsequent centripetal flow during the portal venous phase.

MRI (Fig. 5.6) characteristics are variable [60] with nearly all lesions having a heterogenous appearance [61]. The relatively high lipid content is responsible for the hyperintensity on T1- as well as T2-weighted images. Hemorrhagic areas may also be seen within the lesion—up to 17% in one series [61]. Gadolinium administration leads to further enhancement and shows early arterial enhancement relative to liver, a specific appearance of adenoma. The recent addition of gadobenate dimeglumine as a MRI-enhancing agent provides a further useful diagnostic tool. This agent is eliminated through both renal and hepatobiliary excretion, with about 5% of the dose being excreted into the biliary system by intact hepatocytes. Use of this agent has been shown to have a sensitivity and specificity of 97% and 100%, respectively, in differentiating FNH from adenoma [62].

In the past, technetium-99 m sulfur colloid scanning has been useful in differentiation adenomas from FNH. Administration of sulfur colloid reveals adenomas as a cold spot within the liver due to the scanty presence of Kupffer cells within the lesion. This is however neither sensitive nor specific, but may be helpful in circumstances where differentiation between FNH and adenoma is difficult.

Focal Nodular Hyperplasia

Focal nodular hyperplasia (FNH) is the second most common benign hepatic tumor after hemangioma. It represents about 8% of primary liver lesions and is reported in between 0.6% and 3% of the general population [63], with multiple lesions present in about 20% of patients. In referral centers, it is seen about ten times more frequently than hepatic adenoma [64]. FNH occurs about six to nine times more frequently in women than in men and is most common in the third to fifth decade of life. FNH has also been described as solitary hyperplastic nodule, hepatic hamartoma, focal cirrhosis, and hepatic pseudotumor.

FNH is considered to be a nonneoplastic, hyperplastic response to a congenital vascular malformation. Its constituent hepatocytes have a polyclonal origin [65] and are demonstrated to have an elevation in angiopoietin1/angiopoeitin2 mRNA ratio [66], which differentiates it from the unchanged ratio seen in hepatic adenoma [50]. Additionally, hepatocytes within FNH demonstrate activation of the b-catenin pathway without b-catenin mutation [67], features useful in diagnosis (see below).

Anomalous dystrophic arterial malformations are hypothesized to be central to the pathogenesis of these lesions. Local hyperperfusion of the liver parenchyma is thought to lead to hepatocellular hyperplasia [68–70]. The subsequent polyclonal nature of FNH is consistent with the indolent clinical course followed by lesions and absence of malignant transformation. Additionally, FNH is associated with vascular abnormalities within the liver, including hepatic hemangioma present in 20% of patients. This further supports the concept of a vascular component involved in the pathogenesis of this lesion [63]. FNH does not appear to have any relationship to estrogen [71] though the relationship is controversial [72].

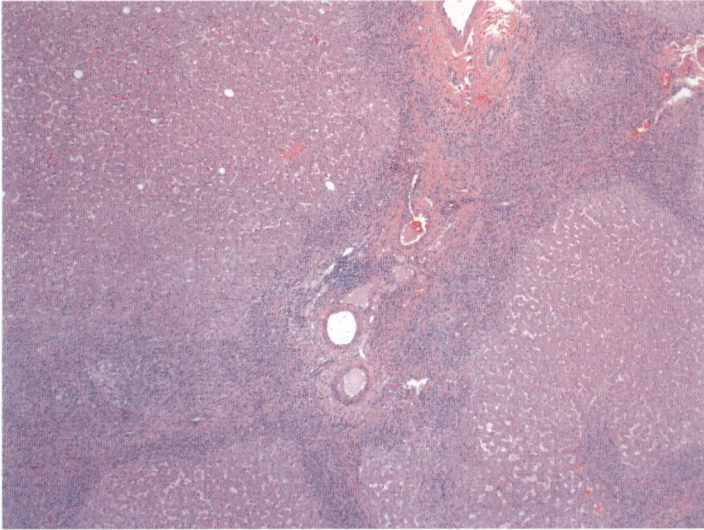

Fig. 5.7 Focal nodular hyperplasia (×20)

Pathology

FNH is usually solitary and rarely greater than 5 cm in diameter, although reports of very large hyperplasias exist with lesions reaching 19 cm being reported [73, 74]. Grossly, FNH may be pedunculated and is characteristically well delineated but unencapsulated. Classically, a central stellate scar is present. This contains a large artery from which multiple branches radiate peripherally through fibrous septae. Review of histology (Fig. 5.7) shows benign-appearing hepatocytes arranged in nodules that are delineated by the fibrous septae. Within the fibrous septa, large and dystrophic vessels, ductular proliferation, and inflammatory cells are observed [70, 75]. Sinusoids and Kupffer cells are present, a feature which assists in differentiating FNH from hepatic adenoma [1, 73, 74, 76]. The presence of perturbed architecture, vascular lesions, and proliferation of bile ductules fulfills minimal histologic criteria for classical FNH [73].

Variants of FNH have been recognized in the past and included telangiectatic FNH. Through clinical and molecular evidence, this is now recognized as a variant of hepatic adenoma and is now designated as inflammatory adenoma or telangiectatic adenoma [50, 51]. Additional variants include a mixed hyperplastic and adenomatous form of FNH with subtle vascular and bile duct differences from hepatic adenoma. A further variant is characterized by cytologic atypia. These variants often fail to show the macroscopically visible scar. In cases lacking key features of FNH such as stellate scar, fibrous bands, and ductular reaction, or in those exhibiting features usually present in HCA such as sinusoidal dilatation, molecular characteristics are useful in differentiating FNH from HCA. Overexpression of glutamine synthase, a target gene of b-catenin, has been successfully used to identify FNH [77].

Presentation

Most lesions are identified incidentally [74] after imaging, with symptoms usually attributable to other disease. Complications such as bleeding are rare. Alpha-fetoprotein is normal, and liver function tests may be elevated nonspecifically.

Radiologic Appearance

Ultrasound is useful in detecting lesions which may appear hyperechoic, isoechoic, or hypoechoic [78]. Use of power Doppler ultrasound may demonstrate arterial flow and assist in differentiation from hepatic adenoma, characterized by venous flow, while contrast-enhanced ultrasound is highly sensitive, specific, and accurate in the identification of FNH [79].

Noncontrast CT will demonstrate a hypo- or isoattenuating lesion relative to normal liver. The central scar is present in approximately 1/3 patients [78]. Larger lesions may be visualized through mass effect with distortion of liver contour and displacement of adjacent vessels, whereas small lesions may be difficult to see. The prominent arterial supply is responsible for the typical hyperattenuating appearance on arterial phase contrast. On portal venous phase imaging, most lesions become isoattenuating, although about 20% remain hyperattenuating [80–82]. During the arterial phase, differences in attenuation between the lesion and the surrounding liver can be used to differentiate FNH from hepatocellular adenoma: A relative enhancement of the lesion 1.6 times greater than that of the surrounding liver is highly accurate in differentiating FNH from adenoma [83, 84]. At imaging, the presence of the central scar is not pathognomic. A similar feature may be present in fibrolamellar hepatocellular carcinoma, hepatic adenoma, and cavernous hemangioma. Central scars are initially hypo- to isoattenuating relative to the liver prior to contrast administration. On arterial and portal venous phase, the scar is usually hypoattenuating compared to the surrounding lesion. Scars become hyperattenuating on delayed phase as contrast moves from the artery into the venous structures within the scar [80].

MRI appearance (Figs. 5.8–5.10): T1-weighted imaging shows these homogenous lesions to be hypo- or isointense, while T2-weighted images will demonstrate lesions to be iso- to hyperintense [85]. The relatively aqueous consistency of the scar results in a hyperintense appearance on T2-weighted images. Early enhancement occurs during the arterial phase with gadolinium administration and subsequent persistent enhancement of the scar on delayed imaging. A sensitivity of 70% and specificity of 98% of gadolinium-enhanced MRI in demonstrating

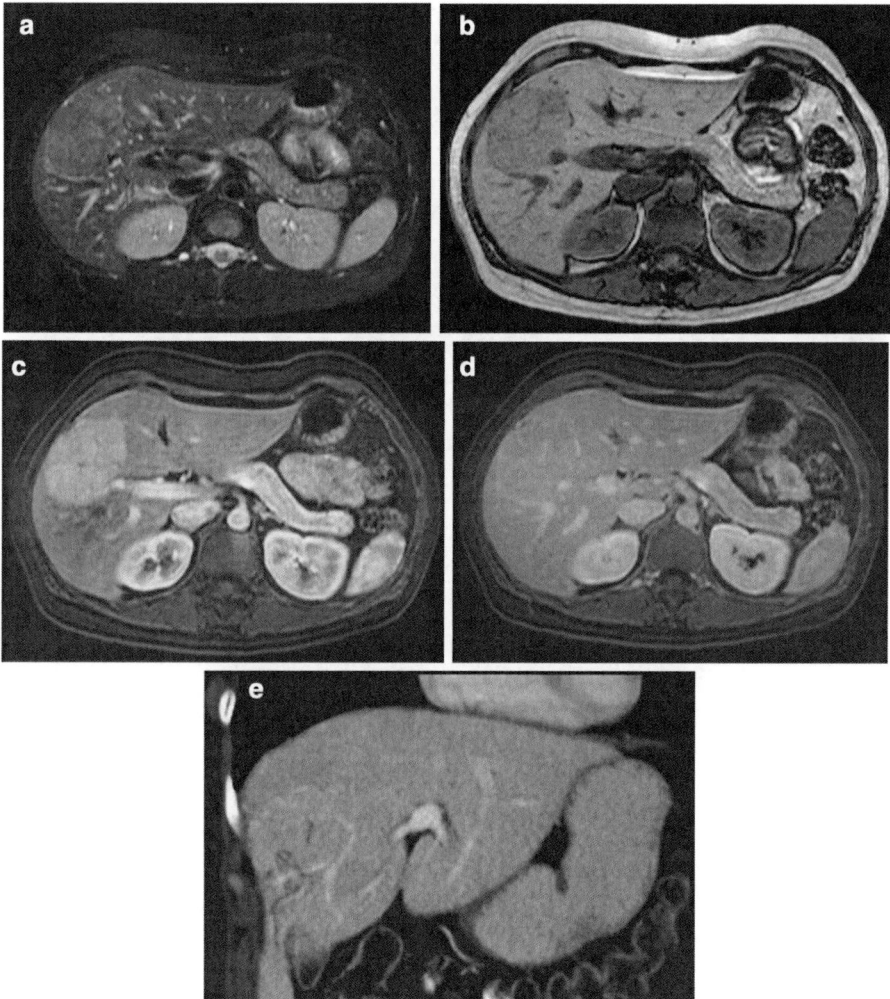

Fig. 5.8 MRI—focal nodular hyperplasia seen as a smooth well-marginated mass isointense on (**a**) T1-weighted and (**b**) T2-weighted images in the right liver lobe, (**c**) homogeneous arterial enhancement with (**d**) delayed enhancement of central scar, (**e**) isodense, well-defined mass within segment VI–VII, hyperdense central scar shown on coronal plane

FNH has been reported [42]. Agents with hepatobiliary elimination (Fig. 5.10) (including manganese, gadolinium, and paramagnetic iron oxide-based contrast agents) target Kupffer cells and hepatocytes and assist in differentiating lesions where doubt persists [86]. These agents have largely replaced the technetium sulfur colloid scan: The presence of Kupffer cells within FNH enables technetium sulfur colloid scans to demonstrate active uptake of colloid approximately 80% of the time [81, 87, 88]. However, occasional hepatic adenomas also demonstrate uptake.

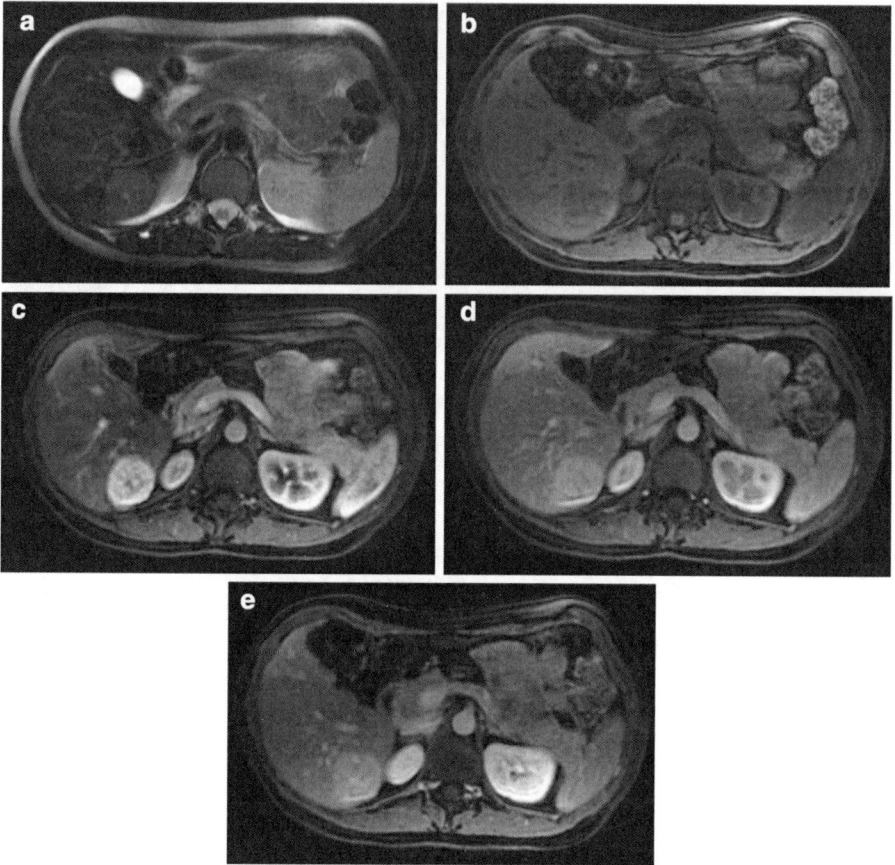

Fig. 5.9 MRI—focal nodular hyperplasia. (**a**) Segment VI contains a slightly hyperintense mass well defined with hyperintense signal of central scar, (**b**) hypointense mass with (**c**) avid enhancement after contrast administration, (**d**) persistent enhancement in venous, and (**e**) delayed image, in addition to delayed enhancement of the central scar

Where imaging is not diagnostic of FNH, biopsy can assist in a histologic diagnosis. A scoring system exists and has proved to be useful [89]. Histologic and molecular characteristics as described above are useful in diagnosis.

Hepatocellular Carcinoma

Hepatocellular carcinoma (HCC) is the most common primary hepatic malignancy. More than 80% of all cases of HCC develop in the setting of cirrhosis. It is the third leading cause of death from cancer worldwide and the ninth leading cause of cancer deaths in the United States [90, 91]. Geographically, those areas with the highest rates are Asia and sub-Saharan Africa where annual rates exceed 20 per 100,000

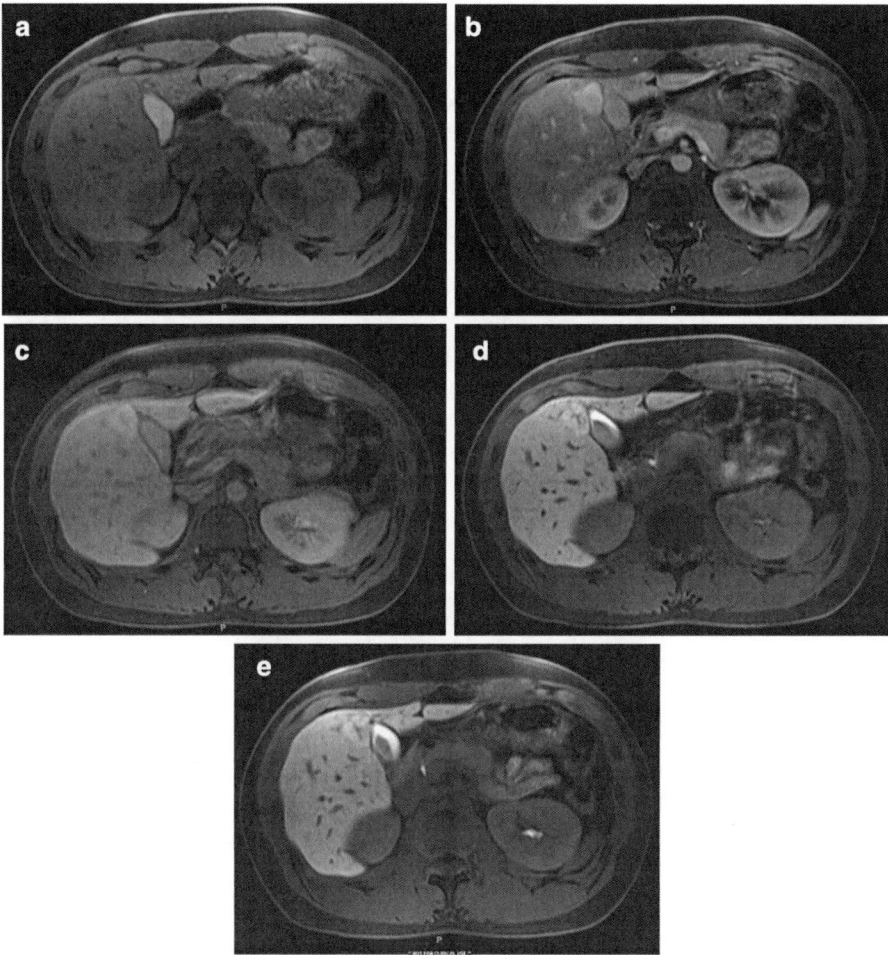

Fig. 5.10 MRI—focal nodular hyperplasia with gadoxetate disodium. (**a**) Hypointense lesion in segment V with (**b**) arterial enhancement with hypointense central branching representing central scar. (**c**) Venous phase shows homogenous enhancement, (**d**) whereas delayed images with hepatobiliary MR contrast at 20 min and (**e**) at 30 min did not show enhancement of the mass but slight enhancement of the scar

people. Rates are lower in Southern Europe and Japan, and lowest in Australia, New Zealand, Northern Europe, and North America [92, 93].

Evidence from different countries shows that the incidence of HCC is rising [92–97]. This reflects the incidence of risk factors—including infection with hepatitis C virus [98] as well as hepatitis B virus [99]. Other risk factors include aflatoxin B1 uptake [100], cigarette smoking, and heavy alcohol consumption [101]. Tyrosinemia, glycogen storage disease, hereditary hemochromatosis, nonalcoholic fatty liver disease, and α_1-antitrypsin deficiency also predispose to liver disease and HCC.

Presentation

Without early detection through screening, HCC is usually asymptomatic until late in its course. HCC diagnosed after the onset of cancer-related symptoms has a dismal prognosis with less than 6 months' life expectancy and no survival benefit from treatment [99]. Advanced lesions may present with upper abdominal pain, fullness, anorexia, weight loss, and early satiety or as a palpable mass. If tumor invasion extends into the hepatic or portal veins, decompensation of residual liver function in the cirrhotic individual may occur with the development of ascites, encephalopathy, or jaundice.

Occasionally, presentation through paraneoplastic syndromes occurs. Mild hypoglycemia—thought to be due to tumor's high metabolic demand—may occur [102]. Reports of severe hypoglycemia due to the secretion of insulin-like growth factor II exist [103]. Erythrocytosis from tumor secretion of erythropoietin has been demonstrated in between 3% and 12% of patients [104, 105]. Hypercalcemia occurs through parathyroid hormone-related peptide and osteolytic metastases [106]. Presentation may occasionally involve severe diarrhea due to the secretion of peptides such as vasoactive intestinal peptide [107]. Cutaneous manifestations of HCC can also occur.

Radiologic Appearance

Ultrasound is commonly used in screening programs for HCC, and the majority of HCC lesions will be diagnosed in patients with cirrhosis. Of lesions evaluated after discovery at screening in cirrhotics, approximately two thirds of de novo liver nodules are HCC [108–111]. At ultrasound, small HCC lesions have margins which are poorly defined and are usually hypoechoic with heterogenous echogenicity. Larger lesions may be iso- to hyperechoic and can be difficult to distinguish from surrounding liver if they are infiltrative [112]. Occlusion of portal veins may be visualized and usually represent direct tumor infiltration of the vessel [113–115]. Through systematic review, the sensitivity and specificity of ultrasound compared to pathologic exam of resected or explanted liver have been placed at 60% and 97%, respectively [116]. Contrast-enhanced ultrasound provides greater sensitivity. This modality is currently unavailable in the United States [117].

CT and MRI

Performance of these studies is critical to the noninvasive diagnosis of HCC and should be performed in expert centers. Both MRI and CT may fulfill a diagnostic role after lesion detection at ultrasound.

On CT, typical HCCs are described as hypervascular and hyperdense on arterial phase. Occasionally, tumors are isodense and are missed on arterial and portal venous phase and appear hypodense on delayed phase [118]. Sensitivity depends on

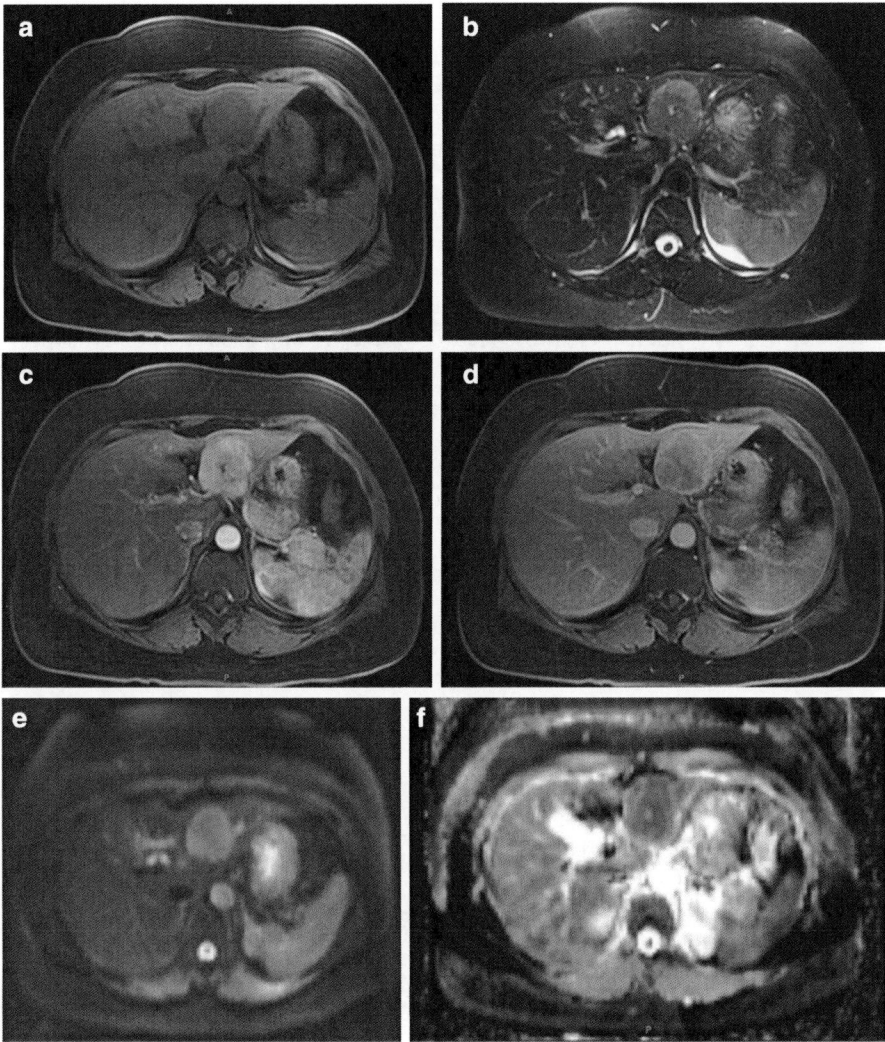

Fig. 5.11 MRI—hepatocellular carcinoma of the left liver lobe—a well-defined nodular mass, (**a**) T1 hypointense, (**b**) T2 hyperintense. (**c**) After contrast administration, there is arterial enhancement (**d**) with rapid washout on venous phase. (**e**) The lesion is characterized by high signal intensity in diffusion-weighted image and (**f**) low signal at ADC map ($1.02 \times 10^{-3}\,mm^2/s$)

the size of lesions. Isolated study suggests CT may have a sensitivity as high as 90% in detecting lesions greater than or equal to 1.5 cm [119, 120]. Using pathological examination of resected or explanted liver, systematic review places the sensitivity and specificity at 68% and 93%, respectively [116].

MRI (Fig. 5.11) shows typical HCC on T1-weighted images as hypointense, with a hyperintense appearance on T2-weighted imaging. Systematic review of MRI compared to pathologic examination of livers shows sensitivity to be 81% and specificity to be 85% [116]. MR imaging with superparamagnetic iron oxide has been shown to have high sensitivity in detecting HCC with a diagnostic accuracy higher than multiphasic CT scan [121, 122].

For HCC to be diagnosed radiologically and avoid the need for biopsy, the typical imaging features should be present. This requires a contrast-enhanced dynamic CT scan or MRI [108, 123, 124]. On arterial phase imaging using either modality, the neoplastic vascularization of HCC is responsible for hyperintense appearance. As contrast perfuses the liver from the portal circulation in the venous phase, arterial contrast leaves the lesion which subsequently becomes relatively hypointense. This "washout" (Fig. 5.11) is highly specific for HCC [108, 109, 125]. Among screened cirrhotic patients, the presence of delayed hypointensity on MRI has been shown to have a sensitivity of 80% and a specificity of 95% for lesions less than 2 cm [126]. "Washout" has been shown to be absent from intrahepatic cholangiocarcinoma confirming the specificity of this appearance on delayed imaging [127]. Occasionally, some small lesions appear hypovascular due to the presence of a dual blood supply and require biopsy. Additionally, at imaging, vascular invasion may be present (Figs. 5.12 and 5.13).

Lesions That May Mimic HCC on Imaging

Nontumor arterioportal shunts are the most common mimics of HCC in a cirrhotic liver [128]. Typically, arterioportal shunts appear as small, peripherally located wedge-shaped enhancing lesions on arterial phase CT [129] or MR scanning [130]. They are different from HCC in that these lesions never show negative enhancement compared with the adjacent liver parenchyma during the portal and delayed phases.

Small hemangiomas may also be confused as HCC. The peripheral globular enhancement with gradual central filling on contrast-enhanced US/CT/MR imaging is virtually pathognomonic of a hemangioma. Additionally, the intensity of contrast enhancement is usually stronger in hemangioma than HCC. MRI will also show the typical bright hyperintensity of hemangiomas on T2-weighted imaging [131].

Pathology and Biopsy

The American Association for the Study of Liver Disease (2010 update) (http://www.aasld.org/practiceguidelines/Pages/NewUpdatedGuidelines.aspx) makes the following recommendations: Nodules found on ultrasound surveillance that are smaller than 1 cm should be followed with ultrasound at intervals from 3 to 6 months. If there has been no growth over a period of up to 2 years, one can revert to routine surveillance (recommendation 6). The majority of nodules smaller than 1 cm are not HCC. Nodules larger than 1 cm found on ultrasound screening of a cirrhotic liver

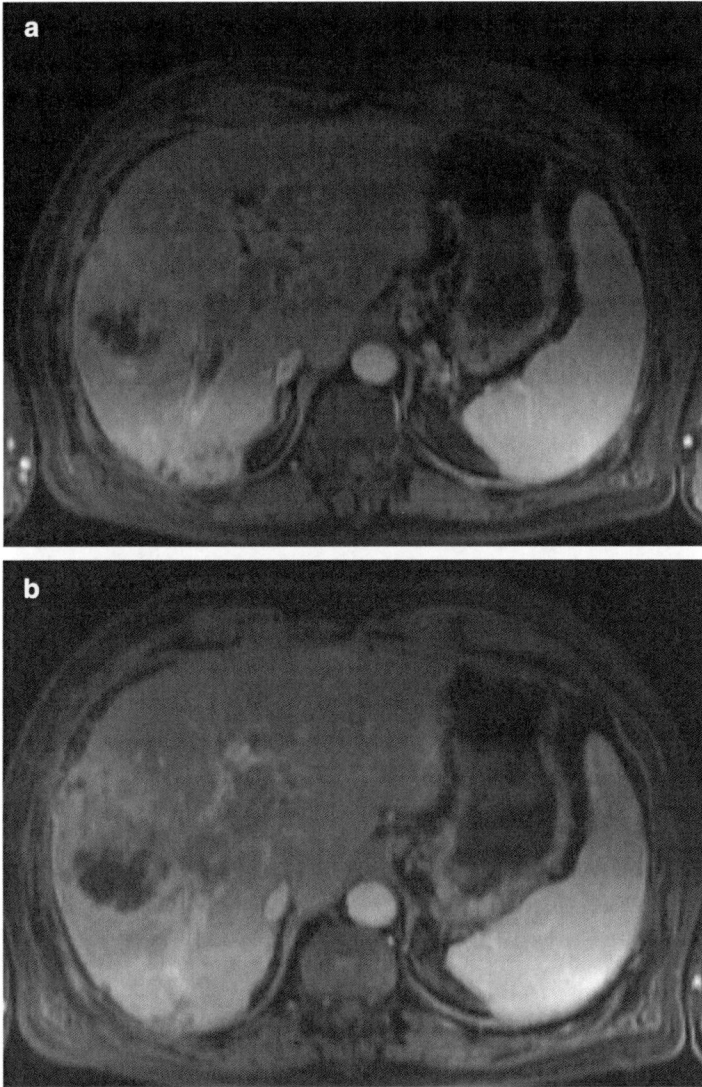

Fig. 5.12 MRI—hepatocellular carcinoma infiltrative into portal vein, (**a**) arterial and (**b**) venous phase

should be investigated further with either four-phase multidetector CT scan or dynamic contrast-enhanced MRI. If the appearance is typical of HCC (Fig. 5.11) (i.e., hypervascular in the arterial phase with washout in the portal venous or delayed phase), the lesion should be treated as HCC. If the findings are not characteristic or the vascular profile is not typical, a second contrast-enhanced study with the other imaging modality should be performed, or the lesion should be biopsied (recommendation 7). It should be noted that at contrast-enhanced ultrasound, intrahepatic

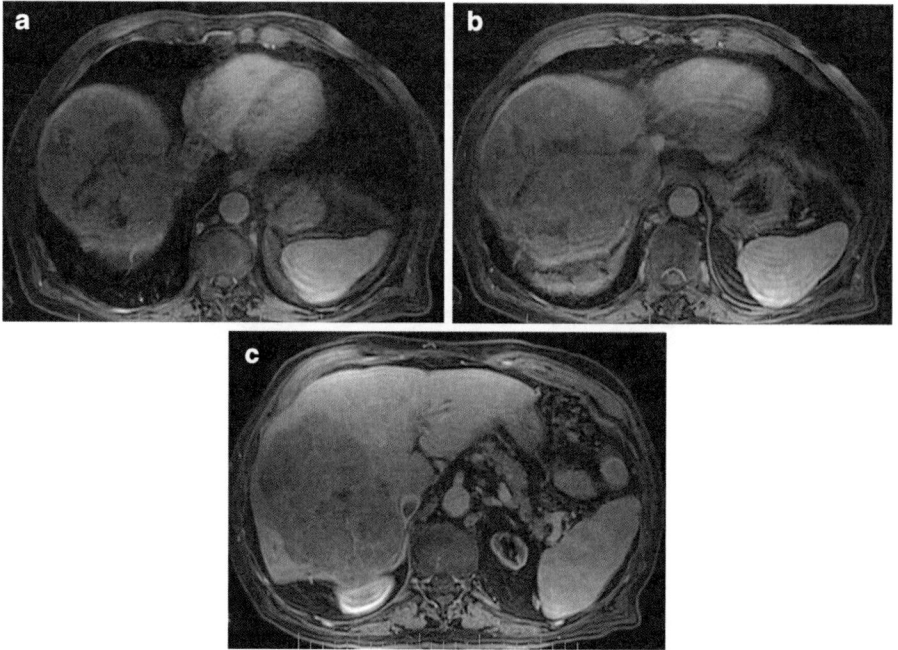

Fig. 5.13 MRI—infiltrative hepatocellular carcinoma—(**a**) and (**b**) extension into right atrium. (**c**) Postcontrast images showing tumor thrombus extending to inferior vena cava and right atrium

cholangiocarcinoma in a cirrhotic liver may display a vascular pattern indistinguishable from HCC, with homogeneous contrast uptake followed by washout. This would lead to misdiagnosis and could have major therapeutic implications [132]. The major risk of biopsy is tumor seeding along the needle tract. Through systematic review, the incidence of seeding following biopsy of a tumor is 2.7% overall [133]. Puncture-related seeding appears restricted to poorly differentiated tumors and peripheral tumors that cannot be approached through a rim of nontumoral liver [134, 135].

Grossly, HCC are usually pale tumors varying from unifocal to multifocal or diffusely infiltrative. Intrahepatic metastases and invasion into and extension within portal venous and vascular structures may occur. Hematologic spread to the lungs and other organs occurs late in the disease and is the major mechanism of metastasis. Lymph node metastases to the perihilar, peripancreatic, and para-aortic nodes above and below the diaphragm are found in fewer than half of HCCs with hematologic spread beyond the liver.

Histologically (Figs. 5.14–5.16), HCCs range from well-differentiated to highly anaplastic and undifferentiated lesions. Vascular invasion may be *seen* (Fig. 5.17). HCC cells have an elevated nuclear-to-cytoplasmic ratio, trabecular architecture, atypical naked nuclei, and peripheral wrapping [136]. Cells may closely resemble hepatocytes with architecture similar to normal liver plates or may be arranged in an

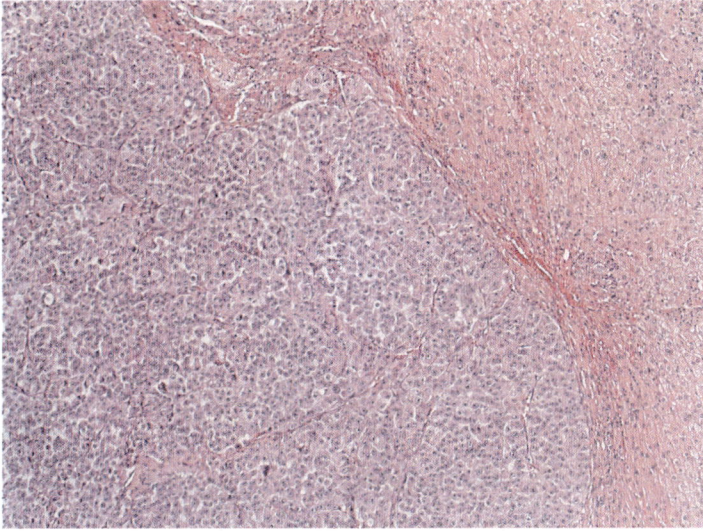

Fig. 5.14 Hepatocellular carcinoma, moderately differentiated (×40)

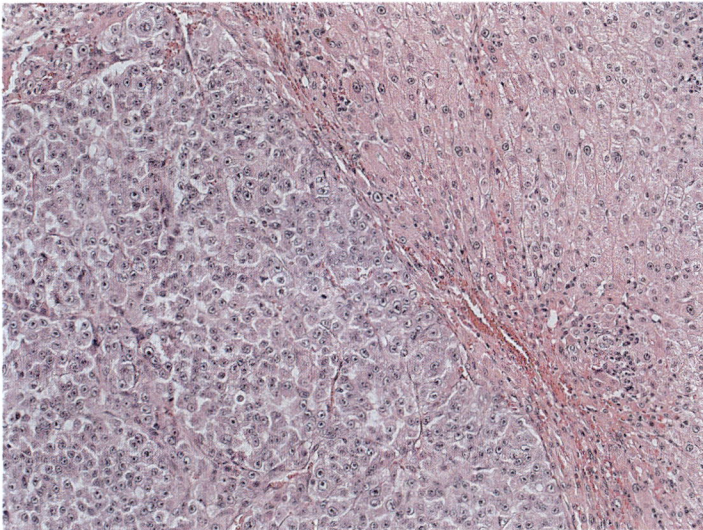

Fig. 5.15 Hepatocellular carcinoma, moderately differentiated (×64)

acinar, pseudoglandular pattern. Poorly differentiated forms show pleomorphic tumor cells with numerous anaplastic giant cells that are small and undifferentiated with necrosis often present [137].

Fibrolamellar carcinoma (Figs. 5.18 and 5.19) is a variant of HCC, often occurring in normal liver and carrying a better prognosis. The etiology is unknown, but it

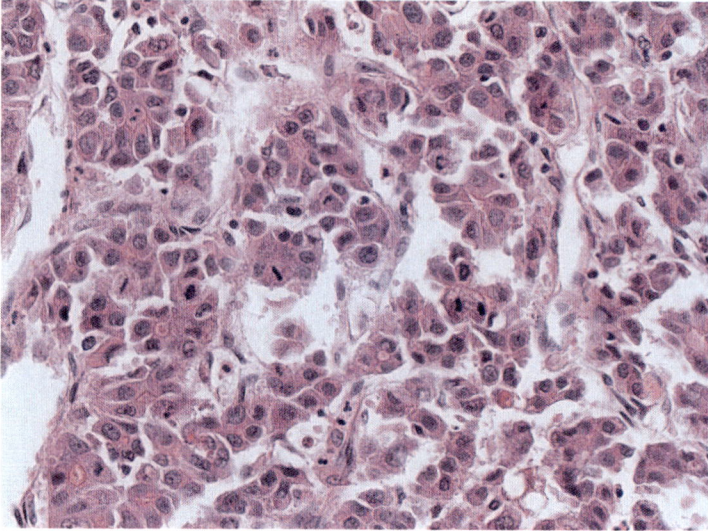

Fig. 5.16 Hepatocellular carcinoma, moderately to poorly differentiated (×160)

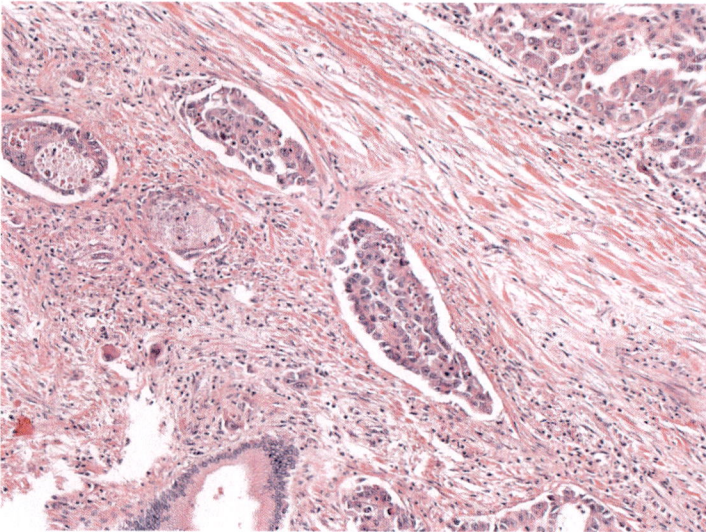

Fig. 5.17 Hepatocellular carcinoma with vascular invasion (×64)

occurs with equal incidence in young male and female adults (20–40 years of age) and constitutes about 5% of HCC [138]. It usually presents as single large, hard scirrhous tumor with fibrous bands coursing through it. Histologically, it is composed of well-differentiated cells growing in nests or cords separated by parallel lamellae of dense collagen bundles. The tumor cells have abundant eosinophilic cytoplasm and prominent nucleoli.

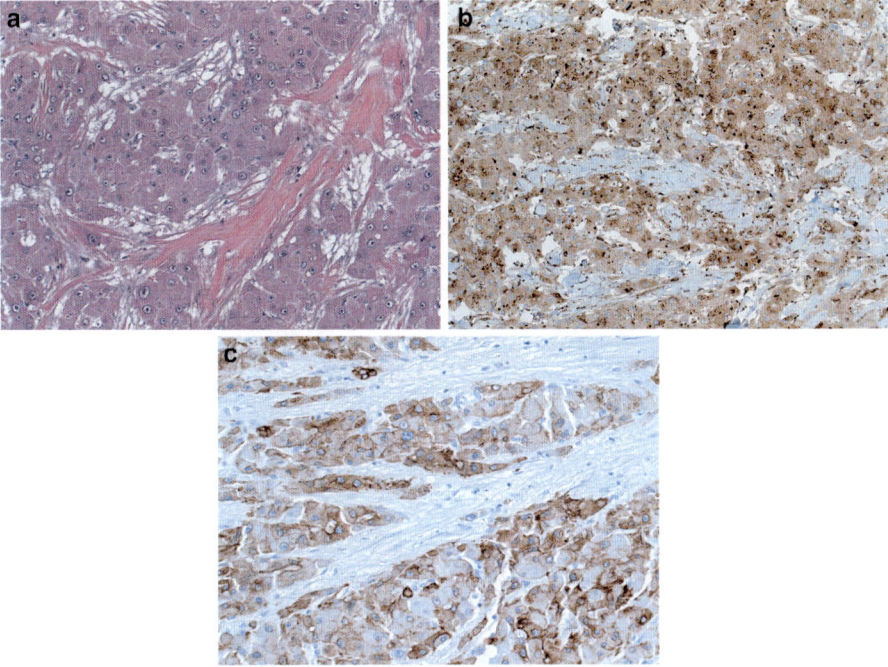

Fig. 5.18 (**a**) Fibrolamellar carcinoma (×64) (**b**) with CD68 staining (×64) (**c**) and CD7 staining (×100) (all fibrolamellar carcinomas should be confirmed with CK7 and CD68 stains)

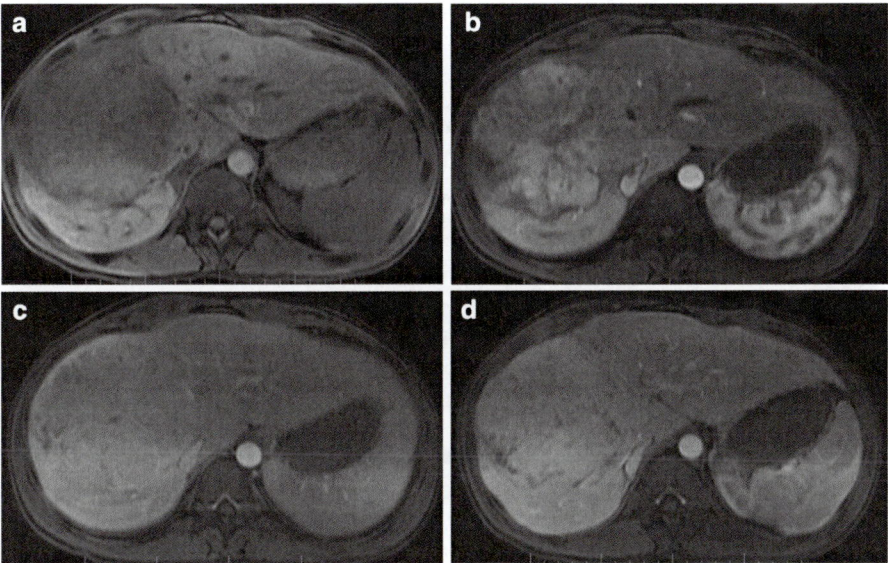

Fig. 5.19 MRI—fibrolamellar variant of hepatocellular carcinoma, (**a**) arterial, (**b**) venous, (**c**) and (**d**) delayed phases

Spectrum of Nodules in Cirrhosis

Diagnosis of HCC is made more challenging by the spectrum of smaller nodules that occur in cirrhosis. In cirrhotics, evidence supports the existence of precursors evolving into HCC. The development of a *regenerative nodule* may be the first step in hepatocarcinogenesis, subsequently developing into HCC through *dysplastic nodules* (DN) in a multistep fashion [137]. Nomenclature and diagnostic criteria now revolve around the now widely adopted 1995 International Working Party of the World Congresses of Gastroenterology nomenclature [139]. Nodular lesions found in chronic liver disease are classified into *large regenerative nodules, low-grade dysplastic nodules* (L-DN), *high-grade dysplastic nodules* (H-DN), and HCC. Additionally, the entity of *dysplastic focus* is defined as a cluster of hepatocytes with features of early neoplasia measuring less than 0.1 cm. *Small HCC* was defined as a tumor measuring less than 2 cm and may now be divided into two groups. The first group, *early HCC*, is well differentiated and distinguished by a vaguely nodular appearance; the second group, *progressed HCC*, is distinctly nodular, mostly moderately differentiated and often with microvascular invasion [140]. *Early HCC* has a longer time to recurrence and a higher 5-year survival than *progressed HCC* [141]. *Early HCC* is defined by Japanese pathologists and is similar to *very early HCC* as termed in the Barcelona Clinic Liver Cancer staging scheme [109]. It is generally hypovascular with ill-defined margins and has a vague outline on ultrasound [142]. On contrast imaging, it is hypovascular with few unpaired arteries (without bile ducts) histologically, and cells showing varying grades of dysplasia [143]. Invasion of the portal space by hepatocytes may be present, but vessel invasion is absent. Several studies show small foci of typical HCC within these lesions as well as invasion of the portal space by hepatocytes. This suggests that they are precursors of typical HCC lesions [137, 144, 145]. In contrast, *small* or *progressed* HCC are well defined on ultrasound with a typical appearance on CT and with typical histologic features. Microvascular invasion is present (Fig. 5.17) (in contrast to "early HCC" where invasion is absent) [137, 143, 144].

Given the complexity and difficulty of histologic diagnosis, as well as the possible consequences of erroneous diagnosis, biopsies of small lesions should be evaluated by expert pathologists. Tissue that is not clearly HCC should be stained with all currently available markers including CD34, CK7, glypican 3, HSP-70, and glutamine synthetase to improve diagnostic accuracy (AASLD recommendation 8).

Serum Markers

Alpha-fetoprotein (AFP) in the past has played a role in the diagnosis of and screening for HCC. However, the low positive predictive value [146, 147] and low sensitivity [148] when used in screening underscore the limitation of using the AFP as a screening test for HCC. The AFP test for HCC has a sensitivity of 39%–65% and a specificity of 76%–94%. AFP may not be elevated in up to 30% of patients with HCC [149]. Elevated serum AFP levels are seen in patients with intrahepatic cholangiocarcinoma (more common in cirrhotics than in individuals without cirrhosis) as well as in patients with gastric cancer. An elevated AFP has also been documented in colorectal metastases [150, 151]. Although a higher cutoff value (>400 ng/mL) improves the specificity of AFP testing, it reduces its sensitivity to less than 20%, making the test of borderline useful in screening. Lower cutoff values (>20 ng/mL) reduce the specificity to less than 20%. Levels of AFP greater than 400 ng/mL should be highly suspicious for HCC, and further imaging studies with CT scan or MRI should be performed immediately [149, 152]. The AASLD guidelines recommend that AFP is not used in the diagnosis of HCC.

Further data are needed to confirm the benefits of other serum markers, such as glypican 3, protein induced by vitamin K absence (PIVKA or des-gamma-carboxy prothrombin), and alpha-fetoprotein fractions in conventional clinical practice.

Intrahepatic Cholangiocarcinoma

Intrahepatic cholangiocarcinoma is a highly malignant cancer of biliary epithelium origin with an annual incidence of approximately 5,000 cases in the United States. It accounts for about 3% of gastrointestinal cancers and portends a poor prognosis, with a 3-year survival of 15%–55% after resection [153]. The anatomic margins for distinguishing intra- and extrahepatic cholangiocarcinomas are the second-order bile ducts. About 6% of tumors involve the intrahepatic biliary tree [154]. The incidence and mortality of intrahepatic cholangiocarcinoma (ICC) across different geographical regions including North America appear to be increasing [155].

Data from the National Cancer Institute's Surveillance, Epidemiology and End Results program (SEER) indicate that approximately 15% of primary liver tumors in the United Stated are ICCs, making it the second most common primary liver tumor [156]. Since ICC is found in patients with cirrhosis, its correct differentiation from HCC is a major clinical issue given that prognosis and treatment options differ significantly.

Risk Factors

Several risk factors predispose to ICC which is in more common in males with an incidence that increases with age. Primary biliary cirrhosis, primary sclerosing cholangitis, hepatolithiasis, choledochal cyst disease, hepatitis B, hepatitis C, and the use of the radiological contrast agent Thorotrast are considered to contribute to increased risk. The high disease prevalence in parts of Southeast and Eastern Asia has resulted in the identification of chronic biliary tract infestation with the parasitic liver flukes, Opisthorchis viverrini, and Clonorchis sinensis, as causative for cholangiocarcinoma [157]. The rising ICC incidence reported in the United States, Europe, and Asia appears to be associated with the increasing prevalence of hepatitis C, an important risk factor [156, 158–160]. Obesity-related nonalcoholic fatty liver disease has also recently been recognized to contribute to risk for ICC and may be associated with the observed rising incidence of ICC in North America [161].

Presentation

ICC most commonly is detected as an incidental liver mass on imaging. Occasionally, workup of nonspecifically deranged liver function tests may reveal a lesion, while presentation may also involve the discovery of an indeterminate liver mass as part of a workup for vague gastrointestinal complaints or other unrelated symptoms. Less often, patients with advanced disease may present with symptoms that include right upper quadrant abdominal pain or constitutional symptoms such as fatigue, anorexia, and weight loss [162]. Jaundice is observed in a significant proportion of patients and generally indicates compression or invasion of the biliary confluence by centrally located tumors.

Diagnosis

Presentation is usually with an isolated liver lesion found on imaging, or after referral with an imaged lesion and subsequent biopsy showing adenocarcinoma. In either situation, further workup needs to be performed. Since metastatic disease is more common in a normal liver than ICC, diagnostic workup should include a chest, abdomen and pelvic CT, upper and lower endoscopy, and mammography to exclude a primary malignancy at these common sites. Where these studies do not demonstrate disease, a PET/CT may be useful, although the exact role of this modality is still being determined (see below).

Serology

Alpha-fetoprotein, cancer antigen (CA) 19-9, CA 125, and carcinoembryonic antigen (CEA) are among the tumor markers that have been evaluated for an association with ICC. CA-19-9 has been most studied, but remains nonspecific and is of limited value. This marker has been evaluated most extensively in the setting of primary sclerosing cholangitis (PSC). A level greater than 100 U/mL has been reported to have a sensitivity of 75% and a specificity of 80% for the presence of cholangiocarcinoma [163, 164], while a serum level greater than 129 U/mL has a sensitivity of 78.6% and specificity of 98.5% for cholangiocarcinoma in PSC [165], although this level was associated with advanced, unresectable cholangiocarcinoma. In a series of 103 patients without PSC, the sensitivity of a serum CA 19-9 level of >100 U/mL in diagnosing cholangiocarcinoma was 53%, with true negative rates for nonmalignant liver disease and benign bile duct stricture of 76% and 92%, respectively [166]. Cholangitis and cholestasis decrease the sensitivity and specificity of CA 19-9, while CA 19-9 is virtually undetectable in patients with the Lewis antigen [167]. Baseline values of CEA and CA 19-9 if elevated may be useful in following response to treatment.

Imaging

The Liver Cancer Study Group of Japan (LCSGJ) classifies ICC into three types: "mass-forming," "periductal-infiltrating," and "intraductal-growing type" [168]. The "mass-forming type" is associated with a better overall survival compared with the "periductal-infiltrating" type [169] and constitutes about 85% of ICC. As anticipated, it forms a definite mass located in the liver parenchyma. The "periductal-infiltrating" type extends longitudinally along the bile duct, often resulting in dilatation of the peripheral bile duct. The "intraductal growth" type proliferates toward the biliary lumen like a papillary lesion or a tumor thrombus [168].

Ultrasound: This modality is generally insensitive for the detection of ICC. When a "mass-forming" cholangiocarcinoma is visualized at US, it is seen as a homogeneous mass with an irregular but well-defined margin. As sometimes seen surrounding other malignant tumors, a thin peripheral hypoechoic rim may be present [170]. Contrast-enhanced ultrasound of ICC in cirrhotic patients may display a vascular pattern that is indistinguishable from HCC, with homogeneous contrast uptake followed by washout [132]. Further diagnostic information should be obtained prior to treatment decisions.

CT: The typical CT features of "mass-forming" cholangiocarcinoma include homogeneous attenuation, irregular rim-like peripheral enhancement on arterial phase, followed by gradual centripetal enhancement on delayed phase. Some tumors are seen only on delayed-phase images and may be missed if this phase is not performed. Ductal dilatation may be seen peripheral to the tumor [171] and is a feature that has been shown at MRI to be useful in differentiating mass-forming ICC from colorectal metastases [172, 173]. ICC may have a fibrotic stroma and show delayed enhancement, whereas tumors without fibrosis do not show this feature [174].

MRI: On MR imaging, similar features are present. The mass shows an irregular margin with hyperintensity on T2-weighted images and with hypointensity on T1-weighted images. Enhancement may be more prominent at MRI than at CT. Hyperattenuating areas in ICC on delayed-phase images may reflect fibrous stroma within a tumor, a feature associated with a poorer prognosis in cirrhotic patients. Various atypical imaging patterns are frequently seen [171].

Several tumors or tumorlike conditions should be included in the differential diagnosis for a mass-forming cholangiocarcinoma [171]. HCC with cirrhotic stroma, sclerosing HCC, and combined HCC-cholangiocarcinoma can all appear nearly identical to ICC and need to be considered, especially in patients with chronic liver disease [175–177].

The rarer "periductal-infiltrating type" cholangiocarcinoma appears on ultrasound as a diffuse, mass-like bile duct thickening with or without obliteration of the bile duct lumen. At CT and MR imaging, diffuse periductal thickening and increased enhancement due to tumor infiltration are present, with an abnormally dilated or irregularly narrowed duct and peripheral ductal dilatation. Findings of a long-segment stricture with an irregular margin, asymmetric narrowing, ductal enhancement, and lymph node enlargement, as well as a periductal soft-tissue lesion suggest an early malignant stricture. This can be a challenging diagnosis to make [171].

"Intraductal" cholangiocarcinoma imaging patterns include diffuse and marked duct ectasia with or without a grossly visible papillary mass. An intraductal polypoid mass within localized ductal dilatation may be visualized. This type may also appear as an intraductal, cast-like lesion within a mildly dilated duct or as a focal, stricture-like lesion with mild proximal ductal dilatation [171].

FDG-PET: The role of FDG-PET in the management of ICC remains to be fully established. Studies suggest that tumors are FDG avid in between 78% and 85% of cases with a nodular morphology, while those with an infiltrating morphology are avid only 18% of the time [173, 178]. By upstaging extent of disease, PET has been shown to change surgical management in between one quarter and one third of patients when compared to CT or MRI [178, 179]. The role of PET scan may therefore assist in the exclusion of an occult primary in addition to delineating disease extent.

Cholangiography and ERCP

Where a malignant biliary stricture is suspected, conventional cytology obtained at percutaneous transhepatic cholangiography or endoscopic retrograde cholangiography is highly specific but limited in confirming the presence of malignancy in one-half of cases. Digital image analysis and fluorescent in situ hybridization testing have been increasingly used to determine the chromosomal alterations of individual cells in malignant biliary strictures. These have been shown to improve sensitivity and positive predictive value in cholangiocarcinoma detection [180, 181]. In patients with PSC, natural history studies suggest an annual incidence of cholangiocarcinoma of 0.5–2.5%. In this setting, screening strategies are evolving, and these emerging techniques are promising.

Pathology and Biopsy

Usually, malignancy is suspected at imaging. After workup, if resection is possible, biopsy should be deferred. If transplantation is considered or the lesion is not considered resectable, a biopsy of the lesion or enlarged nodes may be useful. It may not be possible to distinguish rare primary hepatic tumors from a more common primary lesion or a solitary metastasis solely on the basis of cross-sectional imaging and tumor markers, in which case, image-guided biopsy is also necessary to confirm the diagnosis. (AASLD 2009 guidelines—http://www.aasld.org/practiceguidelines/Pages/NewUpdatedGuidelines.aspx).

Premalignant lesions: It has been hypothesized that cholangiocarcinoma may develop through two key premalignant precursor lesions: biliary intraepithelial neoplasia (BilIN) and intraductal papillary neoplasm of the bile duct (IPNB).

BilIN is characterized by a flat or micropapillary growth of atypical biliary epithelium. It previously was called "atypical biliary epithelia" and "biliary dysplasia." BilIN is characteristically a microscopic lesion that can progress through three grades to tubular adenocarcinoma [182, 183].

IPNB is a macroscopic lesion characterized by prominent papillary growth of atypical biliary epithelium with a fibrovascular core and overproduction of mucin [184]. IPNB, like BilIN, occurs in bile ducts associated with chronic inflammatory conditions and can transform into two types of invasive cancers, each with different biologic behavior and prognosis: mucinous carcinoma or tubular adenocarcinoma [185]. Survival rates in patients who have mucinous carcinoma are considerably better than in patients who have tubular adenocarcinoma [186]. Furthermore, IPNB-associated cholangiocarcinoma has a more favorable outcome than cholangiocarcinoma that develops through the BilIN pathways [183, 187]. Once tubular adenocarcinoma develops from IPNB lesions, however, the reported survival rates are similar to those for nonpapillary cholangiocarcinoma and are worse than those for mucinous biliary cancers [186].

Macroscopic appearance: ICCs are often multilobulated and unencapsulated with a light-tan color at the periphery and a gray-white firm center corresponding to extensive fibrous scarring. Intrahepatic metastases may be seen and carry a poorer prognosis [188].

By macroscopic subtype, the "mass-forming" type corresponds to a solid nodule sharply demarcated from the adjacent liver parenchyma; the "periductal-infiltrating" type shows extensive infiltration along intrahepatic portal structures; and the "intraductal" type in which the tumor is confined within large bile ducts, often with papillary architecture [189].

Histology: ICC may resemble any adenocarcinoma of extrahepatic origin, so that a confident diagnosis depends on the exclusion of other primary sites on clinical grounds. The tumor cells are most often arranged in tubules and glands, which may be cribriform, but can also form nests, solid cords, or papillary structures. There is typically a fibrous stroma, in contrast to most hepatocellular carcinomas. Most cholangiocarcinomas tend to be well differentiated with columnar to cuboidal cells and a moderate amount of clear or slightly granular, lightly eosinophilic cytoplasm. Nuclei are usually small and typically lack the prominent, eosinophilic nucleoli present in HCC. Poorly differentiated tumors are not infrequent. The tumor cells can grow along sinusoids and spread intravascularly throughout the liver, an important prognostic factor. Vascular invasion is considered present when there is either major vessel involvement or microscopic invasion of smaller vascular structures [190]. This forms part of the TNM staging of the seventh edition of the AJCC.

Occasionally, variant tumors are mucinous with copious cytoplasmic and extracellular mucin. Other uncommon variants include adenosquamous, clear cell carcinomas, and spindle cell or sarcomatoid carcinomas. Numerous antigens have been found in cholangiocarcinoma, but none specifically can be used to distinguish ICC from metastatic adenocarcinoma [46]. Finally, a subtype of ICC that exists is cholangiolocellular carcinoma, a rare tumor that frequently is associated with HCV infection and should be differentiated from ICC [191, 192].

Combined Hepatocellular-Cholangiocarcinoma

Liver tumors that contain both HCC and ICC areas are given this term and represent less than 1% of all primary liver carcinomas [188]. Subcategories have been modified into (1) collision type with coincidental occurrence of HCC and ICC; (2) transitional type, with intermediate differentiation and transition between HCC and ICC; and (3) fibrolamellar type resembling the fibrolamellar variant of HCC, but containing mucin-producing glands [193]. The diagnosis of combined HCC/ICC requires unequivocal histologic presence of both hepatocellular and cholangiocellular elements intimately mixed within the same tumor [188].

Distinguishing ICC from HCC and other tumors may represent a difficult problem for the pathologist. Hepatocellular carcinoma may grow in a pseudoglandular pattern, but unlike the true glands of ICC, there is no mucin production by the cells lining the pseudoglands. Differences in architecture, the presence of bile, and characteristic staining pattern of specific markers such as HepPar1, AFP, CEA, CA 19-9, glypican 3, cytoplasmic TTF-1, and the cytokeratins 8, 18, 7, 19, as well as N-cadherin may aid in differentiation [189, 194]. Benign biliary lesions can be mistaken for ICC where reactive atypia from inflammation is present [46].

Metastatic Liver Disease

Metastases are the most common type of malignant liver tumor. It is estimated that between 40% and 50% of all malignancies are complicated by liver metastases [195] with regional lymph nodes the only more common site of metastasis from primary solid tumors [196]. In the presence of cirrhosis, liver metastasis is an unusual finding [197].

Liver metastases are most commonly associated with malignancy from the gastrointestinal tract (commonly the colon, esophagus, and stomach), pancreas (including neuroendocrine tumors), breast, lung, bladder, head and neck, melanoma, and prostate. Traditionally, metastases have been divided into *colorectal, neuroendocrine*, and *noncolorectal nonneuroendocrine origin*.

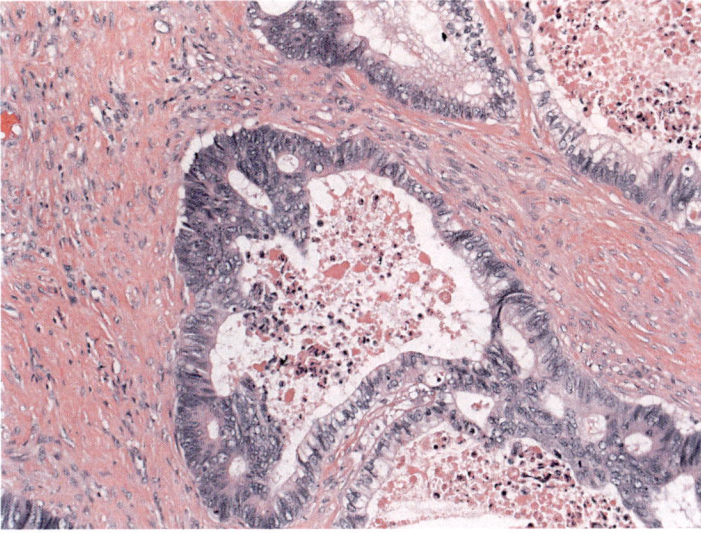

Fig. 5.20 Colon cancer, metastatic (×64)

Colorectal Metastases (Fig. 5.20)

Of patients presenting with colorectal cancer, approximately 25% of patients have synchronous liver metastasis [198]. Furthermore, nearly half of patients who undergo resection of the colorectal primary eventually develop metachronous liver metastasis [199]. Untreated but potentially resectable patients have a median survival of 6–12 months [200, 201]. As approaches to liver resection evolve, metastatic colorectal disease is becoming more treatable. In patients who undergo resection, 5-year survival in the range of 20–40% has been reported [202–204] with one series showing a 10-year survival of 29% for aggressive resection [205]. The volume of future liver remnant and health of remaining liver are prime determinants in selection for an operative approach [206, 207] and decisions concerning resectability now center around what will remain after resection [208].

Neuroendocrine Cancer (Carcinoid Tumors)

Neuroendocrine tumors (Fig. 5.21) are rare neoplasms that typically have an indolent natural history. Arising from the foregut, midgut, hindgut, or pancreas and classified as functional or nonfunctional, hepatic metastases can lead to incapacitating symptoms while resection and debulking can increase long-term survival [209–211]. In a series of 170 patients undergoing resection of hepatic metastases from neuroendocrine tumors between 1977 and 1998 at the Mayo Clinic, overall survival was 61% and 35% at 5 and 10 years, respectively [210]. In evaluating disease extent

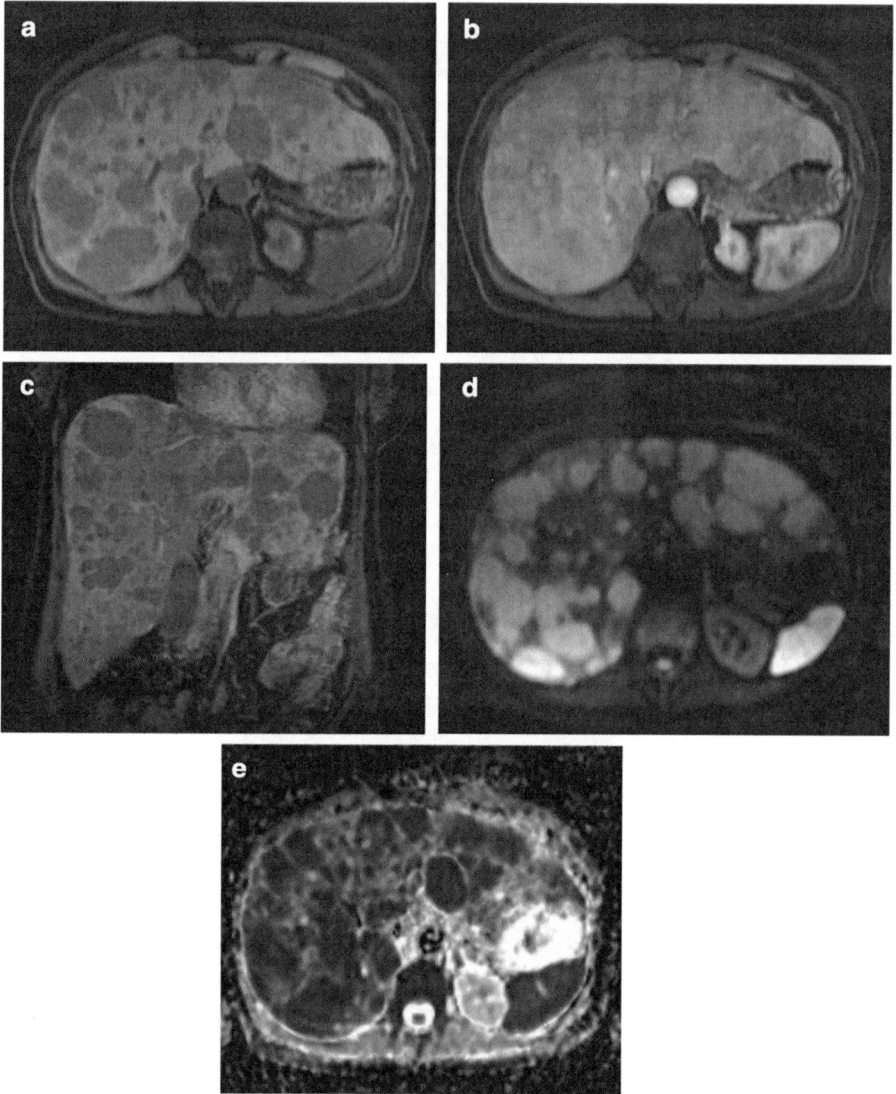

Fig. 5.21 MRI—neuroendocrine tumor metastatic to liver. (**a**) Innumerable nodular hypointense lesions of diffuse distribution within the liver. (**b**) Postcontrast images in arterial phase showed slight enhancement of the lesions. (**c**) Coronal plane demonstrates enlargement of the liver with innumerable hypointense lesions (**d**). Innumerable high signal lesions in diffusion-weighted image (**e**) with low signal intensity at ADC map

and site of the primary, somatostatin receptor scintigraphy is utilized when the lesion is not demonstrated by other studies [212]. Newer somatostatin analogs combined with PET have demonstrated very high sensitivities, specificities, and diagnostic accuracies and appear to improve upon conventional scintigraphy [213].

Nonneuroendocrine, Noncolorectal Tumors

Almost all cancers have been associated with the ability to metastasize to the liver. Five-year survival rates in the 20%–40% range after hepatic resection of metastases from breast, renal, and gastrointestinal tumors have been demonstrated [214, 215].

Clinical Presentation

Most liver metastases are asymptomatic, while a minority of patients may report abdominal pain, jaundice, or pruritus. Examination may reveal hepatomegaly, a friction rub over hepatic metastases, or ascites caused by hepatic venous obstruction or peritoneal carcinomatosis. Liver metastases from neuroendocrine tumors can lead to significant symptoms caused by the production of functioning hormones. Hepatic metastases from gastrointestinal carcinoid tumors are associated with release of vasoactive peptides and serotonin into the systemic circulation and can result in hot flushes, bronchospasms, arrhythmias, and diaphoresis. Carcinoid syndrome occurs when the liver is not able to metabolize the active substances produced by the carcinoid tumor. This problem usually results when tumors are either bulky or metastatic or when their venous drainage bypasses the liver.

Radiologic Appearance

At ultrasound, metastases typically appear as space-occupying lesions with distortion of the internal anatomy or surface. Frequently, a hypoechoic halo surrounds the lesion [216, 217]. Similar to hepatocellular carcinoma, they may be echo-poor or echogenic with mixed patterns and cystic regions after necrosis. Although false positives are rare, false negatives occur in 15% due to failure to detect small lesions (<1 cm). Even when performed by experienced radiologists, the sensitivity of unenhanced US for detection of liver lesions measuring 1–2 cm is between 36% and 61% [218, 219]. Contrast-enhanced ultrasound improves sensitivity [220] with reports ranging from 50% to 8% [221, 222]. Intraoperative ultrasound has the highest sensitivity for lesion detection, ranging between 93% and 94%, and may alter operative strategy [223, 224].

CT: Appearance of metastases is variable on CT. It is of benefit in providing information for staging metastatic lesions. Tumor borders may be sharp, ill-defined, or nodular, and lesions may be round, ovoid, or irregular. On unenhanced CT, metastases are usually hypodense with contrast showing peripheral ring enhancement and hypervascular metastases most clearly visualized during the arterial phase. Cystic metastases are clearly differentiated from simple liver cysts by the presence of mural nodules, fluid–fluid levels, or septations. Multifocal HCC appearing in a normal liver may be difficult to differentiate from multiple metastases, but metastases rarely protrude prominently from the liver surface, a feature that is commonly seen with HCC [225]. Metastases which appear hypervascular include renal cell carcinoma, thyroid carcinoma in addition to carcinoids, and neuroendocrine tumors.

CT is sensitive in detecting metastasis. One of the largest studies evaluating the overall preoperative CT detection of resected colorectal cancer metastases showed a detection rate of 85.1% with a positive predictive value of 96.1 [226] Others report sensitivities ranging from 73% to 87% [227, 228], while a recent meta-analysis reported a sensitivity of CT at 74.8% on a per-patient basis and 82.6% on a per-lesion basis [229]. For lesions which are hypo-enhancing compared to the background liver parenchyma, portal phase CT is more sensitive in detecting lesions than unenhanced or arterial phase CT [230]. However, it should be noted that hepatic steatosis can significantly limit the ability of CT to detect focal liver lesions [231]. MRI is also useful in this setting.

MRI (Fig. 5.21): Numerous studies have now demonstrated the superiority of liver MRI over CT in the evaluation of metastatic disease [29]. Semelka et al. demonstrated that liver MRI detected significantly more lesions than CT and was also better able to characterize lesions once detected. Recent meta-analysis demonstrates this superiority across studies and multiple institutions reporting an overall sensitivity and specificity of MRI for the identification of liver lesions of 81.1% and 97.2%, respectively [229].

Most metastases are hypo- to isointense on T1- and iso- to hyperintense on T2-weighted images [232]. Liver metastases are not as bright as hemangiomas or simple cysts on T2-weighted images. However, neuroendocrine tumors, sarcoma and melanoma, and metastases with cystic change due to liquefactive necrosis may be hyperintense on T2-weighted imaging [233]. Metastases are also described as showing a "doughnut sign" (a hypointense rim surrounding an irregular or ovoid center of even lower signal intensity) on T1-weighted images as well as a "target sign" (a hyperintense center due to necrosis surrounded by a relatively less intense rim of viable tumor) on T2-weighted imaging [234].

Dynamic contrast-enhanced MRI contributes further information. Hypovascular liver metastases are generally from lung, breast, stomach, and colorectum and are visualized most effectively in the portal venous phase. Breast carcinoma metastases are generally hypovascular, although occasionally hypervascular. Neuroendocrine tumors, renal cell, breast, melanoma, and thyroid carcinoma are tumors most commonly causing hypervascular hepatic metastases. These may develop early enhancement with variable degrees of washout and peripheral rim enhancement [232]. The appearance of rim enhancement that is hypointense to the center of the lesion ("peripheral washout" sign) on delay is highly specific, but insensitive for the diagnosis of malignancy [235]. The advent of new hepatobiliary contrast agents is promising. With improving hardware and pulse sequences, as well as these new hepatocyte-specific contrast agents, there is mounting evidence that the diagnostic yield and accuracy of MRI will continue to expand [232].

Positron Emission Tomography (PET) and Fusion PET/CT: In patients with colorectal cancer, PET/CT has shown high sensitivity (95% on a per-patient basis, 76% on a per-lesion basis) in liver metastases [236]. Two studies which directly compared PET/CT and contrast-enhanced MRI reported sensitivities and specificities of MRI of 81–85%, 100% and PET/CT of 69–71%, 93.7% [221, 237]. PET/CT has the additional advantage of being able to detect local and regional disease in addition to evaluating the liver [238] and has been also been shown to be valuable in restaging patients with a presumed solitary metastatic lesion [239] and has been shown to alter management in patients with colorectal cancer metastases [240, 241] as well as in patients with noncolorectal liver metastases [242]. PET combined with a somatostatin analog has demonstrated a very high sensitivity, specificity, and diagnostic accuracy and improves upon convention scintigraphy in the detection of neuroendocrine tumors [213].

Acknowledgments Dr Michael Torbenson, Department of Pathology, Johns Hopkins Hospital *for pathology images.* Dr Ihab Kamel, Department of Radiology, Johns Hopkins Hospital *for radiological imaging.*

References

1. Ishak KG, Rabin L. Benign tumors of the liver. Med Clin North Am. 1975;59(4):995–1013.
2. Gandolfi L, Leo P, Solmi L, Vitelli E, Verros G, Colecchia A. Natural history of hepatic haemangiomas: clinical and ultrasound study. Gut. 1991;32(6):677–80.
3. Farges O, Daradkeh S, Bismuth H. Cavernous hemangiomas of the liver: are there any indications for resection? World J Surg. 1995;19(1):19–24.
4. Nichols 3 FC, van Heerden JA, Weiland LH. Benign liver tumors. Surg Clin North Am. 1989;69(2):297–314.
5. Yoon SS, Charny CK, Fong Y, et al. Diagnosis, management, and outcomes of 115 patients with hepatic hemangioma. J Am Coll Surg. 2003;197(3):392–402.
6. Saegusa T, Ito K, Oba N, et al. Enlargement of multiple cavernous hemangioma of the liver in association with pregnancy. Intern Med. 1995;34(3):207–11.
7. Graham E, Cohen AW, Soulen M, Faye R. Symptomatic liver hemangioma with intra-tumor hemorrhage treated by angiography and embolization during pregnancy. Obstet Gynecol. 1993;81(5(Pt 2)):813–6.
8. Winkfield B, Vuillemin E, Rousselet MC, Bellec V, Aube C, Cales P. Progression of a hepatic hemangioma under progestins. Gastroenterol Clin Biol. 2001;25(1):108–10.
9. Conter RL, Longmire Jr WP. Recurrent hepatic hemangiomas. Possible association with estrogen therapy. Ann Surg. 1988;207(2):115–9.
10. Glinkova V, Shevah O, Boaz M, Levine A, Shirin H. Hepatic haemangiomas: possible association with female sex hormones. Gut. 2004;53(9):1352–5.
11. Adam YG, Huvos AG, Fortner JG. Giant hemangiomas of the liver. Ann Surg. 1970;172(2):239–45.
12. Grieco MB, Miscall BG. Giant hemangiomas of the liver. Surg Gynecol Obstet. 1978;147(5):783–7.
13. Zimmerman A. Tumors of the liver—pathologic aspects. In: Blumgart LH, editor. Surgery of the liver, biliary tract, and pancreas, vol. 2. 4th ed. Philadelphia: Saunders Elsevier; 2006.
14. Tait N, Richardson AJ, Muguti G, Little JM. Hepatic cavernous haemangioma: a 10 year review. Aust N Z J Surg. 1992;62(7):521–4.
15. Cappellani A, Zanghi A, Di Vita M, Zanghi G, Tomarchio G, Petrillo G. Spontaneous rupture of a giant hemangioma of the liver. Ann Ital Chir. 2000;71(3):379–83.

16. Hall GW. Kasabach-Merritt syndrome: pathogenesis and management. Br J Haematol. 2001;112(4):851–62.

17. Lehmann FS, Beglinger C, Schnabel K, Terracciano L. Progressive development of diffuse liver hemangiomatosis. J Hepatol. 1999;30(5):951–4.

18. Moon WS, Yu HC, Lee JM, Kang MJ. Diffuse hepatic hemangiomatosis in an adult. J Korean Med Sci. 2000;15(4):471–4.

19. Mungovan JA, Cronan JJ, Vacarro J. Hepatic cavernous hemangiomas: lack of enlargement over time. Radiology. 1994;191(1):111–3.

20. Okano H, Shiraki K, Inoue H, et al. Natural course of cavernous hepatic hemangioma. Oncol Rep. 2001;8(2):411–4.

21. Pietrabissa A, Giulianotti P, Campatelli A, et al. Management and follow-up of 78 giant haemangiomas of the liver. Br J Surg. 1996;83(7):915–8.

22. Perkins AB, Imam K, Smith WJ, Cronan JJ. Color and power Doppler sonography of liver hemangiomas: a dream unfulfilled? J Clin Ultrasound. 2000;28(4):159–65.

23. Ohnishi K, Nomura F. Ultrasonic Doppler studies of hepatocellular carcinoma and comparison with other hepatic focal lesions. Gastroenterology. 1989;97(6):1489–97.

24. Dietrich CF, Mertens JC, Braden B, Schuessler G, Ott M, Ignee A. Contrast-enhanced ultrasound of histologically proven liver hemangiomas. Hepatology. 2007;45(5):1139–45.

25. Yamashita Y, Ogata I, Urata J, Takahashi M. Cavernous hemangioma of the liver: pathologic correlation with dynamic CT findings. Radiology. 1997;203(1):121–5.

26. Nino-Murcia M, Olcott EW, Jeffrey Jr RB, Lamm RL, Beaulieu CF, Jain KA. Focal liver lesions: pattern-based classification scheme for enhancement at arterial phase CT. Radiology. 2000;215(3):746–51.

27. Kim T, Federle MP, Baron RL, Peterson MS, Kawamori Y. Discrimination of small hepatic hemangiomas from hypervascular malignant tumors smaller than 3 cm with three-phase helical CT. Radiology. 2001;219(3):699–706.

28. Yun EJ, Choi BI, Han JK, et al. Hepatic hemangioma: contrast-enhancement pattern during the arterial and portal venous phases of spiral CT. Abdom Imag. 1999;24(3):262–6.

29. Semelka RC, Martin DR, Balci C, Lance T. Focal liver lesions: comparison of dual-phase CT and multisequence multiplanar MR imaging including dynamic gadolinium enhancement. J Magn Reson Imag. 2001;13(3):397–401.

30. Stark DD, Felder RC, Wittenberg J, et al. Magnetic resonance imaging of cavernous hemangioma of the liver: tissue-specific characterization. Am J Roentgenol. 1985;145(2):213–22.

31. McFarland EG, Mayo-Smith WW, Saini S, Hahn PF, Goldberg MA, Lee MJ. Hepatic hemangiomas and malignant tumors: improved differentiation with heavily T2-weighted conventional spin-echo MR imaging. Radiology. 1994;193(1):43–7.

32. Lee MG, Baker ME, Sostman HD, et al. The diagnostic accuracy/efficacy of MRI in differentiating hepatic hemangiomas from metastatic colorectal/breast carcinoma: a multiple reader ROC analysis using a jackknife technique. J Comput Assist Tomogr. 1996;20(6):905–13.

33. Tamm EP, Rabushka LS, Fishman EK, Hruban RH, Diehl AM, Klein A. Intrahepatic, extramedullary hematopoiesis mimicking hemangioma on technetium-99 m red blood cell SPECT examination. Clin Imag. 1995;19(2):88–91.

34. Belli L, De Carlis L, Beati C, Rondinara G, Sansalone V, Brambilla G. Surgical treatment of symptomatic giant hemangiomas of the liver. Surg Gynecol Obstet. 1992;174(6):474–8.

35. Terriff BA, Gibney RG, Scudamore CH. Fatality from fine-needle aspiration biopsy of a hepatic hemangioma. Am J Roentgenol. 1990;154(1):203–4.

36. Davies R. Haemorrhage after fine-needle aspiration biopsy of an hepatic haemangioma. Med J Aust. 1993;158(5):364.

37. Sherlock S. Hepatic adenomas and oral contraceptives. Gut. 1975;16(9):753–6.

38. Baum JK, Bookstein JJ, Holtz F, Klein EW. Possible association between benign hepatomas and oral contraceptives. Lancet. 1973;2(7835):926–9.

39. Klatskin G. Hepatic tumors: possible relationship to use of oral contraceptives. Gastroenterology. 1977;73(2):386–94.

40. Edmondson HA, Henderson B, Benton B. Liver-cell adenomas associated with use of oral contraceptives. N Engl J Med. 1976;294(9):470–2.
41. Rooks JB, Ory HW, Ishak KG, et al. Epidemiology of hepatocellular adenoma. The role of oral contraceptive use. J Am Med Assoc. 1979;242(7):644–8.
42. Cherqui D, Rahmouni A, Charlotte F, et al. Management of focal nodular hyperplasia and hepatocellular adenoma in young women: a series of 41 patients with clinical, radiological, and pathological correlations. Hepatology. 1995;22(6):1674–81.
43. Benhamou JP. Diagnostic approach to a liver mass: diagnosis of an asymptomatic liver tumor in a young woman. J Hepatol. 1996;25 Suppl 1:30–4.
44. Labrune P, Trioche P, Duvaltier I, Chevalier P, Odievre M. Hepatocellular adenomas in glycogen storage disease type I and III: a series of 43 patients and review of the literature. J Pediatr Gastroenterol Nutr. 1997;24(3):276–9.
45. Talente GM, Coleman RA, Alter C, et al. Glycogen storage disease in adults. Ann Intern Med. 1994;120(3):218–26.
46. Goodman ZD. Neoplasms of the liver. Mod Pathol. 2007;20 Suppl 1:S49–60.
47. Scheuer P, Lefkowitch J. Liver Biopsy Interpretation. 6th ed. London, Edimburgh, New York, Philadelphia, St Louis, Sidney, Toronto: W.B. Saunders. 2000:191–227.
48. Zucman-Rossi J, Jeannot E, Nhieu JT, et al. Genotype-phenotype correlation in hepatocellular adenoma: new classification and relationship with HCC. Hepatology. 2006;43(3):515–24.
49. Laumonier H, Bioulac-Sage P, Laurent C, Zucman-Rossi J, Balabaud C, Trillaud H. Hepatocellular adenomas: magnetic resonance imaging features as a function of molecular pathological classification. Hepatology. 2008;48(3):808–18.
50. Bioulac-Sage P, Rebouissou S, Sa Cunha A, et al. Clinical, morphologic, and molecular features defining so-called telangiectatic focal nodular hyperplasias of the liver. Gastroenterology. 2005;128(5):1211–8.
51. Paradis V, Benzekri A, Dargere D, et al. Telangiectatic focal nodular hyperplasia: a variant of hepatocellular adenoma. Gastroenterology. 2004;126(5):1323–9.
52. Leese T, Farges O, Bismuth H. Liver cell adenomas. A 12-year surgical experience from a specialist hepato-biliary unit. Ann Surg. 1988;208(5):558–64.
53. Nagorney DM. Benign hepatic tumors: focal nodular hyperplasia and hepatocellular adenoma. World J Surg. 1995;19(1):13–8.
54. Rubin RA, Mitchell DG. Evaluation of the solid hepatic mass. Med Clin North Am. 1996;80(5):907–28.
55. Kerlin P, Davis GL, McGill DB, Weiland LH, Adson MA, Sheedy 2 PF. Hepatic adenoma and focal nodular hyperplasia: clinical, pathologic, and radiologic features. Gastroenterology. 1983;84(5 Pt 1):994–1002.
56. Foster JH, Berman MM. The malignant transformation of liver cell adenomas. Arch Surg. 1994;129(7):712–7.
57. Ribeiro A, Burgart LJ, Nagorney DM, Gores GJ. Management of liver adenomatosis: results with a conservative surgical approach. Liver Transplant Surg. 1998;4(5):388–98.
58. Golli M, Van Nhieu JT, Mathieu D, et al. Hepatocellular adenoma: color Doppler US and pathologic correlations. Radiology. 1994;190(3):741–4.
59. Grazioli L, Federle MP, Brancatelli G, Ichikawa T, Olivetti L, Blachar A. Hepatic adenomas: imaging and pathologic findings. Radiographics. 2001;21(4):877–92. discussion 892–4.
60. Chung KY, Mayo-Smith WW, Saini S, Rahmouni A, Golli M, Mathieu D. Hepatocellular adenoma: MR imaging features with pathologic correlation. Am J Roentgenol. 1995;165(2):303–8.
61. Paulson EK, McClellan JS, Washington K, Spritzer CE, Meyers WC, Baker ME. Hepatic adenoma: MR characteristics and correlation with pathologic findings. Am J Roentgenol. 1994;163(1):113–6.
62. Grazioli L, Morana G, Kirchin MA, Schneider G. Accurate differentiation of focal nodular hyperplasia from hepatic adenoma at gadobenate dimeglumine-enhanced MR imaging: prospective study. Radiology. 2005;236(1):166–77.

63. Vilgrain V, Uzan F, Brancatelli G, Federle MP, Zappa M, Menu Y. Prevalence of hepatic hemangioma in patients with focal nodular hyperplasia: MR imaging analysis. Radiology. 2003;229(1):75–9.
64. Cherqui D, Mathieu D, Zafrani ES, Dhumeaux D. Focal nodular hyperplasia and hepatocellular adenoma in women. Current data. Gastroenterol Clin Biol. 1997;21(12):929–35.
65. Paradis V, Laurent A, Flejou JF, Vidaud M, Bedossa P. Evidence for the polyclonal nature of focal nodular hyperplasia of the liver by the study of X-chromosome inactivation. Hepatology. 1997;26(4):891–5.
66. Paradis V, Bieche I, Dargere D, et al. A quantitative gene expression study suggests a role for angiopoietins in focal nodular hyperplasia. Gastroenterology. 2003;124(3):651–9.
67. Rebouissou S, Couchy G, Libbrecht L, et al. The beta-catenin pathway is activated in focal nodular hyperplasia but not in cirrhotic FNH-like nodules. J Hepatol. 2008;49(1):61–71.
68. Wanless IR, Mawdsley C, Adams R. On the pathogenesis of focal nodular hyperplasia of the liver. Hepatology. 1985;5(6):1194–200.
69. Fukukura Y, Nakashima O, Kusaba A, Kage M, Kojiro M. Angioarchitecture and blood circulation in focal nodular hyperplasia of the liver. J Hepatol. 1998;29(3):470–5.
70. Kondo F, Nagao T, Sato T, et al. Etiological analysis of focal nodular hyperplasia of the liver, with emphasis on similar abnormal vasculatures to nodular regenerative hyperplasia and idiopathic portal hypertension. Pathol Res Pract. 1998;194(7):487–95.
71. Mathieu D, Kobeiter H, Maison P, et al. Oral contraceptive use and focal nodular hyperplasia of the liver. Gastroenterology. 2000;118(3):560–4.
72. Giannitrapani L, Soresi M, La Spada E, Cervello M, D'Alessandro N, Montalto G. Sex hormones and risk of liver tumor. Ann N Y Acad Sci. 2006;1089:228–36.
73. Nguyen BN, Flejou JF, Terris B, Belghiti J, Degott C. Focal nodular hyperplasia of the liver: a comprehensive pathologic study of 305 lesions and recognition of new histologic forms. Am J Surg Pathol. 1999;23(12):1441–54.
74. Goodman ZD. Benign tumors of the liver. In: Okuda K, Ishak KG, editors. Neoplasms of the liver. Tokyo: Springer; 1987.
75. Belghiti J, Vilgrain V, Paradis V. Benign liver lesions. In: Blumgart LH, editor. Surgery of the liver, biliary tract and pancreas. 4th ed. Philadelphia: Saunders Elsevier; 2006.
76. Klatskin G, Conn H. Neoplasms of the liver and intrahepatic bile ducts. In: histopathology of the liver. Oxford: Oxford University Press; 1993.
77. Bioulac-Sage P, Laumonier H, Rullier A, et al. Over-expression of glutamine synthetase in focal nodular hyperplasia: a novel easy diagnostic tool in surgical pathology. Liver Int. 2009;29(3):459–65.
78. Shamsi K, De Schepper A, Degryse H, Deckers F. Focal nodular hyperplasia of the liver: radiologic findings. Abdom Imag. 1993;18(1):32–8.
79. Trillaud H, Bruel JM, Valette PJ, et al. Characterization of focal liver lesions with SonoVue-enhanced sonography: international multicenter-study in comparison to CT and MRI. World J Gastroenterol. 2009;15(30):3748–56.
80. Brancatelli G, Federle MP, Grazioli L, Blachar A, Peterson MS, Thaete L. Focal nodular hyperplasia: CT findings with emphasis on multiphasic helical CT in 78 patients. Radiology. 2001;219(1):61–8.
81. Mergo PJ, Ros PR. Benign lesions of the liver. Radiol Clin North Am. 1998;36(2):319–21.
82. Carlson SK, Johnson CD, Bender CE, Welch TJ. CT of focal nodular hyperplasia of the liver. Am J Roentgenol. 2000;174(3):705–12.
83. Ruppert-Kohlmayr AJ, Uggowitzer MM, Kugler C, Zebedin D, Schaffler G, Ruppert GS. Focal nodular hyperplasia and hepatocellular adenoma of the liver: differentiation with multiphasic helical CT. Am J Roentgenol. 2001;176(6):1493–8.
84. Buetow PC, Pantongrag-Brown L, Buck JL, Ros PR, Goodman ZD. Focal nodular hyperplasia of the liver: radiologic-pathologic correlation. Radiographics. 1996;16(2):369–88.
85. Vilgrain V, Flejou JF, Arrive L, et al. Focal nodular hyperplasia of the liver: MR imaging and pathologic correlation in 37 patients. Radiology. 1992;184(3):699–703.

86. Ba-Ssalamah A, Schima W, Schmook MT, et al. Atypical focal nodular hyperplasia of the liver: imaging features of nonspecific and liver-specific MR contrast agents. Am J Roentgenol. 2002;179(6):1447–56.

87. Drane WE, Krasicky GA, Johnson DA. Radionuclide imaging of primary tumors and tumor-like conditions of the liver. Clin Nucl Med. 1987;12(7):569–82.

88. Rogers JV, Mack LA, Freeny PC, Johnson ML, Sones PJ. Hepatic focal nodular hyperplasia: angiography, CT, sonography, and scintigraphy. Am J Roentgenol. 1981;137(5):983–90.

89. Fabre A, Audet P, Vilgrain V, et al. Histologic scoring of liver biopsy in focal nodular hyperplasia with atypical presentation. Hepatology. 2002;35(2):414–20.

90. Parkin DM, Bray F, Ferlay J, Pisani P. Global cancer statistics, 2002. CA Cancer J Clin. 2005;55(2):74–108.

91. Altekruse SF, McGlynn KA, Reichman ME. Hepatocellular carcinoma incidence, mortality, and survival trends in the United States from 1975 to 2005. J Clin Oncol. 2009;27(9):1485–91.

92. Bosch FX, Ribes J, Diaz M, Cleries R. Primary liver cancer: worldwide incidence and trends. Gastroenterology. 2004;127(5 Suppl 1):S5–16.

93. Parkin DM, Bray F, Ferlay J, Pisani P. Estimating the world cancer burden: Globocan 2000. Int J Cancer. 2001;94(2):153–6.

94. El-Serag HB, Mason AC. Rising incidence of hepatocellular carcinoma in the United States. N Engl J Med. 1999;340(10):745–50.

95. Deuffic S, Poynard T, Buffat L, Valleron AJ. Trends in primary liver cancer. Lancet. 1998;351(9097):214–5.

96. Stroffolini T, Andreone P, Andriulli A, et al. Characteristics of hepatocellular carcinoma in Italy. J Hepatol. 1998;29(6):944–52.

97. Taylor-Robinson SD, Foster GR, Arora S, Hargreaves S, Thomas HC. Increase in primary liver cancer in the UK, 1979–94. Lancet. 1997;350(9085):1142–3.

98. Tanaka Y, Hanada K, Mizokami M, et al. A comparison of the molecular clock of hepatitis C virus in the United States and Japan predicts that hepatocellular carcinoma incidence in the United States will increase over the next two decades. Proc Natl Acad Sci USA. 2002;99(24):15584–9.

99. Llovet JM, Burroughs A, Bruix J. Hepatocellular carcinoma. Lancet. 2003;362(9399):1907–17.

100. Chen CJ, Wang LY, Lu SN, et al. Elevated aflatoxin exposure and increased risk of hepatocellular carcinoma. Hepatology. 1996;24(1):38–42.

101. Jee SH, Ohrr H, Sull JW, Samet JM. Cigarette smoking, alcohol drinking, hepatitis B, and risk for hepatocellular carcinoma in Korea. J Natl Cancer Inst. 2004;96(24):1851–6.

102. Eastman RC, Carson RE, Orloff DG, et al. Glucose utilization in a patient with hepatoma and hypoglycemia. Assessment by a positron emission tomography. J Clin Invest. 1992;89(6):1958–63.

103. Tietge UJ, Schofl C, Ocran KW, et al. Hepatoma with severe non-islet cell tumor hypoglycemia. Am J Gastroenterol. 1998;93(6):997–1000.

104. Kew MC, Fisher JW. Serum erythropoietin concentrations in patients with hepatocellular carcinoma. Cancer. 1986;58(11):2485–8.

105. Sakisaka S, Watanabe M, Tateishi H, et al. Erythropoietin production in hepatocellular carcinoma cells associated with polycythemia: immunohistochemical evidence. Hepatology. 1993;18(6):1357–62.

106. Yen TC, Hwang SJ, Wang CC, Lee SD, Yeh SH. Hypercalcemia and parathyroid hormone-related protein in hepatocellular carcinoma. Liver. 1993;13(6):311–5.

107. Steiner E, Velt P, Gutierrez O, Schwartz S, Chey W. Hepatocellular carcinoma presenting with intractable diarrhea. A radiologic-pathologic correlation. Arch Surg. 1986;121(7):849–51.

108. Burrel M, Llovet JM, Ayuso C, et al. MRI angiography is superior to helical CT for detection of HCC prior to liver transplantation: an explant correlation. Hepatology. 2003;38(4):1034–42.

109. Forner A, Vilana R, Ayuso C, et al. Diagnosis of hepatic nodules 20 mm or smaller in cirrhosis: Prospective validation of the noninvasive diagnostic criteria for hepatocellular carcinoma. Hepatology. 2008;47(1):97–104.

110. Dai Y, Chen MH, Fan ZH, Yan K, Yin SS, Zhang XP. Diagnosis of small hepatic nodules detected by surveillance ultrasound in patients with cirrhosis: Comparison between contrast-enhanced ultrasound and contrast-enhanced helical computed tomography. Hepatol Res. 2008;38(3):281–90.

111. Sangiovanni A, Manini MA, Iavarone M, et al. The diagnostic and economic impact of contrast imaging techniques in the diagnosis of small hepatocellular carcinoma in cirrhosis. Gut. 2010;59(5):638–44.

112. Ishiguchi T, Shimamoto K, Fukatsu H, Yamakawa K, Ishigaki T. Radiologic diagnosis of hepatocellular carcinoma. Semin Surg Oncol. 1996;12(3):164–9.

113. Okuda K, Ohnishi K, Kimura K, et al. Incidence of portal vein thrombosis in liver cirrhosis. An angiographic study in 708 patients. Gastroenterology. 1985;89(2):279–86.

114. Cedrone A, Rapaccini GL, Pompili M, et al. Portal vein thrombosis complicating hepatocellular carcinoma. Value of ultrasound-guided fine-needle biopsy of the thrombus in the therapeutic management. Liver. 1996;16(2):94–8.

115. De Sio I, Castellano L, Calandra M, Romano M, Persico M, Del Vecchio-Blanco C. Ultrasound-guided fine needle aspiration biopsy of portal vein thrombosis in liver cirrhosis: results in 15 patients. J Gastroenterol Hepatol. 1995;10(6):662–5.

116. Colli A, Fraquelli M, Casazza G, et al. Accuracy of ultrasonography, spiral CT, magnetic resonance, and alpha-fetoprotein in diagnosing hepatocellular carcinoma: a systematic review. Am J Gastroenterol. 2006;101(3):513–23.

117. Whittingham TA. New and future developments in ultrasonic imaging. Br J Radiol. 1997;70(Spec No):S119 32.

118. Lim JH, Choi D, Kim SH, et al. Detection of hepatocellular carcinoma: value of adding delayed phase imaging to dual-phase helical CT. Am J Roentgenol. 2002;179(1):67–73.

119. Hollett MD, Jeffrey Jr RB, Nino-Murcia M, Jorgensen MJ, Harris DP. Dual-phase helical CT of the liver: value of arterial phase scans in the detection of small (< or = 1.5 cm) malignant hepatic neoplasms. Am J Roentgenol. 1995;164(4):879–84.

120. Bolondi L, Gaiani S, Celli N, et al. Characterization of small nodules in cirrhosis by assessment of vascularity: the problem of hypovascular hepatocellular carcinoma. Hepatology. 2005;42(1):27–34.

121. Kang BK, Lim JH, Kim SH, et al. Preoperative depiction of hepatocellular carcinoma: ferumoxides-enhanced MR imaging versus triple-phase helical CT. Radiology. 2003;226(1):79–85.

122. Kim SK, Kim SH, Lee WJ, et al. Preoperative detection of hepatocellular carcinoma: ferumoxides-enhanced versus mangafodipir trisodium-enhanced MR imaging. Am J Roentgenol. 2002;179(3):741–50.

123. Levy I, Greig PD, Gallinger S, Langer B, Sherman M. Resection of hepatocellular carcinoma without preoperative tumor biopsy. Ann Surg. 2001;234(2):206–9.

124. Mueller GC, Hussain HK, Carlos RC, Nghiem HV, Francis IR. Effectiveness of MR imaging in characterizing small hepatic lesions: routine versus expert interpretation. Am J Roentgenol. 2003;180(3):673–80.

125. Yu JS, Kim KW, Kim EK, Lee JT, Yoo HS. Contrast enhancement of small hepatocellular carcinoma: usefulness of three successive early image acquisitions during multiphase dynamic MR imaging. Am J Roentgenol. 1999;173(3):597–604.

126. Marrero JA, Hussain HK, Nghiem HV, Umar R, Fontana RJ, Lok AS. Improving the prediction of hepatocellular carcinoma in cirrhotic patients with an arterially-enhancing liver mass. Liver Transplant. 2005;11(3):281–9.

127. Rimola J, Forner A, Reig M, et al. Cholangiocarcinoma in cirrhosis: absence of contrast washout in delayed phases by magnetic resonance imaging avoids misdiagnosis of hepatocellular carcinoma. Hepatology. 2009;50(3):791–8.

128. Kim TK, Jang HJ, Wilson SR. Imaging diagnosis of hepatocellular carcinoma with differentiation from other pathology. Clin Liver Dis. 2005;9(2):253–79.

129. Kim TK, Choi BI, Han JK, Chung JW, Park JH, Han MC. Nontumorous arterioportal shunt mimicking hypervascular tumor in cirrhotic liver: two-phase spiral CT findings. Radiology. 1998;208(3):597–603.
130. Yu JS, Kim KW, Jeong MG, Lee JT, Yoo HS. Nontumorous hepatic arterial-portal venous shunts: MR imaging findings. Radiology. 2000;217(3):750–6.
131. Jang HJ, Kim TK, Lim HK, et al. Hepatic hemangioma: atypical appearances on CT, MR imaging, and sonography. Am J Roentgenol. 2003;180(1):135–41.
132. Vilana R, Forner A, Bianchi L, et al. Intrahepatic peripheral cholangiocarcinoma in cirrhosis patients may display a vascular pattern similar to hepatocellular carcinoma on contrast-enhanced ultrasound. Hepatology. 2010;51(6):2020–9.
133. Silva MA, Hegab B, Hyde C, Guo B, Buckels JA, Mirza DF. Needle track seeding following biopsy of liver lesions in the diagnosis of hepatocellular cancer: a systematic review and meta-analysis. Gut. 2008;57(11):1592–6.
134. Livraghi T, Solbiati L, Meloni MF, Gazelle GS, Halpern EF, Goldberg SN. Treatment of focal liver tumors with percutaneous radio-frequency ablation: complications encountered in a multicenter study. Radiology. 2003;226(2):441–51.
135. Llovet JM, Vilana R, Bru C, et al. Increased risk of tumor seeding after percutaneous radiofrequency ablation for single hepatocellular carcinoma. Hepatology. 2001;33(5):1124–9.
136. Gomaa AI, Khan SA, Leen EL, Waked I, Taylor-Robinson SD. Diagnosis of hepatocellular carcinoma. World J Gastroenterol. 2009;15(11):1301–14.
137. The International Consensus Group for Hepatocellular Neoplasia. Pathologic diagnosis of early hepatocellular carcinoma: a report of the international consensus group for hepatocellular neoplasia. Hepatology. 2009;49(2):658–4.
138. Torbenson M. Review of the clinicopathologic features of fibrolamellar carcinoma. Adv Anat Pathol. 2007;14(3):217–23.
139. International Working Party. Terminology of nodular hepatocellular lesions. Hepatology. 1995;22(3):983–93.
140. Kojiro M, Nakashima O. Histopathologic evaluation of hepatocellular carcinoma with special reference to small early stage tumors. Semin Liver Dis. 1999;19(3):287–96.
141. Takayama T, Makuuchi M, Hirohashi S, et al. Early hepatocellular carcinoma as an entity with a high rate of surgical cure. Hepatology. 1998;28(5):1241–6.
142. Kojiro M. Focus on dysplastic nodules and early hepatocellular carcinoma: an Eastern point of view. Liver Transpl. 2004;10(2 Suppl 1):S3–8.
143. Nakashima Y, Nakashima O, Tanaka M, Okuda K, Nakashima M, Kojiro M. Portal vein invasion and intrahepatic micrometastasis in small hepatocellular carcinoma by gross type. Hepatol Res. 2003;26(2):142–7.
144. Sakamoto M, Hirohashi S. Natural history and prognosis of adenomatous hyperplasia and early hepatocellular carcinoma: multi-institutional analysis of 53 nodules followed up for more than 6 months and 141 patients with single early hepatocellular carcinoma treated by surgical resection or percutaneous ethanol injection. Jpn J Clin Oncol. 1998;28(10):604–8.
145. Takayama T, Makuuchi M, Hirohashi S, et al. Malignant transformation of adenomatous hyperplasia to hepatocellular carcinoma. Lancet. 1990;336(8724):1150–3.
146. Sherman M, Peltekian KM, Lee C. Screening for hepatocellular carcinoma in chronic carriers of hepatitis B virus: incidence and prevalence of hepatocellular carcinoma in a North American urban population. Hepatology. 1995;22(2):432–8.
147. Trevisani F, D'Intino PE, Morselli-Labate AM, et al. Serum alpha-fetoprotein for diagnosis of hepatocellular carcinoma in patients with chronic liver disease: influence of HBsAg and anti-HCV status. J Hepatol. 2001;34(4):570–5.
148. Gupta S, Bent S, Kohlwes J. Test characteristics of alpha-fetoprotein for detecting hepatocellular carcinoma in patients with hepatitis C. A systematic review and critical analysis. Ann Intern Med. 2003;139(1):46–50.
149. McClune AC, Tong MJ. Chronic hepatitis B and hepatocellular carcinoma. Clin Liver Dis. 2010;14(3):461–76.

150. Sato Y, Sekine T, Ohwada S. Alpha-fetoprotein-producing rectal cancer: calculated tumor marker doubling time. J Surg Oncol. 1994;55(4):265–8.
151. Adachi Y, Tsuchihashi J, Shiraishi N, Yasuda K, Etoh T, Kitano S. AFP-producing gastric carcinoma: multivariate analysis of prognostic factors in 270 patients. Oncology. 2003;65(2):95–101.
152. Maheshwari A, Kantsevoy S, Jagannath S, Thuluvath PJ. Endoscopic ultrasound and fine-needle aspiration for the diagnosis of hepatocellular carcinoma. Clin Liver Dis. 2010;14(2):325–32.
153. Weber SM, Jarnagin WR, Klimstra D, DeMatteo RP, Fong Y, Blumgart LH. Intrahepatic cholangiocarcinoma: resectability, recurrence pattern, and outcomes. J Am Coll Surg. 2001;193(4):384–91.
154. Nakeeb A, Pitt HA, Sohn TA, et al. Cholangiocarcinoma. A spectrum of intrahepatic, perihilar, and distal tumors. Ann Surg. 1996;224(4):463–73. discussion 473–5.
155. Patel T. Increasing incidence and mortality of primary intrahepatic cholangiocarcinoma in the United States. Hepatology. 2001;33(6):1353–7.
156. Shaib YH, El-Serag HB, Davila JA, Morgan R, McGlynn KA. Risk factors of intrahepatic cholangiocarcinoma in the United States: a case-control study. Gastroenterology. 2005;128(3):620–6.
157. Flavell DJ. Liver-fluke infection as an aetiological factor in bile-duct carcinoma of man. Trans R Soc Trop Med Hyg. 1981;75(6):814–24.
158. El-Serag HB, Engels EA, Landgren O, et al. Risk of hepatobiliary and pancreatic cancers after hepatitis C virus infection: A population-based study of U.S. veterans. Hepatology. 2009;49(1):116–23.
159. Donato F, Gelatti U, Tagger A, et al. Intrahepatic cholangiocarcinoma and hepatitis C and B virus infection, alcohol intake, and hepatolithiasis: a case-control study in Italy. Cancer Causes Control. 2001;12(10):959–64.
160. Kobayashi M, Ikeda K, Saitoh S, et al. Incidence of primary cholangiocellular carcinoma of the liver in japanese patients with hepatitis C virus-related cirrhosis. Cancer. 2000;88(11):2471–7.
161. Welzel TM, Graubard BI, El-Serag HB, et al. Risk factors for intrahepatic and extrahepatic cholangiocarcinoma in the United States: a population-based case-control study. Clin Gastroenterol Hepatol. 2007;5(10):1221–8.
162. Poultsides GA, Zhu AX, Choti MA, Pawlik TM. Intrahepatic cholangiocarcinoma. Surg Clin North Am. 2010;90(4):817–37.
163. Ramage JK, Donaghy A, Farrant JM, Iorns R, Williams R. Serum tumor markers for the diagnosis of cholangiocarcinoma in primary sclerosing cholangitis. Gastroenterology. 1995;108(3):865–9.
164. Hultcrantz R, Olsson R, Danielsson A, et al. A 3-year prospective study on serum tumor markers used for detecting cholangiocarcinoma in patients with primary sclerosing cholangitis. J Hepatol. 1999;30(4):669–73.
165. Levy C, Lymp J, Angulo P, Gores GJ, Larusso N, Lindor KD. The value of serum CA 19-9 in predicting cholangiocarcinomas in patients with primary sclerosing cholangitis. Dig Dis Sci. 2005;50(9):1734–40.
166. Patel AH, Harnois DM, Klee GG, LaRusso NF, Gores GJ. The utility of CA 19-9 in the diagnoses of cholangiocarcinoma in patients without primary sclerosing cholangitis. Am J Gastroenterol. 2000;95(1):204–7.
167. Nichols JC, Gores GJ, LaRusso NF, Wiesner RH, Nagorney DM, Ritts Jr RE. Diagnostic role of serum CA 19-9 for cholangiocarcinoma in patients with primary sclerosing cholangitis. Mayo Clin Proc. 1993;68(9):874–9.
168. Yamasaki S. Intrahepatic cholangiocarcinoma: macroscopic type and stage classification. J Hepatobiliary Pancreat Surg. 2003;10(4):288–91.
169. Yamamoto J, Kosuge T, Takayama T, et al. Surgical treatment of intrahepatic cholangiocarcinoma: four patients surviving more than five years. Surgery. 1992;111(6):617–22.

170. Wernecke K, Henke L, Vassallo P, et al. Pathologic explanation for hypoechoic halo seen on sonograms of malignant liver tumors: an in vitro correlative study. Am J Roentgenol. 1992;159(5):1011–6.
171. Lim JH. Cholangiocarcinoma: morphologic classification according to growth pattern and imaging findings. Am J Roentgenol. 2003;181(3):819–27.
172. Maetani Y, Itoh K, Watanabe C, et al. MR imaging of intrahepatic cholangiocarcinoma with pathologic correlation. Am J Roentgenol. 2001;176(6):1499–507.
173. Anderson CD, Rice MH, Pinson CW, Chapman WC, Chari RS, Delbeke D. Fluorodeoxyglucose PET imaging in the evaluation of gallbladder carcinoma and cholangiocarcinoma. J Gastrointest Surg. 2004;8(1):90–7.
174. Valls C, Guma A, Puig I, et al. Intrahepatic peripheral cholangiocarcinoma: CT evaluation. Abdom Imag. 2000;25(5):490–6.
175. Lee WJ, Lim HK, Jang KM, et al. Radiologic spectrum of cholangiocarcinoma: emphasis on unusual manifestations and differential diagnoses. Radiographics. 2001;21(Spec No):S97–116.
176. Zuo HQ, Yan LN, Zeng Y, et al. Clinicopathological characteristics of 15 patients with combined hepatocellular carcinoma and cholangiocarcinoma. Hepatobiliary Pancreat Dis Int. 2007;6(2):161–5.
177. Nishie A, Yoshimitsu K, Asayama Y, et al. Detection of combined hepatocellular and cholangiocarcinomas on enhanced CT: comparison with histologic findings. Am J Roentgenol. 2005;184(4):1157–62.
178. Kim YJ, Yun M, Lee WJ, Kim KS, Lee JD. Usefulness of 18 F-FDG PET in intrahepatic cholangiocarcinoma. Eur J Nucl Med Mol Imag. 2003;30(11):1467–72.
179. Corvera CU, Blumgart LH, Akhurst T, et al. 18 F-fluorodeoxyglucose positron emission tomography influences management decisions in patients with biliary cancer. J Am Coll Surg. 2008;206(1):57–65.
180. Moreno Luna LE, Kipp B, Halling KC, et al. Advanced cytologic techniques for the detection of malignant pancreatobiliary strictures. Gastroenterology. 2006;131(4):1064–72.
181. Boberg KM, Jebsen P, Clausen OP, Foss A, Aabakken L, Schrumpf E. Diagnostic benefit of biliary brush cytology in cholangiocarcinoma in primary sclerosing cholangitis. J Hepatol. 2006;45(4):568–74.
182. Zen Y, Adsay NV, Bardadin K, et al. Biliary intraepithelial neoplasia: an international interobserver agreement study and proposal for diagnostic criteria. Mod Pathol. 2007;20(6):701–9.
183. Chen MF, Jan YY, Chen TC. Clinical studies of mucin-producing cholangiocellular carcinoma: a study of 22 histopathology-proven cases. Ann Surg. 1998;227(1):63–9.
184. Shimonishi T, Zen Y, Chen TC, et al. Increasing expression of gastrointestinal phenotypes and p53 along with histologic progression of intraductal papillary neoplasia of the liver. Hum Pathol. 2002;33(5):503–11.
185. Nakanishi Y, Zen Y, Kondo S, Itoh T, Itatsu K, Nakanuma Y. Expression of cell cycle-related molecules in biliary premalignant lesions: biliary intraepithelial neoplasia and biliary intraductal papillary neoplasm. Hum Pathol. 2008;39(8):1153–61.
186. Zen Y, Sasaki M, Fujii T, et al. Different expression patterns of mucin core proteins and cytokeratins during intrahepatic cholangiocarcinogenesis from biliary intraepithelial neoplasia and intraductal papillary neoplasm of the bile duct--an immunohistochemical study of 110 cases of hepatolithiasis. J Hepatol. 2006;44(2):350–8.
187. Higashi M, Yonezawa S, Ho JJ, et al. Expression of MUC1 and MUC2 mucin antigens in intrahepatic bile duct tumors: its relationship with a new morphological classification of cholangiocarcinoma. Hepatology. 1999;30(6):1347–55.
188. Theise ND, Nakashima O, Park YN, Nakanuma Y. Combined hepatocellular-cholangiocarcinoma. In: Bosman FT, Carneiro F, Hruban RH, Theise ND, editors. WHO classification of tumours of the digestive system. Lyon: IARC Press; 2010. pp. 225–7.
189. Sempoux C, Jibara G, Ward SC, et al. Intrahepatic cholangiocarcinoma: new insights in pathology. Semin Liver Dis. 2011;31(1):49–60.

190. Nathan H, Aloia TA, Vauthey JN, et al. A proposed staging system for intrahepatic cholangiocarcinoma. Ann Surg Oncol. 2009;16(1):14–22.
191. Shiota K, Taguchi J, Nakashima O, Nakashima M, Kojiro M. Clinicopathologic study on cholangiolocellular carcinoma. Oncol Rep. 2001;8(2):263–8.
192. Kanamoto M, Yoshizumi T, Ikegami T, et al. Cholangiolocellular carcinoma containing hepatocellular carcinoma and cholangiocellular carcinoma, extremely rare tumor of the liver: a case report. J Med Invest. 2008;55(1–2):161–5.
193. Goodman ZD, Ishak KG, Langloss JM, Sesterhenn IA, Rabin L. Combined hepatocellular-cholangiocarcinoma. A histologic and immunohistochemical study. Cancer. 1985;55(1): 124–35.
194. Mosnier JF, Kandel C, Cazals-Hatem D, et al. N-cadherin serves as diagnostic biomarker in intrahepatic and perihilar cholangiocarcinomas. Mod Pathol. 2009;22(2):182–90.
195. Choti MA, Bulkley GB. Management of metastatic disease. In: Schiff ER, Sorrell MF, Maddrey WC, editors. Disease of the liver. Philadelphia: Lippincott-Raven; 1999. pp. 1319–33.
196. Baker ME, Pelley R. Hepatic metastases: basic principles and implications for radiologists. Radiology. 1995;197(2):329–37.
197. Seitz G. Why are metastases in cirrhotic livers so rare? Ultraschall Med. 1989;10(3):123–6.
198. Bengmark S, Hafstrom L. The natural history of primary and secondary malignant tumors of the liver I. The prognosis for patients with hepatic metastases from colonic and rectal carcinoma by laparotomy. Cancer. 1969;23(1):198–202.
199. Bozzetti F, Doci R, Bignami P, Morabito A, Gennari L. Patterns of failure following surgical resection of colorectal cancer liver metastases. Rationale for a multimodal approach. Ann Surg. 1987;205(3):264–70.
200. Wood CB, Gillis CR, Blumgart LH. A retrospective study of the natural history of patients with liver metastases from colorectal cancer. Clin Oncol. 1976;2(3):285–8.
201. Wagner JS, Adson MA, Van Heerden JA, Adson MH, Ilstrup DM. The natural history of hepatic metastases from colorectal cancer. A comparison with resective treatment. Ann Surg. 1984;199(5):502–8.
202. Scheele J, Stang R, Altendorf-Hofmann A, Paul M. Resection of colorectal liver metastases. World J Surg. 1995;19(1):59–71.
203. Sugarbaker PH. Surgical decision making for large bowel cancer metastatic to the liver. Radiology. 1990;174(3 Pt 1):621–6.
204. Fong Y, Cohen AM, Fortner JG, et al. Liver resection for colorectal metastases. J Clin Oncol. 1997;15(3):938–46.
205. Minagawa M, Makuuchi M, Torzilli G, et al. Extension of the frontiers of surgical indications in the treatment of liver metastases from colorectal cancer: long-term results. Ann Surg. 2000;231(4):487–99.
206. Charnsangavej C, Clary B, Fong Y, Grothey A, Pawlik TM, Choti MA. Selection of patients for resection of hepatic colorectal metastases: expert consensus statement. Ann Surg Oncol. 2006;13(10):1261–8.
207. Abdalla EK, Adam R, Bilchik AJ, Jaeck D, Vauthey JN, Mahvi D. Improving resectability of hepatic colorectal metastases: expert consensus statement. Ann Surg Oncol. 2006;13(10): 1271–80.
208. Pawlik TM, Schulick RD, Choti MA. Expanding criteria for resectability of colorectal liver metastases. Oncologist. 2008;13(1):51–64.
209. Chen H, Hardacre JM, Uzar A, Cameron JL, Choti MA. Isolated liver metastases from neuroendocrine tumors: does resection prolong survival? J Am Coll Surg. 1998;187(1):88–92. discussion 92–3.
210. Sarmiento JM, Heywood G, Rubin J, Ilstrup DM, Nagorney DM, Que FG. Surgical treatment of neuroendocrine metastases to the liver: a plea for resection to increase survival. J Am Coll Surg. 2003;197(1):29–37.
211. Chamberlain RS, Canes D, Brown KT, et al. Hepatic neuroendocrine metastases: does intervention alter outcomes? J Am Coll Surg. 2000;190(4):432–45.

212. Slooter GD, Mearadji A, Breeman WA, et al. Somatostatin receptor imaging, therapy and new strategies in patients with neuroendocrine tumours. Br J Surg. 2001;88(1):31–40.
213. Gabriel M, Decristoforo C, Kendler D, et al. 68 Ga-DOTA-Tyr3-octreotide PET in neuroendocrine tumors: comparison with somatostatin receptor scintigraphy and CT. J Nucl Med. 2007;48(4):508–18.
214. Weitz J, Blumgart LH, Fong Y, et al. Partial hepatectomy for metastases from noncolorectal, nonneuroendocrine carcinoma. Ann Surg. 2005;241(2):269–76.
215. Adam R, Aloia T, Krissat J, et al. Is liver resection justified for patients with hepatic metastases from breast cancer? Ann Surg. 2006;244(6):897–907. discussion 907–8.
216. Bruneton JN, Raffaelli C, Balu-Maestro C, Padovani B, Chevallier P, Mourou MY. Sonographic diagnosis of solitary solid liver nodules in cancer patients. Eur Radiol. 1996;6(4):439–42.
217. Paley MR, Ros PR. Hepatic metastases. Radiol Clin North Am. 1998;36(2):349–63.
218. Wernecke K, Rummeny E, Bongartz G, et al. Detection of hepatic masses in patients with carcinoma: comparative sensitivities of sonography, CT, and MR imaging. Am J Roentgenol. 1991;157(4):731–9.
219. Hagspiel KD, Neidl KF, Eichenberger AC, Weder W, Marincek B. Detection of liver metastases: comparison of superparamagnetic iron oxide-enhanced and unenhanced MR imaging at 1.5 T with dynamic CT, intraoperative US, and percutaneous US. Radiology. 1995;196(2):471–8.
220. Albrecht T, Hohmann J, Oldenburg A, Skrok J, Wolf KJ. Detection and characterisation of liver metastases. Eur Radiol. 2004;14 Suppl 8:P25–33.
221. Mainenti PP, Mancini M, Mainolfi C, et al. Detection of colo-rectal liver metastases: prospective comparison of contrast enhanced US, multidetector CT, PET/CT, and 1.5 Tesla MR with extracellular and reticulo-endothelial cell specific contrast agents. Abdom Imag. 2010;35(5):511–21.
222. Quaia E, D'Onofrio M, Palumbo A, Rossi S, Bruni S, Cova M. Comparison of contrast-enhanced ultrasonography versus baseline ultrasound and contrast-enhanced computed tomography in metastatic disease of the liver: diagnostic performance and confidence. Eur Radiol. 2006;16(7):1599–609.
223. Wildi SM, Gubler C, Hany T, et al. Intraoperative sonography in patients with colorectal cancer and resectable liver metastases on preoperative FDG-PET-CT. J Clin Ultrasound. 2008;36(1):20–6.
224. Sahani DV, Kalva SP, Tanabe KK, et al. Intraoperative US in patients undergoing surgery for liver neoplasms: comparison with MR imaging. Radiology. 2004;232(3):810–4.
225. Winston C, Teitcher J. Computed tomography of the liver, biliary tract, and pancreas. In: Blumgart LH, ed. Surgery of the liver, biliary tract and pancreas. 4th ed. 2006.
226. Valls C, Andia E, Sanchez A, et al. Hepatic metastases from colorectal cancer: preoperative detection and assessment of resectability with helical CT. Radiology. 2001;218(1):55–60.
227. Bhattacharjya S, Bhattacharjya T, Baber S, Tibballs JM, Watkinson AF, Davidson BR. Prospective study of contrast-enhanced computed tomography, computed tomography during arterioportography, and magnetic resonance imaging for staging colorectal liver metastases for liver resection. Br J Surg. 2004;91(10):1361–9.
228. Kamel IR, Choti MA, Horton KM, et al. Surgically staged focal liver lesions: accuracy and reproducibility of dual-phase helical CT for detection and characterization. Radiology. 2003;227(3):752–7.
229. Floriani I, Torri V, Rulli E, et al. Performance of imaging modalities in diagnosis of liver metastases from colorectal cancer: a systematic review and meta-analysis. J Magn Reson Imag. 2010;31(1):19–31.
230. Soyer P, Poccard M, Boudiaf M, et al. Detection of hypovascular hepatic metastases at triple-phase helical CT: sensitivity of phases and comparison with surgical and histopathologic findings. Radiology. 2004;231(2):413–20.
231. Adams LA, Talwalkar JA. Diagnostic evaluation of nonalcoholic fatty liver disease. J Clin Gastroenterol. 2006;40 Suppl 1:S34–8.

232. Namasivayam S, Martin DR, Saini S. Imaging of liver metastases: MRI. Cancer Imag. 2007;7:2–9.
233. Imam K, Bluemke DA. MR imaging in the evaluation of hepatic metastases. Magn Reson Imag Clin North Am. 2000;8(4):741–56.
234. Wittenberg J, Stark DD, Forman BH, et al. Differentiation of hepatic metastases from hepatic hemangiomas and cysts by using MR imaging. Am J Roentgenol. 1988;151(1):79–84.
235. Mahfouz AE, Hamm B, Wolf KJ. Peripheral washout: a sign of malignancy on dynamic gadolinium-enhanced MR images of focal liver lesions. Radiology. 1994;190(1):49–52.
236. Bipat S, van Leeuwen MS, Comans EF, et al. Colorectal liver metastases: CT, MR imaging, and PET for diagnosis–meta-analysis. Radiology. 2005;237(1):123–31.
237. Yang M, Martin DR, Karabulut N, Frick MP. Comparison of MR and PET imaging for the evaluation of liver metastases. J Magn Reson Imag. 2003;17(3):343–9.
238. Kantorova I, Lipska L, Belohlavek O, Visokai V, Trubac M, Schneiderova M. Routine (18) F-FDG PET preoperative staging of colorectal cancer: comparison with conventional staging and its impact on treatment decision making. J Nucl Med. 2003;44(11):1784–8.
239. Grassetto G, Fornasiero A, Bonciarelli G, et al. Additional value of FDG-PET/CT in management of "solitary" liver metastases: preliminary results of a prospective multicenter study. Mol Imag Biol. 2010;12(2):139–44.
240. Huguet EL, Old S, Praseedom RK, Balan KK, Gibbs P, Jamieson NV. F18-FDG-PET evaluation of patients for resection of colorectal liver metastases. Hepatogastroenterology. 2007;54(78):1667–71.
241. Sorensen M, Mortensen FV, Hoyer M, Vilstrup H, Keiding S. Liver Tumour Board at Aarhus University Hospital. FDG-PET improves management of patients with colorectal liver metastases allocated for local treatment: a consecutive prospective study. Scand J Surg. 2007;96(3):209–13.
242. Chua SC, Groves AM, Kayani I, et al. The impact of 18 F-FDG PET/CT in patients with liver metastases. Eur J Nucl Med Mol Imag. 2007;34(12):1906–14.

Chapter 6
Paraneoplastic Syndromes

Po-Hung Chen and Ayman Koteish

Paraneoplastic (literally "alongside cancer") syndromes are the consequences of malignancy that cannot be attributed to local tumor invasion, distant metastases, or adverse effects from cancer therapy. Occasionally, these are the herald signs and symptoms that prompt the workup toward the eventual identification of the primary malignancy. Paraneoplastic syndromes may possess significant or even life-threatening clinical implications, sometimes more so than local effects of the cancer itself. They may even mimic metastatic disease and thus alter treatment plan [1]. The timely recognition of these relatively infrequent entities is therefore clinically vital; they are more likely to respond favorably to the effective treatment of the underlying cancer than to efforts toward direct symptomatic management.

This chapter aims to highlight the various paraneoplastic manifestations associated with primary malignancies of the hepatobiliary system (Table 6.1). A section is included to describe a paraneoplastic hepatic dysfunction of nonhepatic malignancies without liver metastases. Finally, there is a brief discussion on the malignant transformation potential of benign hepatic adenomas.

P.-H. Chen, MD (✉)
Fellow, Division of Gastroenterology and Hepatology, The Johns Hopkins Hospital,
600 N. Wolfe Street, Baltimore, MD 21287, USA
e-mail: victor.chen@jhmi.edu

A. Koteish, MD
Department of Medicine, The Johns Hopkins Hospital, 600 N. Wolfe Street,
Baltimore, MD 21287, USA
e-mail: akoteish@jhmi.edu

N. Reau and F.F. Poordad (eds.), *Primary Liver Cancer: Surveillance, Diagnosis and Treatment*, Clinical Gastroenterology, DOI 10.1007/978-1-61779-863-4_6,
© Springer Science+Business Media New York 2012

Hepatocellular Carcinoma

Paraneoplastic syndromes associated with hepatocellular carcinoma (HCC) occur relatively infrequently but often portend poor prognosis. Patients with paraneoplastic syndromes are more likely to have main portal vein thrombosis and tumor metastasis. High serum alpha-fetoprotein levels, large tumor sizes, and hepatitis B-related HCC (as opposed to hepatitis C-related cancer) are all risk factors for the development of paraneoplastic syndromes. On the other hand, the different grades of cellular differentiation of HCC have little apparent correlation with these syndromes [2].

Table 6.1 Primary malignancies of the hepatobiliary system

Neoplasm	Paraneoplastic manifestation	% of patients affected
Hepatocellular carcinoma	Hypoglycemia	30%; Type B (severe) <5%
	Hypercalcemia	1.5–40%
	Hypercholesterolemia	~10%
	Erythrocytosis	1–3%
	Watery diarrhea	20–50%; Severe <5 %
	Cutaneous findings 　1. Pityriasis rotunda 　2. Dermatomyositis 　3. Acanthosis nigricans 　4. Disseminated superficial 　　　porokeratosis	n/d[a]
	Feminization	n/d
	Neurological findings 　1. Chronic inflammatory demyelinating 　　　polyradiculoneuropathy (CIDP) 　2. Myasthenia gravis	Uncommon
Cholangiocarcinoma	Hypercalcemia	~20%
	Cutaneous findings 　1. Erythema multiforme 　2. Acute febrile neutrophilic 　　　dermatosis (Sweet's syndrome) 　3. Acrokeratosis paraneoplastica 　　　(Bazex's syndrome) 　4. Acanthosis nigricans 　5. Disseminated superficial 　　　porokeratosis 　6. Porphyria cutanea tarda	Uncommon
	Thrombophlebitis migrans 　(Trousseau's syndrome)	Uncommon
Primary hepatic lymphoma	Hypercalcemia	n/d
	Immune thrombocytopenic 　purpura (ITP)	n/d
Primary hepatic carcinoid	Carcinoid syndrome	Less common than 　in carcinoid liver 　metastases
	Zollinger–Ellison syndrome	n/d

[a]"n/d" denotes "no data"

Hypoglycemia is commonly associated with pancreatic tumors (e.g., insulinoma). In non-islet cell tumors such as HCC, paraneoplastic hypoglycemia occurs somewhat less frequently, yet remains a well-recognized entity. Indeed, affecting up to 30% of the patients, hypoglycemia is among the more prevalent paraneoplastic syndromes associated with HCC. Several case reports in the literature have explored this phenomenon, which at times may be the only clinical manifestation for months prior to the diagnosis of HCC. Patients may present with recurrent seizures as a result of the low serum glucose. Two classic types of hypoglycemia have been described in HCC (types A and B) [3]. Type A is a mild-to-moderate hypoglycemia in the terminal stages of a rapidly growing, poorly differentiated tumor when native gluconeogenesis can no longer keep up with the metabolic demands of the cancer and the rest of the body. The fact that HCC frequently occurs in cirrhotic livers with impaired gluconeogenesis only exacerbates the matter. The less common (under 5%) type B is a severe hypoglycemia that manifests early in the course of well-differentiated HCC; plasma glucose levels of <30 mg/dl have been reported [4]. A proposed mechanism for the hypoglycemia is the production of big insulin-like growth factor II (big IGF-II), which results from the incomplete conversion of pro-IGF-II to IGF-II. Unlike its fully converted counterpart, big IGF-II does not complex well with binding proteins. The end result is a higher concentration of free IGF-II that readily gains access to target tissues causing hypoglycemia [5]. Growth hormone and IGF-I levels consequently may be low due to negative feedback. With both type A and B hypoglycemia, plasma levels of insulin, C-peptide, and proinsulin are suppressed, and serum cortisol level is elevated. This is in contrast to insulinoma-induced hypoglycemia, where plasma concentrations of insulin, C-peptide, and proinsulin are increased above baseline.

Various treatments for hypoglycemia have been proposed. The optimal treatment is tumor eradication—or, failing that, reduction of tumor burden. Conservative treatment options that have been reported include frequent high carbohydrate meals, supportive glucose infusions, corticosteroids, growth hormone, glucagon, and somatostatin analogues.

Malignancy-associated **hypercalcemia** is well documented. However, the pathophysiologic mechanism is variable depending on the primary cancer. In solid tumors of squamous cell origin (e.g., lung) and renal cell carcinoma, hypercalcemia is attributed to the paraneoplastic production of parathyroid hormone-related peptide (PTH-rP), which mimics many of the actions of parathyroid hormone (PTH), including renal calcium reabsorption and bone resorption. Serum testing finds PTH-rP concentration to be elevated and PTH level suppressed. On the other hand, multiple myeloma causes elevated serum calcium by way of osteolytic bone metastases. Increased production of 1,25-dihydroxyvitamin D also leads to hypercalcemia and is associated with certain lymphomas. Finally, the ectopic secretion of intact parathyroid hormone (iPTH) offers yet another possible explanation. Tumors such as breast cancer can even employ more than one pathway (PTH-rP and bony metastases in this case) [6].

In hepatocellular carcinoma, the prevalence of hypercalcemia varies widely between 1.5% and 40% in different reports [7, 8]. Somnolence and disorientation have been reported at extreme levels of serum calcium [9]. PTH-rP production is most commonly implicated as the pathogenic mechanism [10]. However, at least three reports to date have described patients with markedly elevated serum iPTH levels along with normal PTH-rP concentrations. Sestamibi scan with single-photon emission computed tomographic (SPECT) imaging has been used successfully to localize the ectopic iPTH source in the liver [11]. Direct tumor therapy such as transcatheter arterial chemoembolization (TACE) led to an improvement of serum iPTH and calcium, supporting the idea that the tumor was the offending source [12]. The basic principles behind the various therapies for hypercalcemia of malignancy include volume expansion, induction of calciuria, inhibition of 1,25-dihydroxyvitamin D synthesis, prevention of bone resorption, and tumor reduction. Dialysis is occasionally needed in severe hypercalcemia.

With most malignancies, patients develop hypocholesterolemia along with marked weight loss. This is in contrast with HCC, where **hypercholesterolemia** may develop even while the patient appears wasted and cachectic. The levels of serum cholesterol seen in these patients may rival those with homozygous familial hypercholesterolemia [13]. Paraneoplastic hypercholesterolemia was reported in 11.4% of the HCC patients in a Taiwanese study [14]. Defined in the study as serum cholesterol levels above 250 mg/dl, the hypercholesterolemia resolved to normal levels after the treatment of HCC but again rose when tumors recurred or progressed. The exact mechanism for this is not yet known. One proposed explanation is a decrease in the uptake of cholesterol by HCC cells due to an abnormal LDL gene that leads to the reduced expression of the membrane LDL receptor protein [15].

Erythrocytosis or polycythemia is an uncommon paraneoplastic syndrome in HCC, found in 1–3% of patients in recent literature (older studies from 1950s to 1970s reported slightly higher prevalence ranging from 3% to 12%) [16–18]. The actual prevalence may be higher; however, as HCC is associated with advanced liver disease particularly in the United States, several confounding factors exist that may hinder the manifestation of high hemoglobin levels. These include ongoing gastrointestinal bleeding, volume expansion, and abnormal iron metabolism (i.e., anemia of chronic disease). Erythrocytosis is associated with large hepatoma size and markedly abnormal alpha-fetoprotein levels. Hemoglobin levels as high as 21.5 mg/dl without hemoconcentration from decreased plasma volume have been documented [19]. The underlying pathogenesis is increased erythropoietin production. The body's major source of erythropoietin is the kidneys, which may respond to focal hypoxia and necrosis found in an enlarging hepatic tumor. HCC cells are also able to synthesize erythropoietin, with or without the presence of ongoing tissue hypoxia. A 1993 Japanese study illustrated this when erythropoietin was identified in the rough endoplasmic reticulum of HCC cells, but not the surrounding normal liver cells. In the study, erythropoietin level was higher in the hepatic vein than in the hepatic artery, supporting the notion that it originated from the liver. Erythropoietin level then dropped drastically after the patient received cisplatin [20].

Watery diarrhea is a common paraneoplastic finding in HCC, affecting 20–50% of the patients [21]. However, <5% of HCC patients report diarrhea as their chief complaint. The severity of illness varies from patient to patient, ranging from intermittent symptoms to five bowel movements or more per day for >10 weeks [22]. There may be nocturnal occurrences, and the presence of blood is rare. The mechanism for HCC-associated diarrhea may be the production of secretagogues by the tumor, a process similar to that of pancreatic neuroendocrine tumors. Specifically, Steiner et al., used immunohistochemistry and radioimmunoassay to uncover the presence of vasoactive intestinal peptide, gastrin, and prostaglandin E2 in HCC tumor cells [23]. Aside from the usual battery of antidiarrheal therapies such as somatostatin analogues or deodorized tincture of opium, symptom suppression also has been achieved via the surgical removal of the tumor as well as the use of nonsteroidal anti-inflammatory drugs (which inhibit prostaglandin synthesis) [24].

A number of **cutaneous** paraneoplastic findings have been reported in HCC. These include pityriasis rotunda, dermatomyositis, acanthosis nigricans, and disseminated superficial porokeratosis.

Pityriasis rotunda has been described in Japanese and African patients suffering various infections (e.g., Mycobacterium, Entamoeba), cirrhosis, or malignancies. A 1986 series raised the possibility of using these skin lesions as a marker for HCC in black Africans [25]. These lesions are round, flat, and scaly, with or without changes to the native pigmentation. Their sizes may vary from 1 to >30 cm, and they occur on the body, the shoulders, and the thighs. There is no associated pain or pruritus.

Dermatomyositis is a systemic inflammatory state. It presents with a progressive weakening of proximal muscles as well as characteristic skin lesions. These may include Gottron's papules (scaly rash over the metacarpophalangeal and interphalangeal joints), heliotrope rash (violaceous eruption on the top eyelids), shawl and V signs (erythema over the chest and shoulders in a V-shaped pattern), and erythroderma (large areas of erythema elsewhere on the body) [26].

The association between dermatomyositis and cancer is well known. Population-based studies have shown ovarian, pancreatic, and lung cancers to exhibit particularly robust correlations [27, 28]. While much less common, there also have been reports on the association between dermatomyositis and HCC. In many cases, advanced HCC (at least 6.0 cm in diameter or metastatic disease) was found at the time of dermatomyositis diagnosis [29]. Several mechanisms have been proposed, including paraneoplastic syndrome, cross-reactivity of antibodies against tumor and skin/muscle, and common carcinogenic triggers [30]. One account from Taiwan supported the notion of a paraneoplastic relationship by demonstrating the improvement of dermatomyositis after treatment with oral corticosteroids and TACE. Any residual symptoms then completely resolved following the surgical resection of HCC, without requiring further maintenance corticosteroids [31]. However, the overall clinical course remained unfavorable as the patient eventually died from the complications of HCC. This was consistent with the other reports of HCC and dermatomyositis in the literature.

Acanthosis nigricans is a characteristic skin finding usually associated with benign systemic states such as insulin resistance and obesity. It is characterized by velvety, thickened plaques usually with a brownish hue and occurs most commonly—but not exclusively—in the flexural areas of the body. It is frequently asymptomatic, though on occasion may present with pain or pruritus. Malignancy should be considered when rapid progression or mucosal involvement is observed. While less common than its benign counterpart, malignant acanthosis nigricans can herald the presence of an internal cancer and often evolves in parallel with the clinical status of the said neoplasm [32]. In a series of 277 cases of malignant acanthosis nigricans, the association was strongest with gastric adenocarcinoma (55%), but lung and liver cancers were also reported [33].

Porokeratosis is a disorder in epidermal keratinization, described as atrophic patches surrounded by annular hyperkeratinized borders. One variant, disseminated superficial porokeratosis (DSP), is sometimes associated with immunosuppression and hematologic malignancies, though rarely with solid tumors. Kono et al., in 2000 presented the first three reported cases of DSP in HCC, all of which were hepatitis C-related [34]. In all three cases, the interval between the development of DSP and the diagnosis of HCC was <6 months. DSP has since been described in cholangio-carcinoma and ovarian adenocarcinoma as well. One proposed pathogenic pathway is the overexpression of p53 in certain keratinocytes, causing abnormal differentiation in these cells and eventually creating porokeratosis lesions. The p53 gene plays a vital oncogenic role in the development of various solid organ tumors, including HCC, cholangiocarcinoma, and ovarian adenocarcinoma [35].

Porphyria cutanea tarda, characterized by vesicles and bullae in response to light sensitivity and minor trauma, was at one time also thought to be a paraneoplastic finding of HCC [36]. However, more recent studies have suggested the converse to be more likely that patients with porphyria cutanea tarda are at an increased risk for developing HCC [37].

Men with HCC occasionally develop **feminization**, with signs and symptoms such as gynecomastia, prepubescent testes, decreased libido, and feminine hair distribution [38, 39]. These are hardly foreign findings in chronic liver diseases especially cirrhosis and are attributable to hyperestrogenism. However, feminization can occur in HCC without the presence of background liver cirrhosis. Patients' serum and urinary estrogens are typically elevated, while testosterone and pituitary hormone (follicle-stimulating hormone, luteinizing hormone, and prolactin) levels are low or low normal. One proposed mechanism for the hyperestrogenism is the conversion of circulating androgens to estrogens by the HCC, a process that is also seen in normal placental tissues. Kew et al., demonstrated the in vitro aromatization by HCC of dehydroepiandrosterone sulfate to estrone and estradiol [40]. Like many other paraneoplastic syndromes, feminization often improves or resolves with the treatment of the HCC.

Paraneoplastic **neurological** disorders are highly variable and can arise anywhere in the nervous system. Immunologic processes—possibly from molecular mimicry that occurs during tumor formation—underlie most if not all of these disorders. It is therefore standard practice to measure certain key antibodies if there is clinical suspicion for paraneoplastic neurological entities. The association is classically strongest with small cell lung cancer, breast cancer, and gynecological cancers; neurological syndromes are much less often reported in the setting of HCC [41]. Two such examples are described here.

Chronic inflammatory demyelinating polyradiculoneuropathy (CIDP) is characterized by slowly progressive, diffuse muscle weakness with hyporeflexia and variable sensory deficits. Another name sometimes used for the disorder is chronic relapsing Guillain–Barré syndrome, as CIDP is considered the chronic form of the acute disease. As the name implies, the diffuse loss of the myelin sheath insulating the nerves is the underlying mechanism responsible for CIDP. The diagnosis is made by a combination of clinical findings, cerebrospinal fluid tests, nerve conduction study, and possibly sural nerve biopsy. CIDP is associated with a number of benign and malignant diseases, including inflammatory bowel disease, various connective tissue disorders, Hodgkin's lymphoma, and the osteosclerotic form of plasmacytoma. While there are several published cases arguing in favor of the notion of the possible paraneoplastic CIDP in HCC, this remains an extremely uncommon relationship [42]. Treatment of CIDP consists of immunosuppression, typically starting with corticosteroids, but may also include plasmapheresis and intravenous immunoglobulin [43].

Another well-described paraneoplastic neurological disorder is myasthenia gravis (MG), a disease of dysfunctional neuromuscular junctions; MG occurs when acetylcholine molecules are unable to reach their target receptors across the synapse. MG is most commonly linked to thymoma and much less so to extrathymic malignancies. Vautravers et al., reported one of the first cases of pathologically proven HCC presenting with paraneoplastic MG [44]. The patient had complained of postexercise muscle fatigue, ptosis, and dysphagia. The diagnosis of MG was made when the electromyogram showed a >10% decrease in compound muscle action potential after a train of low-frequency stimulations. The serum level of antiacetylcholine receptor antibody was also elevated. His malignancy workup was negative for a thymic tumor but instead revealed a 15-cm liver mass. Biopsies of the mass revealed HCC without background cirrhosis; viral hepatitides were negative. The patient's symptoms first improved with neostigmine, a parasympathomimetic that inhibits the breakdown of acetylcholine. He then underwent Lipiodol chemoembolization with pirarubicin and ultimately surgical resection of the tumor. Neostigmine was stopped at that point, with no recurrence of neurological symptoms.

Other HCC-associated neurological disorders that have been published in the literature include Guillain—Barré syndrome, vasculitic demyelinating polyneuropathy, and subacute encephalomyeloneuritis (involvement of both the central and the peripheral nervous systems) [45–47]. However, given the limited overall information from the isolated reports, the jury is still out on whether these are true paraneoplastic processes.

Cholangiocarcinoma

Cholangiocarcinoma is the second most common primary hepatic malignancy, accounting for 3% of gastrointestinal malignancies [48].

As is with HCC above, **hypercalcemia of malignancy** has also been reported in cholangiocarcinoma. In the series by Oldenburg et al. [7], hypercalcemia was found in 18% of the patients. Most of these patients had elevated serum PTH levels, suggesting that ectopic iPTH secretion was likely the offending mechanism [7]. Between the isolation of PTH-rP in 1987 and 2010, nine cases of cholangiocarcinoma-associated hypercalcemia have been reported in the literature. In the majority of these cases, the cancer already had progressed to advanced stages when the paraneoplastic syndrome manifested [49]. The adjusted serum calcium has been reported to be as high as 16.4 mg/dl, in a patient who presented with lethargy and confusion. The patient rebounded favorably with the treatment of his hypercalcemia and survived sufficiently long to receive six subsequent courses of chemotherapy for his tumor [50].

Like HCC, paraneoplastic **cutaneous** manifestations have been reported in patients with cholangiocarcinoma. These are uncommon associations overall; several made their first appearance in the medical literature after the year 2000.

Frequently associated with infections especially herpes simplex virus, erythema multiforme (EM) is usually a self-limited skin disorder that resolves within weeks. Persistent EM is rare and may be associated with viral infections, inflammatory bowel disease, or malignancy. Tzovaras et al., provided in 2007 the first description of persistent EM in a patient with extrahepatic cholangiocarcinoma [51]. The skin lesions improved alongside tumor response to chemotherapy but reappeared when the tumor relapsed. Classically, EM has a target-like appearance with a dusky center that may possibly blister, a dark red surrounding zone of inflammation, and a lighter erythematous ring on the periphery. However, true to its name "multiforme," frequently there are additional lesions that do not fit the classic description. EM can involve both mucosal and cutaneous sites [52].

First described in 1964 as acute febrile neutrophilic dermatosis, Sweet's syndrome is characterized by painful cutaneous plaques, fever, and neutrophilic leukocytosis [53]. Approximately one fifth of the cases are cancer-related; most of these patients have hematopoietic malignancies, but still 15% suffer from solid tumors [54]. The most common of these solid tumors originates from the genitourinary organs, breast, and gastrointestinal tract. A 2006 article reported the first published case of Sweet's syndrome associated with an intrahepatic cholangiocarcinoma [55]. The skin lesions resolved following the administration of oral potassium iodide. Other pharmacologic options include corticosteroids, nonsteroidal anti-inflammatory drugs, colchicine, dapsone, doxycycline, clofazimine, and cyclosporine.

Acrokeratosis paraneoplastica, or Bazex's syndrome, is a rare paraneoplastic psoriasiform eruption. It consists of erythematous to violaceous scaly plaques, which may be pruritic. The nose and the helices of the ears are commonly affected; this marks a departure from the usual patterns of psoriasis. Other sites of involvement include the nails, hands, feet, elbows, and knees; in later stages, even the legs, arms, and the trunk may be affected [56]. Nail changes are reminiscent of psoriasis and may include yellow discoloration, subungual debris, nail plate flattening, and onycholysis [57]. The earliest of the dermatological changes may precede the diagnosis of the neoplasm by up to 1 year [58]. Squamous cell carcinoma of the upper aerodigestive tract is by far the most implicated tumor. However, a case associated with extrahepatic cholangiocarcinoma has been reported in the literature [59]. The successful treatment of the underlying malignancy is generally required to eradicate the rash (though nail changes often persist); conventional dermatological therapies are generally unhelpful.

Other paraneoplastic cutaneous manifestations of cholangiocarcinoma include acanthosis nigricans, disseminated superficial porokeratosis, and porphyria cutanea tarda. All are associated with HCC also; these discussions are elsewhere in this chapter. As mentioned earlier, a rapid progression or mucosal involvement of acanthosis nigricans should raise the suspicion for an occult malignancy. The earliest known report of disseminated superficial porokeratosis in a patient with cholangiocarcinoma appeared in the literature in 2006; a second case was later published in 2010 [35, 60]. Unlike its updated relationship with HCC carcinogenesis, porphyria cutanea tarda remains a paraneoplastic syndrome in cholangiocarcinoma. Sökmen et al., presented the first published case of this in 2007 [61]. In the report, the patient's skin findings resolved after the placement of a biliary duct stent and the administration of chemotherapy.

Trousseau first described the association between **venous thromboembolic events** and malignancy in 1865. A special variant of this is Trousseau's syndrome, where there is recurrent and migratory involvement of the superficial veins. In one series of patients with Trousseau's syndrome, pancreatic cancer was the most commonly implicated, followed by lung, prostate, and gastric malignancies [62]. Typically these are adenocarcinomas, specifically mucin-producing tumors [63]. The prevalence of Trousseau's syndrome in all cancers has been reported to range from 1% to 11% [64]. This has not been characterized specifically in cholangiocarcinoma but is thought to be significantly less common. Several case reports in the literature describe the occurrence of unexplained severe diffuse venous thromboembolism that provided the clue to diagnosis of clinically unsuspected cholangiocarcinoma [65, 66]. The treatment for malignancy-related thromboembolism usually involves heparin products. Vitamin K antagonists are markedly inferior in this setting [67].

Primary Hepatic Lymphoma

First described in 1965 by Ata and Kamel, primary non-Hodgkin's lymphoma of the liver constitutes only about 0.016% of all cases of non-Hodgkin's lymphoma [68, 69]. Fewer than 100 cases had been reported in the literature as of 2004, with a 4:1 male preponderance [70]. On imaging studies, primary hepatic lymphomas (PHL) more often take the form of discrete lesions rather than diffusely infiltrating tumors. However, a definitive diagnosis is only available through histological examination. Approximately 80% of PHLs have B-cell origins; the rest are T-cell tumors [71]. Published cases and reviews support associations with hepatitis C and human immunodeficiency virus [72, 73]. On the other hand, there are conflicting data on whether chronic hepatitis B infection plays a role in the pathogenesis of PHL [74].

Due to the rarity of PHL and the limited information available, relatively few discussions exist in the literature with regard to the potential paraneoplastic manifestations. Hypercalcemia and immune thrombocytopenic purpura are two that have been reported [75, 76]. The vast majority of PHL patients present with nonspecific constitutional symptoms such as fever, night sweats, abdominal pain, and weight loss [77].

Primary Hepatic Carcinoid Tumor

Neuroendocrine cells are those that release hormones into circulation in response to a neural signal. While overall rare, carcinoid tumors represent the most common of the neuroendocrine neoplasms in the gastrointestinal tract. Thirteen thousand seven hundred and fifteen cases in the United States were reported in the half-century between 1950 and 1999. Approximately two-thirds of the carcinoid tumors were found in the gastrointestinal tract, and one fourth were in the bronchopulmonary system. In the gastrointestinal tract, the top three locations were the small intestine (42%), rectum (27%), and stomach (9%). At the time of diagnosis, metastatic disease is most likely with carcinoids originating in the cecum and pancreas, and least likely with rectal, gastric, and bronchopulmonary lesions [78].

Gastrointestinal carcinoids frequently metastasize to the liver, at which point carcinoid syndrome (cutaneous flushing, diarrhea, bronchospasm, and palpitations) may occur. In comparison, primary hepatic carcinoid tumors (PHCT) are extremely rare, comprising 0.3% of all carcinoids. First described in 1958 by Edmondson, only 95 cases of PHCT have been reported in the literature as of 2004 [79, 80]. In one series, the age at diagnosis had a median of 50 years old but ranged from 8 to 83 years [81]. Unlike liver metastatic carcinoid tumors, PHCT are usually solitary, centrally located, and less likely to develop carcinoid syndrome [82]. Concurrent Zollinger–Ellison syndrome has been reported [83].

The proper diagnosis of PHCT necessitates a careful stepwise exclusion of extrahepatic carcinoid sources. One proposed diagnostic algorithm therefore consists of initial computed tomography and magnetic resonance imaging, followed by somatostatin scan, upper and lower endoscopies, bone scintigraphy, and explorative laparotomy. Previously resected specimens should be reexamined with staining for neuroendocrine markers. Finally, an extended long-term follow-up plan should be implemented [84]. The confirmation of PHCT is clinically important, as surgical resection and perhaps liver transplantation are potential therapeutic modalities for PHCT but not for secondary hepatic carcinoids. Ten-year survival approaches 70% for postresection PHCT patients [85].

Stauffer's Syndrome

Originally described by Stauffer as "nephrogenic hepatomegaly" in 1961, Stauffer's syndrome is a paraneoplastic hepatic dysfunction of nonhepatic malignancies that occurs in the absence of liver metastases [86]. Strictly defined Stauffer's syndrome is a paraneoplastic presentation of renal cell carcinoma (RCC); however, its constellation of findings is not unique to RCC but rather has been appreciated in the setting of other malignancies as well including lymphomas, bronchial adenocarcinoma, and prostate cancer [87, 88]. The term "Stauffer's syndrome" is therefore used here in the broad sense of its overall manifestation. Classically, Stauffer's is characterized by elevated alkaline phosphatase (ALP), erythrocyte sedimentation rate, alpha-2-globulin, and gamma-glutamyl transferase; thrombocytosis; prolongation of prothombin time; and hepatosplenomegaly. The original patients described were anicteric on presentation, but a less common variant with cholestatic jaundice has been reported more recently [89, 90].

The incidence of Stauffer's syndrome in RCC is estimated to be 3–20%. On occasion, it may be the singular manifestation of an otherwise occult cancer, and it has been noted as an early signal of tumor recurrence [91]. Specifically in RCC, the elevated ALP may normalize after a radical nephrectomy, while persistent or recurrent elevation may signify residual metastatic disease or tumor relapse. However, it should be stressed that the return of ALP to baseline alone does not imply cure of the disease [92]. The presence of Stauffer's syndrome may foreshadow a less favorable prognosis; in the study by Chuang et al., the 5-year survival rate for RCC patients with normal serum ALP was 71% vs. 51% in patients with isolated ALP elevation.

The pathophysiology of Stauffer's syndrome has been linked to a tumor production of cytokines, the specifics of which may vary between different malignancies. Interleukin-6 (IL-6) has been implicated in RCC, though tumor necrosis factor-alpha (TNF-alpha) or interleukin-1 alpha (IL-1 alpha) may also play a role in the paraneoplastic process [93]. The administration of anti-IL-6 in patients with Stauffer's syndrome often led to a decrease in serum ALP levels.

Malignant Transformation of Benign Hepatic Lesions

Benign liver tumors are relatively uncommon. In the order of decreasing prevalence, the top three diagnoses are hemangioma, focal nodular hyperplasia, and hepatic adenoma (HA). All affect women more often than men. Of these, only hepatic adenoma carries a (small) risk of malignant transformation.

The exact incidence and prevalence of hepatic adenoma are not known, but it is considered to be a rare neoplasm. Only few cases have ever been described in men. In women between ages of 16 and 44 with <24 months of exposure to oral contraceptives, HA develops at an annual rate of 1–1.3 per million [94]. The incidence increases fivefold by year five of oral contraceptive use, and 25- to 40-fold after nine or more years of exposure. High systemic estrogen levels may be the primary risk factor, as reports have illustrated decreases in tumor size when oral contraceptives were withheld and increases in size during pregnancy. Accordingly, the introduction of low-dose estrogen oral contraceptives in recent decades may have attenuated some of the risks mentioned above [95]. Other risk factors for HA include the use of anabolic androgenic steroids, elevated levels of endogenously produced androgens, and glycogen storage disease [96].

Hepatic adenoma may be asymptomatic or may present as intense abdominal pain, fever, and hypotension after spontaneous rupture and hemorrhage (in up to 30% of cases) [97]. The risk for this is particularly increased during pregnancy when HA may increase in size. In one multicenter series by Deneve et al., no ruptured HA was <5 cm in its largest diameter [98]. Histopathologically, hepatic adenomas may reach upward of 30 cm in diameter, are homogeneous, feature minimal portal tracts and biliary ducts, have thin-walled vasculature, and have absent Kupffer cells [99]. However, liver biopsy has a somewhat limited role in the diagnosis of HA. The diagnosis is usually made when a patient lacks clear HCC risk factors, the triphasic CT shows the characteristic appearance of HA, and the serum alpha-fetoprotein level is normal. Other laboratory tests are also generally normal.

Other than tumor rupture and hemorrhage as mentioned above, the most important potential complication of HA is its malignant transformation to HCC. This occurs in ~5% of all HA, and larger tumors appear to be more at risk. In the Deneve et al. series, no HA <8 cm in largest diameter had evidence of malignancy, and the mean size of malignant tumors was 11.6 cm. Elsewhere in the literature is the report of a 4-cm HA with multifocal malignant degeneration on histology; to date, this may be the smallest reported HA that has undergone malignant transformation [100]. In addition to tumor size, tumor number also has been implicated as a risk for malignancy. However, Dokmak et al., suggested otherwise, showing statistically insignificant differences in the rates of cancerous changes between patients with a single HA (11%), those having multiple HA (7%), and polyadenomatosis with more than 10 HA (3%) [101]. Finally, hepatic adenomas associated with type I glycogen storage disease are at an increased risk for malignant transformation [102].

References

1. Rugo HS. Paraneoplastic syndromes and other non-neoplastic effects of cancer. In: Goldman L, Ausiello D, editors. Cecil medicine [Internet]. 23rd ed. Philadelphia, PA: Saunders Elsevier; 2008. [cited 2011 Feb 19]. http://www.mdconsult.com/books/page.do?eid=4-u1.0-B978-1-4160-2805-5..50194-4&isbn=978-1-4160-2805-5&type=bookPage&sectionEid=4-u1.0-B978-1-4160-2805-5..50194-4--cesec2&uniqId=235911090-7#4-u1.0-B978-1-4160-2805-5.50194-4--cesec2.
2. Luo JC, Hwang SJ, Wu JC, et al. Paraneoplastic syndromes in patients with hepatocellular carcinoma in Taiwan. Cancer. 1999;86(5):799–804.
3. McFadzean AJ, Yeung RT. Further observation on hypoglycemia in hepatocellular carcinoma. Am J Med. 1969;47(2):200–35.
4. Thipaporn T, Bubpha P, Varaphon V. Hepatocellular carcinoma with persistent hypoglycemia: successful treatment with corticosteroid and frequent high carbohydrate intake. J Med Assoc Thai. 2005;88(12):1941–6.
5. Jayaprasad N, Anees T, Bijin T, Madhusoodanan S. Severe hypoglycemia due to poorly differentiated hepatocellular carcinoma. J Assoc Physicians India. 2006;54:413–5.
6. Horwitz MJ. Hypercalcemia of malignancy. In: Basow DS, editor. UpToDate [Internet]. Waltham, MA: UpToDate; 2011 [cited 21 Feb 2011]. http://www.uptodate.com/contents/hypercalcemia-of-malignancy?source=search_result&selectedTitle=1%7E150.
7. Oldenburg WA, Van Heerden JA, Sizemore GW. Hypercalcemia and primary hepatic tumors. Arch Surg. 1982;117(10):1363–6.

8. Attali P, Houssin D, Roche A. Hepatic arterial embolization for malignant hypercalcemia in hepatocellular carcinoma. Dig Dis Sci. 1984;29(5):446–9.

9. Tudela P, Soldevila B, Mòdol JM, Domènech E. Hypercalcemic encephalopathy in a patient with hepatocellular carcinoma. Dig Dis Sci. 2007;52(11):3296–7.

10. Ghobrial MW, George J, Mannam S, Henien SR. Severe hypercalcemia as an initial presenting manifestation of hepatocellular carcinoma. Can J Gastroenterol. 2002;16(9):607–9.

11. Mahoney EJ, Monchik JM, Donatini G, De Lellis R. Life-threatening hypercalcemia from a hepatocellular carcinoma secreting intact parathyroid hormone: localization by sestamibi single-photon emission computed tomographic imaging. Endocr Pract. 2006;12(3):302–6.

12. Abe Y, Makiyama H, Fujita Y, et al. Severe hypercalcemia associated with hepatocellular carcinoma secreting intact parathyroid hormone: a case report. Intern Med. 2011;50(4): 329–33.

13. Ariyachaipanich A, Takele T, McFarlane P, et al. The paradox of severe hypercholesterolemia and cachexia as a paraneoplastic manifestation of hepatocellular carcinoma. J Clin Lipidol. 2009;3(6):398–400.

14. Hwang S-J, Lee S-D, Chang C-F, et al. Hypercholesterolemia in patients with hepatocellular carcinoma. J Gastroenterol Hepatol. 1992;7:491–6.

15. Sohda T, Iwata K, Kitamura Y, et al. Reduced expression of low-density lipoprotein receptor in hepatocellular carcinoma with paraneoplastic hypercholesterolemia. J Gastroenterol Hepatol. 2008;23(7 Pt 2):e153–6.

16. Trotter JF, Cohn A, Grant R. Erythrocytosis in a patient with hepatocellular carcinoma. J Clin Gastroenterol. 2002;35(4):365–6.

17. Jacobson RJ, Lowenthal MN, Kew MC. Erythrocytosis in hepatocellular cancer. S Afr Med J. 1978;53(17):658–60.

18. McFadzean AJ, Todd D, Tsang KC. Polycythemia in primary carcinoma of the liver. Blood. 1958;13(5):427–35.

19. Chang PE, Tan CK. Paraneoplastic erythrocytosis as a primary presentation of hepatocellular carcinoma. Indian J Med Sci. 2009;63(5):202–3.

20. Sakisaka S, Watanabe M, Tateishi H, et al. Erythropoietin production in hepatocellular carcinoma cells associated with polycythemia: immunohistochemical evidence. Hepatology. 1993;18(6):1357–62.

21. Lai CL, Lam KC, Wong KP, et al. Clinical features of hepatocellular carcinoma: review of 211 patients in Hong Kong. Cancer. 1981;47(11):2746–55.

22. Bruix J, Castells A, Calvet X, et al. Diarrhea as a presenting symptom of hepatocellular carcinoma. Dig Dis Sci. 1990;35(6):681–5.

23. Steiner E, Velt P, Gutierrez O, et al. Hepatocellular carcinoma presenting with intractable diarrhea. A radiologic-pathologic correlation. Arch Surg. 1986;121(7):849–51.

24. Solinas A, Biscarini L, Morrelli A, Del Favero A. Hepatocellular carcinoma and the watery diarrhea syndrome. Arch Surg. 1988;123(1):124.

25. DiBisceglie AM, Hodkinson HJ, Berkowitz I, Kew MC. Pityriasis rotunda. A cutaneous marker of hepatocellular carcinoma in South African blacks. Arch Dermatol. 1986;122(7):802–4.

26. Miller ML. Clinical manifestations and diagnosis of adult dermatomyositis and polymyositis. In: Basow DS, editor. UpToDate [Internet]. Waltham, MA: UpToDate; 2011 [cited 23 Feb 2011]. http://www.uptodate.com/contents/clinical-manifestations-and-diagnosis-of-adult-dermatomyositis-and-polymyositis?source=preview&selectedTitle=1%7E136&anchor=H7#H7.

27. Sigurgeirsson B, Lindelöf B, Edhag O, Allander E. Risk of cancer in patients with dermatomyositis or polymyositis. A population-based study. N Engl J Med. 1992;326(6):363–7.

28. Hill CL, Zhang Y, Sigurgeirsson B, et al. Frequency of specific cancer types in dermatomyositis and polymyositis: a population-based study. Lancet. 2001;357(9250):96–100.

29. Toshikuni N, Torigoe R, Mitsunaga M, et al. Dermatomyositis associated with hepatocellular carcinoma in an elderly female patient with hepatitis C virus-related liver cirrhosis. World J Gastroenterol. 2006;12(10):1641–4.

30. Kee SJ, Kim TJ, Lee SJ, et al. Dermatomyositis associated with hepatitis B virus-related hepatocellular carcinoma. Rheumatol Int. 2009;29(5):595–9.

31. Cheng TI, Tsou MH, Yang PS, et al. Dermatomyositis and erythrocytosis associated with hepatocellular carcinoma. J Gastroenterol Hepatol. 2002;17(11):1239–40.
32. Fargnoli MC, Frascione P. Images in clinical medicine. *Acanthosis nigricans*. N Engl J Med. 2005;353(26):2797.
33. Rigel DS, Jacobs MI. Malignant *Acanthosis nigricans*: a review. J Dermatol Surg Oncol. 1980;6(11):923–7.
34. Kono T, Kobayashi H, Ishii M, et al. Synchronous development of disseminated superficial porokeratosis and hepatitis C virus-related hepatocellular carcinoma. J Am Acad Dermatol. 2000;43(5 Pt 2):966–8.
35. Torres T, Velho GC, Selores M. Disseminated superficial porokeratosis in a patient with cholangiocarcinoma: a paraneoplastic manifestation? An Bras Dermatol. 2010;85(2):229–31.
36. Thompson RP, Nicholson DC, Farnan T, et al. Cutaneous porphyria due to a malignancy primary hepatoma. Gastroenterology. 1970;59(5):779–83.
37. Fracanzani AL, Taioli E, Sampietro M, et al. Liver cancer risk is increased in patients with porphyria cutanea tarda in comparison to matched control patients with chronic liver disease. J Hepatol. 2001;35(4):498–503.
38. McCloskey JJ, Germain-Lee EL, Perman JA, et al. Gynecomastia as a presenting sign of fibrolamellar carcinoma of the liver. Pediatrics. 1988;82(3):379–82.
39. Aabo K, Dimitrov NV. Feminization in hepatocellular carcinoma corrected by chemotherapy: a case report. Med Pediatr Oncol. 1980;8(3):275–80.
40. Kew MC, Kirschner MA, Abrahams GE, Katz M. Mechanism of feminization in primary liver cancer. N Engl J Med. 1977;296(19):1084–8.
41. Darnell RB, Posner JB. Paraneoplastic syndromes involving the nervous system. N Engl J Med. 2003;349(16):1543–54.
42. Sugai F, Abe K, Fujimoto T, et al. Chronic inflammatory demyelinating polyneuropathy accompanied by hepatocellular carcinoma. Intern Med. 1997;36(1):53–5.
43. Arguedas MR, McGuire BM. Hepatocellular carcinoma presenting with chronic inflammatory demyelinating polyradiculoneuropathy. Dig Dis Sci. 2000;45(12):2369–73.
44. Vautravers C, Rat P, Cercueil JP, et al. Hepatocellular carcinoma presenting as paraneoplastic myasthenia gravis. Eur J Intern Med. 2008;19(8):e86–7.
45. Calvey HD, Melia WM, Williams R. Polyneuropathy: an unreported non-metastatic complication of primary hepatocellular carcinoma. Clin Oncol. 1983;9(3):199–202.
46. Walcher J, Witter T, Rupprecht HD. Hepatocellular carcinoma presenting with paraneoplastic demyelinating polyneuropathy and PR3-antineutrophil cytoplasmic antibody. J Clin Gastroenterol. 2002;35(4):364–5.
47. Hatzis GS, Delladetsima I, Koufos C. Hepatocellular carcinoma presenting with paraneoplastic neurologic syndrome in a hepatitis B surface antigen-positive patient. J Clin Gastroenterol. 1998;26(2):144–7.
48. Vauthey JN, Blumgart LH. Recent advances in the management of cholangiocarcinomas. Semin Liver Dis. 1994;14(2):109–14.
49. Trikudanathan G, Dasanu CA. Cholangiocarcinoma and paraneoplastic hypercalcemia: a lethal combination revisited. South Med J. 2010;103(7):716–6.
50. Davis JM, Sadasivan R, Dwyer T, Van Veldhuizen P. Case report: cholangiocarcinoma and hypercalcemia. Am J Med Sci. 1994;307(5):350–2.
51. Tzovaras V, Liberopoulos EN, Zioga A, et al. Persistent erythema multiforme in a patient with extrahepatic cholangiocarcinoma. Oncology. 2007;73(1–2):127–9.
52. Wetter DA. Pathogenesis, clinical features, and diagnosis of erythema multiforme. In: Basow DS, editor. UpToDate [Internet]. Waltham, MA: UpToDate; 2011. [cited 28 Feb 2011]. http://www.uptodate.com/contents/pathogenesis-clinical-features-and-diagnosis-of-erythema-multiforme?source=preview&anchor=H5&selectedTitle=1~150#H6.
53. von den Driesch P. Sweet's syndrome (acute febrile neutrophilic dermatosis). J Am Acad Dermtol. 1994;31(4):535–56.
54. Cohen PR, Talpaz M, Kurzrock R. Malignancy-associated Sweet's syndrome: review of the world literature. J Clin Oncol. 1988;6(12):1887–97.

55. Shinojima Y, Toma Y, Terui T. Sweet syndrome associated with intrahepatic cholangiocarcinoma producing granulocyte colon-stimulating factor. Br J Dermatol. 2006;155(5):1103–4.
56. Bazex A, Griffiths A. Acrokeratosis paraneoplastica—a new cutaneous marker of malignancy. Br J Dermatol. 1980;103(3):301–6.
57. Bolognia JL. Bazex' syndrome. Clin Dermatol. 1993;11(1):37–42.
58. Bolognia JL, Brewer YP, Cooper DL. Bazex syndrome (acrokeratosis paraneoplastica). An analytic review. Medicine (Baltimore). 1991;70(4):269–80.
59. Karabulut AA, Sahin S, Sahin M, et al. Paraneoplastic acrokeratosis of Bazex (Bazex's syndrome): report of a female case associated with cholangiocarcinoma and review of the published work. J Dermatol. 2006;33(12):850–4.
60. Lee HW, Oh SH, Choi JC, et al. Disseminated superficial porokeratosis in a patient with cholangiocarcinoma. J Am Acad Dermatol. 2006;54(2 Suppl):S56–8.
61. Sökmen M, Demirsoy H, Ersoy O, et al. Paraneoplastic porphyria cutanea tarda associated with cholangiocarcinoma: case report. Turk J Gastroenterol. 2007;18(3):200–5.
62. Sack Jr GH, Levin J, Bell WR. Trousseau's syndrome and other manifestations of chronic disseminated coagulopathy in patients with neoplasms: clinical, pathophysiologic, and therapeutic features. Medicine (Baltimore). 1977;56(1):1–37.
63. Callander N, Rapaport SI. Trousseau's syndrome. West J Med. 1993;158(4):364–71.
64. Walsh-McMonagle D, Green D. Low-molecular-weight heparin in the management of Trousseau's syndrome. Cancer. 1997;80(4):649–55.
65. Hernández JL, Riancho JA, González-Macías J. Cholangiocarcinoma presenting as Trousseau's syndrome. Am J Gastroenterol. 1998;93(5):847–8.
66. Jang JW, Yeo CD, Kim JD, et al. Trousseau's syndrome in association with cholangiocarcinoma: positive tests for coagulation factors and anticardiolipin antibody. J Korean Med Sci. 2006;21(1):155–9.
67. Lee AY, Levine MN, Baker RI, et al. Low-molecular-weight heparin versus a coumarin for the prevention of recurrent venous thromboembolism in patients with cancer. N Engl J Med. 2003;349(2):146–53.
68. Ata AA, Kamel IA. Primary reticulum cell sarcoma of the liver: a case report. J Egypt Med Assoc. 1965;48(7):514–21.
69. Leung VK, Lin SY, Loke TK, et al. Primary hepatic peripheral T-cell lymphoma in a patient with chronic hepatitis B infection. Hong Hong Med J. 2009;15(4):288–90.
70. Kitabayashi K, Hasegawa T, Ueno K, et al. Primary hepatic non-Hodgkin's lymphoma in a patient with chronic hepatitis C: report of a case. Surg Today. 2004;34(4):366–9.
71. Ohsawa M, Aozasa K, Horiuchi K, et al. Malignant lymphoma of the liver. Report of five cases and review of the literature. Dig Dis Sci. 1992;37(7):1105–9.
72. Chowla A, Malhi-Chowla N, Chidambaram A, Surick B. Primary hepatic lymphoma in hepatitis C: case report and review of the literature. Am Surg. 1999;65(9):881–3.
73. Scerpella EG, Villareal AA, Casanova PF, Moreno JN. Primary lymphoma of the liver in AIDS. Report of one new case and review of the literature. J Clin Gastroenterol. 1996;22(1):51–3.
74. Leung VK, Lin SY, Loke TK, et al. Primary hepatic peripheral T-cell lymphoma in a patient with chronic hepatitis B infection. Hong Kong Med J. 2009;15(4):288–90.
75. Hsiao HH, Liu YC, Hsu JF, et al. Primary liver lymphoma with hypercalcemia: a case report. Kaohsiung J Med Sci. 2009;25(3):141–4.
76. Aghai E, Quitt M, Lurie M, et al. Primary hepatic lymphoma presenting as symptomatic immune thrombocytopenic purpura. Cancer. 1987;60(9):2308–11.
77. Schweiger F, Shinder R, Rubin S. Primary lymphoma of the liver: a case report and review. Can J Gastroenterol. 2000;14(11):955–7.
78. Modlin IM, Lye KD, Kidd M. A 5-decade analysis of 13,715 carcinoid tumors. Cancer. 2003;97(4):934–59.
79. Edmondson HA. Carcinoid tumor. In: Tumors of the liver and intrahepatic bile ducts (Atlas of Tumor Pathology). Washington: Armed Forces Institute of Pathology; 1958:105–11.
80. Modlin IM, Shapiro MD, Kidd M. An analysis of rare carcinoid tumors: clarifying these clinical conundrums. World J Surg. 2005;29(1):92–101.

81. Gravante G, De Liguori Carino N, Overton J, et al. Primary carcinoids of the liver: a review of symptoms, diagnosis and treatments. Dig Surg. 2008;25(5):364–8.
82. Shetty PK, Baliga SV, Balaiah K, Gnana PS. Primary hepatic neuroendocrine tumor: an unusual cystic presentation. Indian J Pathol Microbiol. 2010;53(4):760–2.
83. Rascarachi G, Sierra M, Hernando M, et al. Primary liver carcinoid tumour with a Zollinger Ellison syndrome—an unusual diagnosis: a case report. Cases J. 2009;2:6346.
84. Fenwick SW, Wyatt JI, Toogood GJ, Lodge JP. Hepatic resection and transplantation for primary carcinoid tumors of the liver. Ann Surg. 2004;239(2):210–9.
85. Knox CD, Anderson CD, Lamps LW, et al. Long-term survival after resection for primary hepatic carcinoid tumor. Ann Surg Oncol. 2003;10(10):1171–5.
86. Stauffer MH. Nephrogenic hepatomegaly. Gastroenterology. 1961;40:694.
87. Saintigny P, Spano JP, Tcherakian F, et al. Non-metastatic intrahepatic cholestasis associated with bronchial adenocarcinoma. Ann Med Interne (Paris). 2003;154(3):171–5.
88. Karakolios A, Kasapis C, Kallinikidis T, et al. Cholestatic jaundice as a paraneoplastic manifestation of prostate adenocarcinoma. Clin Gastroenterol Hepatol. 2003;1(6):480–3.
89. Dourakis SP, Sinani C, Deutsch M, et al. Cholestatic jaundice as a paraneoplastic manifestation of renal cell carcinoma. Eur J Gastroenterol Hepatol. 1997;9(3):311–4.
90. Morla D, Alazemi S, Lichtstein D. Stauffer's syndrome variant with cholestatic jaundice: a case report. J Gen Intern Med. 2006;21(7):C11–3.
91. Girotra M, Abraham RR, Pahwa M, Arora M. Is Stauffer's syndrome an early indicator of RCC recurrence? ANZ J Surg. 2010;80(12):949–50.
92. Chuang YC, Lin AT, Chen KK, et al. Paraneoplastic elevation of serum alkaline phosphatase in renal cell carcinoma: incidence and implication on prognosis. J Urol. 1997;158(5):1684–7.
93. Blay JY, Rossi JF, Wijdenes J, et al. Role of interleukin-6 in the paraneoplastic inflammatory syndrome associated with renal-cell carcinoma. Int J Cancer. 1997;72(3):424–30.
94. Rooks JB, Ory HW, Ishak KG, et al. Epidemiology of hepatocellular adenoma. The role of oral contraceptive use. J Am Med Assoc. 1979;242(7):644–8.
95. Giannitrapani L, Soresi M, La Spada E, et al. Sex hormones and risk of liver tumor. Ann N Y Acad Sci. 2006;1089:228–36.
96. Maillette de Buy Wenniger L, Terpstra V, Beuers U. Focal nodular hyperplasia and hepatic adenoma: epidemiology and pathology. Dig Surg. 2010;27(1):24–31.
97. Cho SW, Marsh JW, Steel J, et al. Surgical management of hepatocellular adenoma: take it or leave it? Ann Surg Oncol. 2008;15(10):2795–803.
98. Deneve JL, Pawlik TM, Cunningham S, et al. Liver cell adenoma: a multicenter analysis of risk factors for rupture and malignancy. Ann Surg Oncol. 2009;16(3):640–8.
99. Lizardi-Cervera J, Cuéllar-Gamboa L, Motola-Kuba D. Focal nodular hyperplasia and hepatic adenoma: a review. Ann Hepatol. 2006;5(3):206–11.
100. Micchelli ST, Vivekanandan P, Boitnott JK, et al. Malignant transformation of hepatic adenomas. Mod Pathol. 2008;21(4):491–7.
101. Dokmak S, Paradis V, Vilgrain V, et al. A single-center surgical experience of 122 patients with single and multiple hepatocellular adenomas. Gastroenterology. 2009;137(5):1698–705.
102. Labrune P, Trioche P, Duvaltier I, et al. Hepatocellular adenomas in glycogen storage disease type I and III: a series of 43 patients and review of the literature. J Pediatr Gastroenterol Nutr. 1997;24(3):276–9.

Chapter 7
Hepatocellular Carcinoma in Children

Christiane Sokollik, Abha Gupta, and Simon C. Ling

Abbreviations

α1-AT	Alpha-1-antitrypsin
AJCC	American Joint Committee on Cancer
COG	Children's Oncology Group
FAP	Familial adenomatous polyposis
FL-HCC	Fibrolamellar HCC
GSD1	Glycogen storage disease type 1
HB	Hepatoblastoma
HCC	Hepatocellular carcinoma
HBV	Hepatitis B virus
HCV	Hepatitis C virus
HT-1	Hereditary tyrosinemia type 1
L3-AFP	Lectin-reactive alpha-fetoprotein
OLT	Orthotopic liver transplantation
PRETEXT	Pretreatment extent of disease
PFIC	Progressive familial intrahepatic cholestasis
SIOPEL	Societé Internationale d'Oncologie Pédiatrique

C. Sokollik, MD • S.C. Ling, MBChB, MRCP (✉)
Division of Gastroenterology, Hepatology and Nutrition,
Department of Paediatrics, University of Toronto, The Hospital for Sick Children,
Toronto, Canada
e-mail: simon.ling@sickkids.ca

A. Gupta, MD, MSc, FRCPC
Division of Hematology/Oncology, Department of Paediatrics,
University of Toronto, The Hospital for Sick Children, Toronto, Canada

N. Reau and F.F. Poordad (eds.), *Primary Liver Cancer: Surveillance, Diagnosis and Treatment*, Clinical Gastroenterology, DOI 10.1007/978-1-61779-863-4_7,
© Springer Science+Business Media New York 2012

Epidemiology

Incidence and Prevalence

Hepatocellular carcinoma (HCC) is the second most common malignant liver tumor in children after hepatoblastoma (HB) and accounts for approximately 0.3% of all pediatric malignancies [1]. The age-adjusted incidence rate of HCC in the United States in children is 0.41 (0.24–0.65) per 1,000,000 population, with no gender predominance [1]. Children with HCC may present at any age, although the incidence is highest between the ages of 10–19 years [1–3].

The main risk factors for development of HCC in children include the following: perinatally acquired hepatitis B infection, disorders causing neonatal cholestasis and progressive fibrotic liver disease (e.g., biliary atresia, progressive familial intrahepatic cholestasis), and metabolic diseases (e.g., hereditary tyrosinemia) (Table 7.1). These predisposing conditions are identified in only a minority of children with HCC and are largely dependent on the population prevalence of hepatitis B [1].

HCC and Hepatitis B Virus (HBV) and Hepatitis C Virus (HCV) in Children

In populations with a high prevalence of vertically transmitted HBV infection such as Alaska, Taiwan, and Japan, nearly 100% of children with HCC also have hepatitis B infection [4, 5]. Immunization of newborns against HBV in these high-risk populations has led to a reduction in HBV-positive HCC [5–7]. An HBV vaccination program was initiated in Taiwan in 1984, and the incidence of HCC among children 6–14 years of age dropped from 0.70 per 100,000 children in 1981–1986 to 0.36 in 1990–1994 [7]. Boys seemed to have a higher incidence and profited more from vaccination than girls [8]. There was no change in the number of brain tumors

Table 7.1 Risk factors for the development of HCC in children

Underlying liver disease	Hepatitis B infection
	Biliary atresia
	Alagille syndrome
	Progressive familial intrahepatic cholestasis (PFIC) type 1 and 2
	Hereditary tyrosinemia
	Alpha-1 antitrypsin deficiency
	Wilson disease
	Glycogen storage disease, type 1
Exposure to toxins	Arsenic
	Aflatoxin
	Radiation

in the same time period, supporting the causal relationship between hepatitis B status and development of HCC. Similar efficacy of HBV vaccination in preventing HCC was shown for Alaskan children, where 16 HCC cases were reported before the start of a vaccination program in 1984 and none in the 20 years thereafter [5].

Hepatitis C infection in the majority of childhood cases follows a mild clinical course without elevated liver enzymes or significant fibrosis [9]. This may explain the rarity of HCV-related HCC in childhood in comparison to adults. In a histological study with the aim to define the natural history of HCV infection in children, 6 (14%) of 42 liver biopsies showed bridging fibrosis or early cirrhosis after a mean duration of infection of 13.4 years [10]. One of the two patients who underwent liver transplantation for portal hypertension and chronic liver disease had HCC lesions in his native liver [10]. Even immunosuppressive and hepatotoxic therapy at the time of infection with HCV seems not to significantly raise the likelihood of liver disease progression and HCC development during childhood. In a cohort of 148 hepatitis C seropositive survivors of childhood cancer of the St. Jude Children's Research Hospital, only two patients were identified to have developed HCC more than 20 years after treatment of acute lymphocytic leukemia in childhood [11, 12].

Other Liver Diseases in Children and HCC Risk

Hereditary tyrosinemia type 1 (HT-1) is an inborn error of tyrosine catabolism due to a defect of the fumarylacetoacetate hydrolase enzyme. The resulting accumulation of fumarylacetoacetate leads to hepatocellular damage, neonatal cholestasis, and coagulopathy and subsequently increases the risk of HCC through mechanisms that are not yet clear [13]. Treatment with nitisinone became available in 1992 to inhibit the upstream enzyme, 4-hydroxyphenylpyruvate dioxygenase, and thus prevent the accumulation of the toxic metabolites. Without nitisinone therapy, the incidence of HCC in HT-1 patients is between 17% and 37% [13, 14]. This risk is greatly reduced if nitisinone treatment is started in the first months of life, such that none of 41 patients developed HCC during a mean treatment duration of over 4 years [15]. However, HCC has been described in cases where treatment was delayed to 2 years of age, and it is hypothesized that predisposing liver damage had already taken place [15, 16].

Alpha-1-antitrypsin (α1-AT) deficiency primarily manifests as lung disease in adults but is also associated with neonatal liver disease, which may progress to cirrhosis during childhood. In patients with the PiZ allele, the polymeric mutant α1-AT accumulates in the endoplasmic reticulum of hepatocytes and causes cell stress. These damaged cells may chronically stimulate neighboring undamaged cells, which then undergo proliferation [17]. This may explain why the origin of the HCC lesion is not necessarily in a cirrhotic area. Although α1-AT deficiency is one of the more common metabolic diseases in children [18], the development of HCC is mainly described in adults [19–21].

There are single case reports of children with Alagille syndrome who have developed HCC [22, 23]. Alagille syndrome is an autosomal dominant cholestatic disorder due to mutation in the *JAG1* or *NOTCH2* genes [24] and is characterized histologically by a paucity of intrahepatic bile ducts. NOTCH signaling plays a role in cell differentiation and proliferation, and it is unclear whether disruption of this signaling or the presence of cirrhotic liver disease is the main trigger for development of HCC in Alagille syndrome [25].

Focal abnormalities of the liver are found in patients with glycogen storage disease type 1 (GSD1), including fatty infiltration, focal nodular hyperplasia, and hepatic adenomas. In a European multicenter retrospective study of patients with GSD1, hepatic adenomas were detected at a median age of 15 years and had an overall prevalence of 16% [26]. None of the 288 patients in this series had evidence of malignant transformation, and although HCC is estimated to occur in 5% of patients with hepatic adenomas [27], there are likely distinct molecular events responsible for the genesis of the two lesions [28]. Although case reports describe the development of HCC in young adults with glycogen storage disease type 1 [29], the relative risk compared to the general population is difficult to ascertain.

The most common cause for early childhood cirrhosis and consequent liver transplantation is biliary atresia. This fibro-obliterative disorder of the biliary tree may be treated by a surgical portoenterostomy to reestablish bile flow within the first few weeks of life, but typically causes progressive liver disease thereafter with eventual requirement for liver transplantation in the majority of affected children. Previously unrecognized small HCC nodules have rarely been found in explanted livers of infants and children with biliary atresia [30–33].

Progressive familial intrahepatic cholestasis (PFIC) types 1 and 2 are characterized by normal serum concentration of gamma-glutamyl transferase despite a picture of cholestatic neonatal hepatitis. In PFIC type 2, mutations in the ABCB11 gene lead to the disrupted synthesis of functional bile salt export pump (BSEP) [34]. The description of ten children with PFIC type 2 who developed HCC before the age of 5 years highlights the need for close observation of patients with PFIC type 2 for the development of HCC [35]. The mechanism of hepatocarcinogenesis in this case series is unclear, but all had cirrhosis at the time of diagnosis of their HCC [35].

Patients with familial adenomatous polyposis (FAP), which is caused by a germline mutation of the adenomatous polyposis coli (APC) gene, develop multiple colonic polyps with an increased risk of malignant transformation and need for colectomy [36]. Hepatoblastoma has been acknowledged as an extracolonic manifestation of FAP [37, 38]. Single case reports also describe the occurrence of HCC in patients with FAP and mutations in the APC gene [39, 40]. APC interacts with the Wnt/β-catenin pathway in the liver where deletion of APC can lead to β-catenin activation and development of HCC [41]. Already in childhood, aberrant signaling pathways due to mutations in tumor suppressor genes and cirrhosis seem to be mechanisms of hepatocarcinogenesis.

HCC and Exposure to Environmental Toxins

Environmental exposures to inorganic arsenic or aflatoxin have been identified as risk factors for development of HCC through epidemiological studies that rely mostly on the incidence of HCC in adults [42, 43]. Arsenic exposure arises from ingestion of contaminated drinking water or cooking using coal with high arsenic content and has been clearly associated with hepatotoxicity manifesting as elevated liver enzymes, hepatomegaly, noncirrhotic portal hypertension, and cirrhosis. Although multiple studies have explored the association between arsenic exposure and HCC, conflicting results further complicated by the suboptimal quality of some studies have precluded designation of arsenic as a clearly proven hepatic carcinogen [43]. Studies of arsenic exposure and liver cancer in children are scarce. Children in the Antofagasta and Mejillones area of Chile were exposed to high concentrations of arsenic in their drinking water between 1958 and 1970 [44]. When compared to children in other areas without excess arsenic exposure, those children exposed at an early age had an especially high incidence of HCC-related mortality in the 0–19-year age range (relative risk 10.6, 95% CI 2.9–39.2). No difference was found for the incidence of other more common childhood cancers, such as leukemia and brain cancer [44].

Biology of HCC in Children

Only one third of pediatric patients have a history of underlying liver disease that may have predisposed them to developing their tumor [45]; in contrast, 70–90% of HCCs in adults are associated with cirrhosis which is an unfavorable prognostic feature [46, 47].

In addition to the typical histologic HCC, there are two additional distinct types of HCC noted in children: transitional liver cell tumors and fibrolamellar HCC. Prokurat et al. described a unique entity termed "transitional liver cell tumors" in seven patients between the ages of 5–18 years. These tumors were morphologically situated between hepatoblastoma and HCC and were positive immunohistochemically for both AFP and β-catenin [48]. The frequency of this subtype in pediatric studies of HCC is unclear.

Fibrolamellar HCC (FL-HCC) is another entity common in younger patients. Microscopically, the "usual" hepatocellular carcinoma and the fibrolamellar variant present distinctly different features. The usual HCC is composed of small and large trabeculae, the latter of which may display central necrosis, imparting an acinar or pseudoglandular appearance. Individual cells have nuclear hyperchromasia, anisocytosis, multiple nucleoli, cytoplasmic bile staining, and frequent and bizarre mitoses [49]. Initially described by Edmunson et al., the fibrolamellar variant is characterized by large, deeply eosinophilic hepatocytes embedded within lamellar fibrosis [50]. Clusters of these cells are separated by narrow to broad bands of laminated collagen. AFP staining is less frequent in FL compared with the usual HCC cases [51]. A review of the Surveillance, Epidemiology, and End Results (SEER) database, which captures tumors that occur in about 14% of the United States population, revealed 68/7964 (0.9%) of HCCs were of the FL type [52]. A prospective study of pediatric HCC described 10 of 46 cases being of FL type [53]. FL-HCC occurs in younger people with noncirrhotic livers (median age 25–39 years), with an equal gender distribution, unlike common HCC which is male dominated [52, 54]. Patients with FL-HCC were once thought to carry a favorable prognosis compared to standard HCC due to a slower rate of growth and more indolent course [55]. However, despite the possibility of late recurrences, more recent studies fail to confirm a favorable prognosis and rather suggest that complete surgical resection of tumor is essential for cure [53, 54].

In adult HCC, a minimum 20-year latency period is typical for viral-related tumor development, whereas HCC in childhood can develop in as few as 3 years after perinatal HBV exposure. The reason for the short period for malignant transformation in childhood HCC is still undetermined, as is the pathogenesis of non-viral-associated HCC [56, 57]. Alternate molecular events are likely responsible for HCC in younger patients. The MET proto-oncogene encodes a transmembrane tyrosine kinase identified as the receptor of a polypeptide known as HGF/SF3. The HGF/Met signaling pathway regulates multiple cellular and physiological functions and is also a powerful oncogene regulating metastasis formation, tumor invasion, and angiogenesis [58]. A Met-regulated gene expression signature characterizes a subgroup of HCC with aggressive phenotypic traits and poor prognosis [58]. In one small series, three missense mutations in the tyrosine kinase domain were detected exclusively in 10 childhood HCCs, while no mutations were detected in 16 adult HCCs, 21 cholangiocarcinomas, or 28 hepatoblastomas [59]. Cyclin-D1 is a cell cycle regulator, and downregulation of cyclin-D1 has been shown to be associated with high tumor grade and poor prognosis in adult HCC [60]. In a small series of nine pediatric and nine adult HCCs, pediatric HCCs were associated with a greater frequency of cyclin-D1 downregulation by immunohistochemical staining [61].

In summary, pathological examination of pediatric HCC should scrutinize for transitional or fibrolamellar subtypes, but despite the striking differences between the epidemiology and physiology of adult vs. pediatric HCC, no histological nor molecular differences have yet been identified that separates standard pediatric from adult HCC.

Clinical Presentation

The main presenting symptoms of HCC in children include either a painless abdominal mass or abdominal pain, followed by nonspecific symptoms such as weight loss, vomiting, and general weakness [62, 63]. Due to these subtle symptoms and a high "de novo" rate without an underlying liver disease, a majority of children have already developed an advanced stage tumor at diagnosis [64]. Very rarely, biliary obstruction may cause jaundice and pruritus. HCC has a disposition for vascular invasion and metastasis; at diagnosis, vascular involvement is present in one quarter and lung metastasis in one third of cases [64]. Although there is little data to explain this advanced stage at presentation, it may be due to later presentation in children who often have no recognized underlying liver disease who are not undergoing screening tests.

International guidelines recommend screening and surveillance for HCC in high-risk adult patients, especially in adults with cirrhosis [65]. Similar guidelines for children are not available because studies have not been undertaken to quantify the incidence of HCC in children at risk (e.g., those with underlying liver diseases associated with HCC) or to determine the cost-effectiveness of screening techniques in the pediatric age group. In spite of this, many pediatric hepatologists try to detect HCC lesions in a resectable stage to improve survival using ultrasound scan and alpha-fetoprotein as first-line tools, accepting their limitations and the lack of certainty about the optimal frequency of screening. There are no special guidelines for children, and it should be taken into account that an underlying liver disease or cirrhosis is not required for HCC to develop in childhood [45].

Differential Diagnosis and Diagnostic Investigation

The primary differential diagnosis of a liver mass and raised alpha-fetoprotein (AFP) includes hepatoblastoma, which is the most common liver tumor in the pediatric population and accounts for 67% of liver cancers in persons less than 20 years of age in the USA [1]. In contrast to HCC, it occurs mainly in infants and younger children under 3 years of age [1, 3]. Associations have been described between hepatoblastoma and low birth weight, as well as with the genetic disorders, Beckwith–Wiedemann syndrome, and familial adenomatous polyposis coli [38, 66]. Hepatoblastoma usually presents as an asymptomatic abdominal mass, later associated with weight loss, anorexia, vomiting, and abdominal pain. AFP is elevated in almost all children with hepatoblastoma. Diagnosis relies on imaging, AFP, and tissue microscopy of either a biopsy or resection specimen.

Other malignant (rhabdoid, sarcoma) and benign liver masses (regenerative nodule, focal nodular hyperplasia, hepatic adenoma, benign vascular tumors, mesenchymal hamartoma) should also be considered in the differential diagnosis (Table 7.2). Investigation therefore requires appropriate bloodwork, imaging, and liver biopsy.

Bloodwork

Routine laboratory tests in all children with suspected HCC should be undertaken to establish the presence of underlying liver disease or secondary complications such as biliary obstruction.

Table 7.2 Liver tumors in children

Tumor	Age at presentation	Special features
Benign		
Hemangioendothelioma	Infancy and early childhood	Association with skin hemangiomas; presentation with congestive heart failure possible
Mesenchymal hamartoma	Infancy and early childhood	Large, multilocular cysts
Hepatocellular adenoma	Adolescence	Usually solitary lesion; intralesional hemorrhage; teenage girls, hx of oral contraceptives; may be multiple in association with glycogen storage disease
Focal nodular hyperplasia	Late childhood and adolescence	Predominantly in females; central scar
Nodular regenerative hyperplasia	Adolescence	Multiple nodules, may be associated with portal hypertension
Malignant		
Hepatoblastoma	Infancy and early childhood	Presentation with enlarged abdomen; some produce HCG with precocious puberty; association with Beckwith–Wiedemann, familial adenomatous polyposis, low birth weight
Hepatocellular carcinoma	Late childhood and adolescence	Association with underlying liver diseases (see text) and "de novo" in noncirrhotic livers
Fibrolamellar variant	Adolescence	Normal AFP; large, deeply eosinophilic hepatocytes within lamellar fibrosis
Sarcomas		
Undifferentiated embryonal sarcoma	Late childhood	Presentation with abdominal pain or mass; AFP negative
Angiosarcoma	Late childhood	Possibly develops within hemangioendothelioma; hypercellular nodules
Embryonal rhabdomyosarcoma	Early childhood	Jaundice due to obstruction of the biliary tree; botryoid growth pattern
Rhabdoid tumor	Infancy	Mainly affects the kidneys
Germ cell tumor	Infancy	May be mixed with other tumor components (e.g., hepatoblastoma, HCC)
Cholangiocarcinoma	Late childhood	Association with choledochal cyst, PSC

AFP has a low sensitivity for the diagnosis of HCC in younger children and is also nonspecific; however, it is a well-established marker for hepatoblastoma. In a retrospective analysis of 46 children with HCC, one third had AFP levels within the normal range at the time of diagnosis [67]. The situation is still more challenging in children with tyrosinemia, in whom high AFP levels are common at diagnosis and may stay elevated or show a secondary rise after starting nitisinone treatment [15].

Lectin-reactive alpha-fetoprotein (L3-AFP) is an AFP isoform that may have greater potential to discriminate between HCC and other masses in the adult population [68]. In a pediatric study of 12 patients with hereditary tyrosinemia and HCC,

L3-AFP showed an early increase in 50%, but in the rest, the increase was delayed or absent [69]. Therefore, L3-AFP may provide supporting information if raised, but a normal value does not exclude malignant transformation. Further studies of biomarkers to improve the early detection of HCC in children with underlying metabolic or familial liver disease are required.

Imaging Modalities

Ultrasound is a preferred imaging modality in children as it is free of ionizing radiation, can be performed repeatedly and without sedation, and therefore has a significant value in screening and post-therapeutic monitoring. The morphology, location, and distribution of lesions can be characterized, and color Doppler examination enables assessment of the vascularization of a tumor and its relationship to vessels.

CT and MRI images provide additional information during staging and preoperative evaluation of resectability. These imaging modalities are superior to ultrasound for the assessment of bile duct and vessel invasion [70]. On CT and MRI scans, HCC is an arterially enhancing mass with a delayed venous washout phase [71].

A chest CT to rule out lung metastasis should be performed in all HCC patients. Intracranial and skeletal metastases are described in children with HCC and need to be ruled out with brain MRI or bone scan if suspected [62].

Role of Biopsy

The diagnosis of HCC in adults with liver cirrhosis can be made when the AFP level is above 200 ng/ml, the tumor exceeds 2 cm, and the typical vascular patterns of HCC are demonstrated on imaging. A biopsy is only mandatory in noncirrhotic patients, in patients with smaller nodules, or those with atypical imaging [65]. However, biopsy prior to treatment is strongly recommended for children to rule out hepatoblastoma, especially due to the rarity of pediatric HCC and stark differences in treatment approaches between HCC and hepatoblastoma [45].

Staging

The staging of adult HCC is based on the American Joint Committee on Cancer (AJCC) criteria. Certain features are considered to be important when considering liver transplantation in patients with unresectable disease, such as the size and number of lesions and macrovascular invasion [72–74]. In children, the staging of HCC has historically followed the PRETEXT (pretreatment extent of disease) system of the Liver Tumor Strategy Group of the Societe International Oncologie

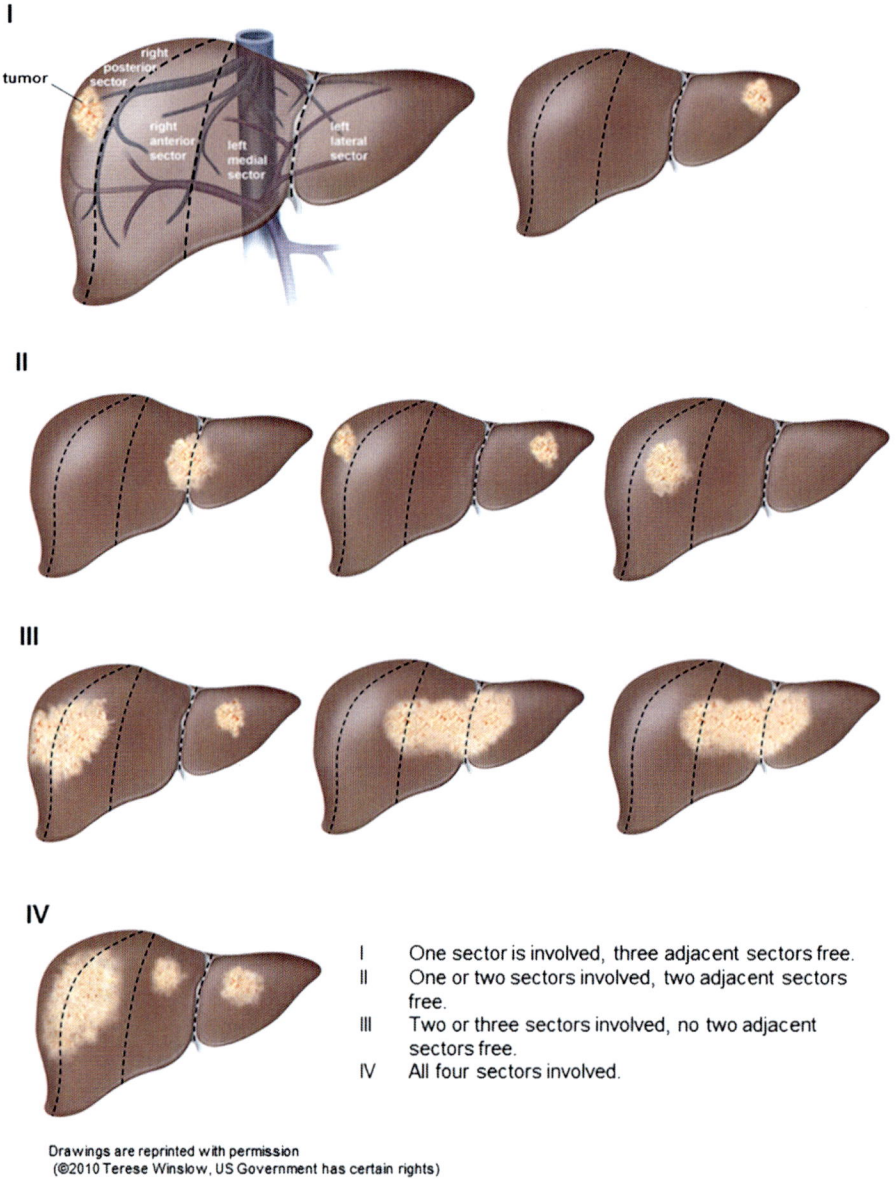

I

II

III

IV

I	One sector is involved, three adjacent sectors free.
II	One or two sectors involved, two adjacent sectors free.
III	Two or three sectors involved, no two adjacent sectors free.
IV	All four sectors involved.

Drawings are reprinted with permission
(©2010 Terese Winslow, US Government has certain rights)

Fig. 7.1 Possible tumor distribution according to the PRETEXT staging

Pediatrique (SIOPEL) or the Children's Oncology Group staging classification, primarily developed for hepatoblastoma (Fig. 7.1). The PRETEXT staging was revised in 2005 with the intention to be applicable to all primary malignant liver tumors of childhood [75]. PRETEXT is a system that objectively defines the extent of the tumor within the liver (PRETEXT I, II, III, and IV) by grouping the liver segments into four surgical sectors [76]. Extrahepatic extensions are indicated by letters: V for hepatic vein, P for portal vein, E for extrahepatic, and M for distant metastasis [75]. The Children's Oncology Group (COG) describes four stages: I, resected disease; II, resected disease with microscopic residual; III, unresectable; and IV, distant metastases. Neither of these pediatric staging systems has been independently validated for HCC, nor have they been correlated with the AJCC system. It is clear, however, that children with distant metastases fair poorly [64, 67].

Treatment

Chemotherapy

Historically, COG and SIOPEL have explored the role of chemotherapy in HCC as an extrapolation of the treatment of hepatoblastoma. Consequently, the outcome of HCC in children has only been reported in the setting of chemotherapy [64, 67]. The response rate of HCC in children treated with cisplatin and doxorubicin (PLADO) or cisplatin/5-fluorouracil/vincristine approaches 50% [64, 67], which is higher than the response rate observed in adult HCC (0–33%) [77, 78]. Regardless of the observed response to chemotherapy, pediatric HCC cannot be cured without complete resection of all sites of disease. The 5-year event-free survival on the COG study for children with completely resected HCC (stage I, $n=8$), partially resected disease (stage III, $n=25$), or those with distant metastases (stage IV, $n=13$) was 88%, 8%, and 0%, respectively [67]. Similarly, 8/40 children reported by SIOPEL were alive (median follow-up 75 months), all of whom had complete surgical resection of their tumor [64]. So far, comparative historical data for pediatric patients in the absence of chemotherapy are lacking, and since documented pediatric survivors of HCC have all had complete resection of their disease, the benefit of additional chemotherapy is questionable. Similar observations were made in the German Pediatric Liver Tumor Group study HEPATOBLASTOMA99 in which all children were treated with carboplatin and etoposide. Tumor-free survival was achieved in 18/20 patients with completely resected disease, whereas only 1/22 patients with advanced disease were alive at the time of reporting [79]. The most recent study from SIOPEL (V) restricts delivery of chemotherapy to those patients who have unresectable disease. Neoadjuvant chemotherapy may be offered to children with unresectable disease to attempt cytoreduction and potentially permit resection. However, it is important to define this goal to the patient and family at the initiation of therapy. In the COG study, only 1 out of 25 patients with unresectable disease successfully underwent complete tumor resection after receiving neoadjuvant chemotherapy [67]. Children with unresectable HCC (with no evidence of extrahepatic disease) should be referred immediately to tertiary care centers with expertise in pediatric transplantation [67].

Sorafenib is a dual-kinase inhibitor targeting both the vascular endothelial growth factor receptor family of proteins and the B-Raf/Met pathway [80]. Sorafenib was the first drug to be shown in a randomized, placebo-controlled trial to improve survival of adults with advanced HCC, leading to FDA approval of this agent in HCC [81]. More recently, sorafenib plus doxorubicin was shown to improve time to disease progression, progression-free survival, and overall survival compared to doxorubicin alone [77]. A trial comparing sorafenib vs. sorafenib plus doxorubicin is ongoing [82]. The phase I study of sorafenib has been completed in children [83] with a maximum tolerated dose of 200 mg/m^2 being identified and may represent a useful alternative to traditional chemotherapy, especially in patients with advanced disease. Further development of clinical trials evaluating sorafenib in pediatric HCC is required.

Transplantation

Orthotopic liver transplantation (OLT) is an important option for patients with a tumor that respects the liver confines but is primarily unresectable. Many believe that the adult Milan criteria (one lesion <5 cm in diameter or <3 lesions less than 3 cm, no macrovascular invasion, no extrahepatic disease) used to outline indications for OLT are too strict for children [84–86]. In one series of ten patients, the actuarial recurrence-free survival at 5 years after OLT was 83.3%, despite that patients had tumors of sizes greater than 5 cm, more than three lesions, or macrovascular invasion [85]. Other studies also suggest that macrovascular invasion does not per se impair the likelihood of survival after OLT in children [87]; however, the absolute denominator of attempted OLT (including those who failed) is unknown. Further, caution should be exercised since macrovascular invasion is considered the strongest predictor of poor outcome in adults [73]. Due to the high risk of tumor recurrence in the setting of limited organ resources, the presence of extrahepatic metastases remains an absolute contraindication for OLT in children with advanced HCC [88]. Data gathered from the United Network for Organ Sharing (UNOS) database further highlight the difficulty of finding the balance between risk of disease recurrence with adverse outcome and increased chance of survival when undergoing OLT. This database prospectively collects data on patients listed for solid organ transplantation in the USA. Between 1997 and 2004, 41 pediatric patients received a liver transplantation for HCC [89]. The 1-, 5-, and 10-year patient survival rate after liver transplantation was 86%, 63%, and 58%, respectively. Recurrence of HCC disease accounted for 86% of the deaths, whereas in the hepatoblastoma group, this was the case in only 56% [89].

The PLUTO registry was formed to establish multicenter and multi-institutional prospective follow-up of pediatric patients undergoing liver transplantation for primary liver malignancies. Data that are recorded and may help in the future to determine appropriate listing criteria for children included PRETEXT grouping, previous therapies, and, e.g., histological subtypes [90, 91]. The first analysis of 16 HCC patients showed a 3-year survival rate of 85% [90]. Four patients had recurrent disease of which one died. Although this registry will begin to outline the international environment of OLT in children with primary liver cancer, rigorous data capture mandated by prospective clinical trials is still required.

Alternative Therapies in Children

Chemoembolization (e.g., transcatheter arterial chemoembolization [TACE] and hepatic arterial chemoembolization [HACE]), which combines the effect of chemotherapy with that of ischemic necrosis induced by arterial embolization, has improved survival in adults with HCC [92, 93]. Several series have demonstrated that chemoembolization is feasible in children and results in tumor responses [24–27]. TACE should be explored as an alternative to systemic chemotherapy in pediatric patients with locally advanced HCC or other liver lesions; however, the paucity of cases and the need for specific technical expertise in large tertiary care pediatric centers likely limit the drive for intense study and general applicability of the technology to children. Similarly, although radiofrequency ablation (RFA, a technique used to destroy hepatic tumors through percutaneous thermocoagulation) is common in the management of adult HCC [94–96], the pediatric RFA experience is limited [97, 98].

Prognosis and Outcomes

The overall survival rate for children with HCC is poor, ranging from 18% to 28% at 5 years after diagnosis [1, 64, 67]. Histopathological features may be helpful in predicting prognosis, as well-differentiated tumors are associated with a better survival [99]. However, the well-differentiated tumors in this study were also smaller, had no capsule formation, and showed less extranodular invasion than poorly differentiated tumors. FL-HCC was assumed to be associated with a better outcome among adult patients, but that could not be confirmed in studies of patients under 21 years of age [53, 64].

Interestingly, in one study, there was a trend to better outcome in patients with a normal AFP level at diagnosis, whereas more children with normal AFP levels had localized disease [67]. In another study, five of six patients who relapsed had normal AFP levels [64]. Prognosis is influenced by the presence of vascular invasion on imaging and the surgical resection success rate, which is greater in unifocal than in multifocal tumors [45]. Complete surgical resection remains essential to achieve a realistic chance of cure. The presence of metastasis is an important adverse predictive factor associated with a 5-year survival of only 9% [64].

Conclusion

HCC occurs in children both with and without underlying chronic liver disease, and its incidence is particularly affected by the population prevalence of vertically acquired HBV infection. Treatment involving chemotherapy, surgical resection, and, when necessary, liver transplantation provides the chance of cure and long-term survival for some affected children. However, there is an important need for prospective multicenter research collaborations to systematically explore treatment strategies in order to further improve clinical outcomes.

References

1. Darbari A, Sabin KM, Shapiro CN, Schwarz KB. Epidemiology of primary hepatic malignancies in U.S. children. Hepatology. 2003;38:560–6.
2. Laiq Z, Bishop JA, Ali SZ. Liver lesions in children and adolescents: Cytopathologic analysis and clinical correlates in 44 cases. Diagn Cytopathol 2011 Feb 9. doi:10.1002/dc.21587. [Epub ahead of print].
3. Meyers RL. Tumors of the liver in children. Surg Oncol. 2007;16:195–203.
4. Wu TC, Tong MJ, Hwang B, Lee SD, Hu MM. Primary hepatocellular carcinoma and hepatitis B infection during childhood. Hepatology. 1987;7:46–8.
5. Lanier AP, Holck P, Ehrsam DG, Key C. Childhood cancer among Alaska Natives. Pediatrics. 2003;112:e396.
6. Tajiri H, Tanaka H, Brooks S, Takano T. Reduction of hepatocellular carcinoma in childhood after introduction of selective vaccination against hepatitis B virus for infants born to HBV carrier mothers. Cancer Causes Control 2011;22(3):523–7.
7. Chang MH, Chen CJ, Lai MS, Hsu HM, Wu TC, Kong MS, et al. Universal hepatitis B vaccination in Taiwan and the incidence of hepatocellular carcinoma in children. Taiwan Childhood Hepatoma Study Group. N Engl J Med. 1997;336:1855–9.
8. Chang MH, Shau WY, Chen CJ, Wu TC, Kong MS, Liang DC, et al. Hepatitis B vaccination and hepatocellular carcinoma rates in boys and girls. J Am Med Assoc. 2000;284:3040–2.
9. Davison SM, Mieli-Vergani G, Sira J, Kelly DA. Perinatal hepatitis C virus infection: diagnosis and management. Arch Dis Child. 2006;91:781–5.
10. Mohan P, Colvin C, Glymph C, Chandra RR, Kleiner DE, Patel KM, et al. Clinical spectrum and histopathologic features of chronic hepatitis C infection in children. J Pediatr. 2007;150:168–74.
11. Strickland DK, Jenkins JJ, Hudson MM. Hepatitis C infection and hepatocellular carcinoma after treatment of childhood cancer. J Pediatr Hematol Oncol. 2001;23:527–9.
12. Castellino S, Lensing S, Riely C, Rai SN, Davila R, Hayden RT, et al. The epidemiology of chronic hepatitis C infection in survivors of childhood cancer: an update of the St Jude Children's Research Hospital hepatitis C seropositive cohort. Blood. 2004;103:2460–6.
13. Weinberg AG, Mize CE, Worthen HG. The occurrence of hepatoma in the chronic form of hereditary tyrosinemia. J Pediatr. 1976;88:434–8.
14. van Spronsen FJ, Thomasse Y, Smit GP, Leonard JV, Clayton PT, Fidler V, et al. Hereditary tyrosinemia type I: a new clinical classification with difference in prognosis on dietary treatment. Hepatology. 1994;20:1187–91.
15. Masurel-Paulet A, Poggi-Bach J, Rolland MO, Bernard O, Guffon N, Dobbelaere D, et al. NTBC treatment in tyrosinaemia type I: long-term outcome in French patients. J Inherit Metab Dis. 2008;31:81–7.

16. van Spronsen FJ, Bijleveld CM, van Maldegem BT, Wijburg FA. Hepatocellular carcinoma in hereditary tyrosinemia type I despite 2-(2 nitro-4-3 trifluoro- methylbenzoyl)-1, 3-cyclohexanedione treatment. J Pediatr Gastroenterol Nutr. 2005;40:90–3.

17. Perlmutter DH. Pathogenesis of chronic liver injury and hepatocellular carcinoma in alpha-1-antitrypsin deficiency. Pediatr Res. 2006;60:233–8.

18. Arnon R, Kerkar N, Davis MK, Anand R, Yin W, Gonzalez-Peralta RP. Liver transplantation in children with metabolic diseases: the studies of pediatric liver transplantation experience. Pediatr Transplant. 2010;14:796–805.

19. Carlson J, Eriksson S. Chronic 'cryptogenic' liver disease and malignant hepatoma in intermediate alpha 1-antitrypsin deficiency identified by a Pi Z-specific monoclonal antibody. Scand J Gastroenterol. 1985;20:835–42.

20. Zhou H, Fischer HP. Liver carcinoma in PiZ alpha-1-antitrypsin deficiency. Am J Surg Pathol. 1998;22:742–8.

21. Elzouki AN, Eriksson S. Risk of hepatobiliary disease in adults with severe alpha 1-antitrypsin deficiency (PiZZ): is chronic viral hepatitis B or C an additional risk factor for cirrhosis and hepatocellular carcinoma? Eur J Gastroenterol Hepatol. 1996;8:989–94.

22. Bhadri VA, Stormon MO, Arbuckle S, Lam AH, Gaskin KJ, Shun A. Hepatocellular carcinoma in children with Alagille syndrome. J Pediatr Gastroenterol Nutr. 2005;41:676–8.

23. Kaufman SS, Wood RP, Shaw Jr BW, Markin RS, Gridelli B, Vanderhoof JA. Hepatocarcinoma in a child with the Alagille syndrome. Am J Dis Child. 1987;141:698–700.

24. McDaniell R, Warthen DM, Sanchez-Lara PA, Pai A, Krantz ID, Piccoli DA, et al. NOTCH2 mutations cause Alagille syndrome, a heterogeneous disorder of the notch signaling pathway. Am J Hum Genet. 2006;79:169–73.

25. Yao Z, Mishra L. Cancer stem cells and hepatocellular carcinoma. Cancer Biol Ther. 2009;8:1691–8.

26. Rake JP, Visser G, Labrune P, Leonard JV, Ullrich K, Smit GP. Glycogen storage disease type I: diagnosis, management, clinical course and outcome. Results of the European Study on Glycogen Storage Disease Type I (ESGSD I). Eur J Pediatr. 2002;161 Suppl 1:S20–34.

27. Farges O, Dokmak S. Malignant transformation of liver adenoma: an analysis of the literature. Dig Surg. 2010;27:32–8.

28. Tward AD, Jones KD, Yant S, Cheung ST, Fan ST, Chen X, et al. Distinct pathways of genomic progression to benign and malignant tumors of the liver. Proc Natl Acad Sci USA. 2007;104:14771–6.

29. Franco LM, Krishnamurthy V, Bali D, Weinstein DA, Arn P, Clary B, et al. Hepatocellular carcinoma in glycogen storage disease type Ia: a case series. J Inherit Metab Dis. 2005;28:153–62.

30. Brunati A, Feruzi Z, Sokal E, Smets F, Fervaille C, Gosseye S, et al. Early occurrence of hepatocellular carcinoma in biliary atresia treated by liver transplantation. Pediatr Transplant. 2007;11:117–9.

31. Tatekawa Y, Asonuma K, Uemoto S, Inomata Y, Tanaka K. Liver transplantation for biliary atresia associated with malignant hepatic tumors. J Pediatr Surg. 2001;36:436–9.

32. Iida T, Zendejas IR, Kayler LK, Magliocca JF, Kim RD, Hemming AW, et al. Hepatocellular carcinoma in a 10-month-old biliary atresia child. Pediatr Transplant. 2009;13:1048–9.

33. Starzl TE, Giles G, Lilly JR, Takagi H, Martineau G, Schroter G, et al. Indications for orthotopic liver transplantation: with particular reference to hepatomas, biliary atresia, cirrhosis, Wilson's disease and serum hepatitis. Transplant Proc. 1971;3:308–12.

34. Strautnieks SS, Bull LN, Knisely AS, Kocoshis SA, Dahl N, Arnell H, et al. A gene encoding a liver-specific ABC transporter is mutated in progressive familial intrahepatic cholestasis. Nat Genet. 1998;20:233–8.

35. Knisely AS, Strautnieks SS, Meier Y, Stieger B, Byrne JA, Portmann BC, et al. Hepatocellular carcinoma in ten children under five years of age with bile salt export pump deficiency. Hepatology. 2006;44:478–86.

36. Bodmer WF, Bailey CJ, Bodmer J, Bussey HJ, Ellis A, Gorman P, et al. Localization of the gene for familial adenomatous polyposis on chromosome 5. Nature. 1987;328:614–6.

37. Giardiello FM, Offerhaus GJ, Krush AJ, Booker SV, Tersmette AC, Mulder JW, et al. Risk of hepatoblastoma in familial adenomatous polyposis. J Pediatr. 1991;119:766–8.

38. Hughes LJ, Michels VV. Risk of hepatoblastoma in familial adenomatous polyposis. Am J Med Genet. 1992;43:1023–5.
39. Su LK, Abdalla EK, Law CH, Kohlmann W, Rashid A, Vauthey JN. Biallelic inactivation of the APC gene is associated with hepatocellular carcinoma in familial adenomatous polyposis coli. Cancer. 2001;92:332–9.
40. Gruner BA, DeNapoli TS, Andrews W, Tomlinson G, Bowman L, Weitman SD. Hepatocellular carcinoma in children associated with Gardner syndrome or familial adenomatous polyposis. J Pediatr Hematol Oncol. 1998;20:274–8.
41. Thompson MD, Monga SP. WNT/beta-catenin signaling in liver health and disease. Hepatology. 2007;45:1298–305.
42. Sun Z, Lu P, Gail MH, Pee D, Zhang Q, Ming L, et al. Increased risk of hepatocellular carcinoma in male hepatitis B surface antigen carriers with chronic hepatitis who have detectable urinary aflatoxin metabolite M1. Hepatology. 1999;30:379–83.
43. Liu J, Waalkes MP. Liver is a target of arsenic carcinogenesis. Toxicol Sci. 2008;105:24–32.
44. Liaw J, Marshall G, Yuan Y, Ferreccio C, Steinmaus C, Smith AH. Increased childhood liver cancer mortality and arsenic in drinking water in northern Chile. Cancer Epidemiol Biomarkers Prev. 2008;17:1982–7.
45. Czauderna P. Adult type vs. Childhood hepatocellular carcinoma—are they the same or different lesions? Biology, natural history, prognosis, and treatment. Med Pediatr Oncol. 2002;39:519–23.
46. Di Bisceglie AM, Rustgi VK, Hoofnagle JH, Dusheiko GM, Lotze MT. NIH conference. Hepatocellular carcinoma. Ann Intern Med. 1988;108:390–401.
47. Kew MC. Hepatocellular carcinoma with and without cirrhosis. A comparison in southern African blacks. Gastroenterology. 1989;97:136–9.
48. Prokurat A, Kluge P, Koscieszia A, Perek D, Kappeler A, Zimmermann A. Transitional liver cell tumors (TLCT) in older children and adolescents: a novel group of aggressive hepatic tumors expressing beta-catenin. Med Pediatr Oncol. 2002;39:510–8.
49. Stocker JT, Husain AN, Dehner LP, Chandra RS. Pediatric pathology. Philadelphia: Lippincott Williams & Wilkins; 2001. p. 773.
50. Edmondson HA. Differential diagnosis of tumors and tumor-like lesions of liver in infancy and childhood. AMA J Dis Child. 1956;91:168–86.
51. Berman MA, Burnham JA, Sheahan DG. Fibrolamellar carcinoma of the liver: an immunohistochemical study of nineteen cases and a review of the literature. Hum Pathol. 1988;19:784–94.
52. El Serag HB, Davila JA. Is fibrolamellar carcinoma different from hepatocellular carcinoma? A US population-based study. Hepatology. 2004;39:798–803.
53. Katzenstein HM, Krailo MD, Malogolowkin MH, Ortega JA, Qu W, Douglass EC, et al. Fibrolamellar hepatocellular carcinoma in children and adolescents. Cancer. 2003;97: 2006–12.
54. Stipa F, Yoon SS, Liau KH, Fong Y, Jarnagin WR, D'Angelica M, et al. Outcome of patients with fibrolamellar hepatocellular carcinoma. Cancer. 2006;106:1331–8.
55. Craig JR, Peters RL, Edmondson HA, Omata M. Fibrolamellar carcinoma of the liver: a tumor of adolescents and young adults with distinctive clinico-pathologic features. Cancer. 1980;46:372–9.
56. Cheah PL, Looi LM, Lin HP, Yap SF. Childhood primary hepatocellular carcinoma and hepatitis B virus infection. Cancer. 1990;65:174–6.
57. Chang MH, Chen DS, Hsu HC, Hsu HY, Lee CY. Maternal transmission of hepatitis B virus in childhood hepatocellular carcinoma. Cancer. 1989;64:2377–80.
58. Kaposi-Novak P, Lee JS, Gomez-Quiroz L, Coulouarn C, Factor VM, Thorgeirsson SS. Met-regulated expression signature defines a subset of human hepatocellular carcinomas with poor prognosis and aggressive phenotype. J Clin Invest. 2006;116:1582–95.
59. Park WS, Dong SM, Kim SY, Na EY, Shin MS, Pi JH, et al. Somatic mutations in the kinase domain of the Met/hepatocyte growth factor receptor gene in childhood hepatocellular carcinomas. Cancer Res. 1999;59:307–10.

60. Peng SY, Chou SP, Hsu HC. Association of downregulation of cyclin D1 and of overexpression of cyclin E with p53 mutation, high tumor grade and poor prognosis in hepatocellular carcinoma. J Hepatol. 1998;29:281–9.
61. Kim H, Lee MJ, Kim MR, Chung IP, Kim YM, Lee JY, et al. Expression of cyclin D1, cyclin E, cdk4 and loss of heterozygosity of 8p, 13q, 17p in hepatocellular carcinoma: comparison study of childhood and adult hepatocellular carcinoma. Liver. 2000;20:173–8.
62. Yu SB, Kim HY, Eo H, Won JK, Jung SE, Park KW, et al. Clinical characteristics and prognosis of pediatric hepatocellular carcinoma. World J Surg. 2006;30:43–50.
63. Bellani FF, Massimino M. Liver tumors in childhood: epidemiology and clinics. J Surg Oncol Suppl. 1993;3:119–21.
64. Czauderna P, Mackinlay G, Perilongo G, Brown J, Shafford E, Aronson D, et al. Hepatocellular carcinoma in children: results of the first prospective study of the International Society of Pediatric Oncology group. J Clin Oncol. 2002;20:2798–804.
65. Bruix J, Sherman M. Management of hepatocellular carcinoma. Hepatology. 2005;42:1208–36.
66. DeBaun MR, Tucker MA. Risk of cancer during the first four years of life in children from The Beckwith-Wiedemann Syndrome Registry. J Pediatr. 1998;132:398–400.
67. Katzenstein HM, Krailo MD, Malogolowkin MH, Ortega JA, Liu-Mares W, Douglass EC, et al. Hepatocellular carcinoma in children and adolescents: results from the Pediatric Oncology Group and the Children's Cancer Group intergroup study. J Clin Oncol. 2002;20:2789–97.
68. Taketa K, Endo Y, Sekiya C, Tanikawa K, Koji T, Taga H, et al. A collaborative study for the evaluation of lectin-reactive alpha-fetoproteins in early detection of hepatocellular carcinoma. Cancer Res. 1993;53:5419–23.
69. Baumann U, Duhme V, Auth MK, McKiernan PJ, Holme E. Lectin-reactive alpha-fetoprotein in patients with tyrosinemia type I and hepatocellular carcinoma. J Pediatr Gastroenterol Nutr. 2006;43:77–82.
70. Saar B, Kellner-Weldon F. Radiological diagnosis of hepatocellular carcinoma. Liver Int. 2008;28:189–99.
71. Marrero JA, Hussain HK, Nghiem HV, Umar R, Fontana RJ, Lok AS. Improving the prediction of hepatocellular carcinoma in cirrhotic patients with an arterially-enhancing liver mass. Liver Transplant. 2005;11:281–9.
72. Mazzaferro V, Regalia E, Doci R, Andreola S, Pulvirenti A, Bozzetti F, et al. Liver transplantation for the treatment of small hepatocellular carcinomas in patients with cirrhosis. N Engl J Med. 1996;334:693–9.
73. Shah SA, Cleary SP, Wei AC, Yang I, Taylor BR, Hemming AW, et al. Recurrence after liver resection for hepatocellular carcinoma: risk factors, treatment, and outcomes. Surgery. 2007;141:330–9.
74. Mazzaferro V, Llovet JM, Miceli R, Bhoori S, Schiavo M, Mariani L, et al. Predicting survival after liver transplantation in patients with hepatocellular carcinoma beyond the Milan criteria: a retrospective, exploratory analysis. Lancet Oncol. 2009;10:35–43.
75. Roebuck DJ, Aronson D, Clapuyt P, Czauderna P, de Ville DG, Gauthier F, et al. PRETEXT: a revised staging system for primary malignant liver tumours of childhood developed by the SIOPEL group. Pediatr Radiol. 2007;37:123–32.
76. Brown J, Perilongo G, Shafford E, Keeling J, Pritchard J, Brock P, et al. Pretreatment prognostic factors for children with hepatoblastoma—results from the International Society of Paediatric Oncology (SIOP) study SIOPEL 1. Eur J Cancer. 2000;36:1418–25.
77. Abou-Alfa GK, Johnson P, Knox JJ, Capanu M, Davidenko I, Lacava J, et al. Doxorubicin plus sorafenib vs doxorubicin alone in patients with advanced hepatocellular carcinoma: a randomized trial. J Am Med Assoc. 2010;304:2154–60.
78. DeVita VTJ TSLaSAR. Cancer: principles & practice of oncology. Philadelphia: Wolters Kluwer/Lippincott Williams & Wilkins; 2008.
79. Von Schweinitz D. International Society of Paediatric Oncology, SIOP XXXVII Annual Congress Meeting: Abstracts. Pediatr Blood Cancer 2005;45:371.

80. Iyer R, Fetterly G, Lugade A, Thanavala Y. Sorafenib: a clinical and pharmacologic review. Expert Opin Pharmacother. 2010;11:1943–55.
81. Llovet JM, Ricci S, Mazzaferro V, Hilgard P, Gane E, Blanc JF, et al. Sorafenib in advanced hepatocellular carcinoma. N Engl J Med. 2008;359:378–90.
82. Phase III Randomized Study of Sorafenib Tosylate With Versus Without Doxorubicin Hydrochloride in Patients With Locally Advanced or Metastatic Hepatocellular Carcinoma. http://www.cancer.gov/clinicaltrials/search/view?cdrid=659348&version=HealthProfessional &protocolsearchid=8987722 . 2011. 31-3-2011 Jul 1;56(7):1013–8.
83. Keir ST, Maris JM, Lock R, Kolb EA, Gorlick R, Carol H, et al. Initial testing (stage 1) of the multi-targeted kinase inhibitor sorafenib by the pediatric preclinical testing program. Pediatr Blood Cancer. 2010;55:1126–33.
84. Otte JB. Should the selection of children with hepatocellular carcinoma be based on Milan criteria? Pediatr Transplant. 2008;12:1–3.
85. Beaunoyer M, Vanatta JM, Ogihara M, Strichartz D, Dahl G, Berquist WE, et al. Outcomes of transplantation in children with primary hepatic malignancy. Pediatr Transplant. 2007;11:655–60.
86. Ismail H, Broniszczak D, Kalicinski P, Markiewicz-Kijewska M, Teisseyre J, Stefanowicz M, et al. Liver transplantation in children with hepatocellular carcinoma. Do Milan criteria apply to pediatric patients? Pediatr Transplant. 2009;13:682–92.
87. Kosola S, Lauronen J, Sairanen H, Heikinheimo M, Jalanko H, Pakarinen M. High survival rates after liver transplantation for hepatoblastoma and hepatocellular carcinoma. Pediatr Transplant. 2010;14:646–50.
88. Gupta AA, Gerstle JT, Ng V, Wong A, Fecteau A, Malogolowkin MH et al. Critical review of controversial issues in the management of advanced pediatric liver tumors. Pediatr Blood Cancer. 2011;56(7):1013–8.
89. Austin MT, Leys CM, Feurer ID, Lovvorn III HN, O'Neill Jr JA, Pinson CW, et al. Liver transplantation for childhood hepatic malignancy: a review of the United Network for Organ Sharing (UNOS) database. J Pediatr Surg. 2006;41:182–6.
90. Otte JB, Meyers R. PLUTO first report. Pediatr Transplant. 2010;14:830–5.
91. Otte JB. Progress in the surgical treatment of malignant liver tumors in children. Cancer Treat Rev. 2010;36:360–71.
92. Llovet JM, Real MI, Montana X, Planas R, Coll S, Aponte J, et al. Arterial embolisation or chemoembolisation versus symptomatic treatment in patients with unresectable hepatocellular carcinoma: a randomised controlled trial. Lancet. 2002;359:1734–9.
93. Lo CM, Ngan H, Tso WK, Liu CL, Lam CM, Poon RT, et al. Randomized controlled trial of transarterial lipiodol chemoembolization for unresectable hepatocellular carcinoma. Hepatology. 2002;35:1164–71.
94. Kudo M. Radiofrequency ablation for hepatocellular carcinoma: updated review in 2010. Oncology. 2010;78 Suppl 1:113–24.
95. Lau WY, Lai EC. The current role of radiofrequency ablation in the management of hepatocellular carcinoma: a systematic review. Ann Surg. 2009;249:20–5.
96. Cho YK, Kim JK, Kim MY, Rhim H, Han JK. Systematic review of randomized trials for hepatocellular carcinoma treated with percutaneous ablation therapies. Hepatology. 2009;49:453–9.
97. Ye J, Shu Q, Li M, Jiang TA. Percutaneous radiofrequency ablation for treatment of hepatoblastoma recurrence. Pediatr Radiol. 2008;38:1021–3.
98. Hoffer FA, Daw NC, Xiong X, Anghelescu D, Krasin M, Yan X, et al. A phase 1/pilot study of radiofrequency ablation for the treatment of recurrent pediatric solid tumors. Cancer. 2009;115:1328–37.
99. Sasaki Y, Imaoka S, Ishiguro S, Nakano H, Kasugai H, Fujita M, et al. Clinical features of small hepatocellular carcinomas as assessed by histologic grades. Surgery. 1996;119:252–60.

Chapter 8
Staging of Hepatocellular Carcinoma

Chalermrat Bunchorntavakul, Maarouf Hoteit, and K. Rajender Reddy

Introduction

Hepatocellular carcinoma (HCC) is a major health problem worldwide and accounts for 80–90% of the cases of primary liver cancer. Although the majority of HCC cases are reported in the developing world, the incidence of HCC has been increasing in several developed countries, including the United States [1]. Globally, between 70% and 90% of cases of HCC are associated with a background of established cirrhosis. HCC can also occur in those without cirrhosis, usually in those with chronic infection with hepatitis B [2–4]. Overall, the diagnosis of hepatocellular carcinoma is associated with a poor long-term survival [5]. However, small HCC tumors, often detected by surveillance, could qualify for curative treatments which are associated with a 5-year survival exceeding 50% [6–8].

Clinical staging of cancers provides a guide to assess prognosis, direct therapeutic intervention, and assist in the evaluation of treatment outcomes. It also provides a method that would allow the consistent dissemination of information and facilitate in design of clinical trials and allow for proper assessment of the data [9]. Unlike other solid tumors in which the prognosis of patients is mostly related to the anatomic extent of tumor, the prognosis in HCC depends largely on the severity of the underlying hepatic dysfunction as well as tumor burden. In fact, the survival of a patient with Child class C cirrhosis is <50% at 1 year, regardless of the presence of

C. Bunchorntavakul, MD • M. Hoteit, MD
Division of Gastroenterology and Hepatology, Department of Medicine,
University of Pennsylvania, Philadelphia, PA, USA
e-mail: dr.chalermrat@gmail.com; maarouf.hoteit@uphs.upenn.edu

K.R. Reddy, MD (✉)
Division of Gastroenterology and Hepatology, Department of Medicine,
University of Pennsylvania, Philadelphia, PA, USA

Hospital of the University of Pennsylvania, Philadelphia, PA 19104, USA
e-mail: rajender.reddy@uphs.upenn.edu

N. Reau and F.F. Poordad (eds.), *Primary Liver Cancer: Surveillance, Diagnosis and Treatment*, Clinical Gastroenterology, DOI 10.1007/978-1-61779-863-4_8,
© Springer Science+Business Media New York 2012

HCC [10]. Thus, liver failure is frequently a competing cause of mortality in patients with HCC, with a potential major impact on prognosis. Further, the severity of hepatic dysfunction often has an important effect on the potential for patients with HCC to tolerate the various modalities of treatment. For example, transarterial chemoembolization is a safe and effective palliative treatment modality only in patients without severe hepatic dysfunction. Accordingly, the ideal clinical staging system for HCC would integrate an evaluation of tumor burden as well as liver function in order to comprehensively define prognosis and determine the optimal treatment options corresponding to each stage.

For a staging system to be universally accepted and practical, it must be prospectively validated and be reproducible in all patient populations. Several staging system have been proposed: the Okuda staging system [11], the cancer of the liver Italian program (CLIP) scoring [12], the Group d'Etude et de Traitement du Carcinome Hépatocellulaire (GRETCH) scoring system [13], the Barcelona clinic liver cancer (BCLC) staging system [14], and the Japan Integrated Staging System (JIS) [15]. The variables used in these systems can be classified into four aspects: (1) tumor factors (e.g., tumor size, number of tumor nodules, alpha fetoprotein (AFP) level, portal vein invasion, nodal or metastatic involvement), (2) global health of the patient (i.e., performance status), (3) underlying liver function (e.g., serum bilirubin, serum albumin, Child–Pugh score, portal hypertension), and (4) the specific intervention recommended for each stage [8, 16, 17]. However, the variables included in each staging system are different, reflecting the various methodologies used in devising the staging schemes, and more importantly, the different patient populations used to construct the models. Although the performance of many of these models has been evaluated extensively, there is no worldwide consensus on the use of a specific HCC staging system.

TNM (Tumor, Node, Metastasis) Staging System

The American Joint Committee on Cancer and the Union Internationale Contre le Cancer (AJCC/UICC) TNM staging system is a histopathology-based system which is widely accepted for solid tumor staging. In HCC, this system recognizes the number and size of tumor(s) as well as the presence of vascular invasion as the most important predictors of prognosis [18–20]. Although the background nonneoplastic liver pathology is not used to assign the final tumor stage, the liver fibrosis score is included as a clinically significant prognostic factor. In this case, F0 designates early stages of hepatic fibrosis and F1 advanced fibrosis and cirrhosis [21, 22]. The prognostic value of the sixth edition AJCC/UICC TNM staging (2002) has been validated in several large surgical cohorts and found to have good accuracy in stratifying postresection and post-transplantation outcomes [23–30]. Five-year survival rates, based upon the TNM staging system in HCC patients who underwent complete resection, are as follows: T1/F0 64%, T1/F1 49%, T2/F0 46%, T2/F1 30%,

Table 8.1 TNM staging by the American Joint Committee on Cancer (AJCC) and the Union Internationale Contre le Cancer (UICC) [35]

Primary tumor (T)	
Tx	Primary tumor cannot be assessed
T0	No evidence of primary tumor
T1	Solitary tumor without vascular invasion
T2	Solitary tumor with vascular invasion or multiple tumors not >5 cm
T3a	Multiple tumors, any >5 cm
T3b	Tumor(s) of any size involving a major branch of portal or hepatic vein
T4	Tumor(s) with direct invasion of adjacent organs other than the gallbladder or with perforation of visceral peritoneum

Regional lymph node (N)	
Nx	Regional lymph node cannot be assessed
N0	No regional lymph node metastasis
N1	Regional lymph node metastasis

Distant metastasis (M)	
M0	No distant metastasis
M1	Distant metastasis

Fibrosis score (F)[a]	
F0	Fibrosis score 0–4 (none to moderated fibrosis)
F1	Fibrosis score 5–6 (severe fibrosis or cirrhosis)

Anatomic stage/prognostic groups			
Stage I	T1	N0	M0
Stage II	T2	N0	M0
Stage IIIA	T3a	N0	M0
Stage IIIB	T3b	N0	M0
Stage IIIC	T4	N0	M0
Stage IVA	Any T	N1	M0
Stage IVB	Any T	Any N	M1

[a]The fibrosis score as defined by Ishak is recommended because of its prognostic value in overall survival. The scoring system uses a 0–6 scale
Modified from Edge et al. [9]

T3/F0 17%, and T3/F1 9% [31]. The TNM system is hence most well suited to evaluate patients in the context of consideration of surgical therapy [32–34]. However, the obvious limitation of the TNM system is that the severity of liver dysfunction, which impacts heavily on outcomes and also in deciding the best choice of therapy, is not taken into consideration.

The AJCC/UICC TNM staging system was revised in 2010 (Table 8.1) [35]. Compared to the 2002 version, intrahepatic cholangiocarcinoma is no longer included, the T3 stage is split into T3a and T3b to highlight the clinical importance of vascular invasion, T4 (invasion of adjacent organs excluding the gallbladder or perforation of the visceral peritoneum) is shifted to Stage IIIC, inferior phrenic lymph node involvement is no longer classified as a distant metastasis, and Stage IV is split into Stages IVA and IVB based on the presence of either nodal involvement or distant metastases. The value of the new TNM staging system needs to be validated.

Table 8.2 TNM staging by Liver Cancer Study Group of Japan (LCSGJ) [36]

Stage I	T1 (fulfilling 3 T factors)	N0	M0
Stage II	T2 (fulfilling 2 T factors)	N0	M0
Stage III	T3 (fulfilling 1 T factor)	N0	M0
Stage IVA	T4 (fulfilling 0 T factor)	N0	M0
	Any T	N1	M0
Stage IVB	Any T	N0–1	M1

T factor: (1) single, (2) <2 cm, and (3) no vascular involvement
Modified from Japan ISGo [36]

The Liver Cancer Study Group of Japan (LCSGJ) also introduced a TNM staging scheme using tumor factors (single tumor, size <2 cm, vascular invasion) as a prognostic predictor upon the tumor (T) stage (Table 8.2) [36]. This system has been validated and utilized in Japan. The performance of the Japanese TNM system has shown to be comparable to that of AJCC/UICC staging system in patients undergoing resection [23, 37–39].

Okuda Staging System

The Okuda staging system is a clinical scheme based on tumor size, presence of ascites, serum bilirubin, and albumin (Table 8.3). It was introduced in 1985 by Okuda et al. [11]. and was the first system that incorporated parameters measuring liver function. A total of 850 patients with HCC were analyzed retrospectively. The median survival in patients who had no specific treatment was 8.3 months for Stage I, 2 months for Stage II, and 0.7 months for Stage III, while the median survival in patients who had liver resection was 25.6 months for Stage I and 12.2 months for Stage II patients [11]. Further prospective validation of the system has not been conducted. When compared with other staging systems, the Okuda system has been shown to have lower predictive capacity [33, 40–44]. Because the Okuda criteria reflect signs of severe disease (bilirubin >3 mg/dl, albumin <3 mg/dl, clinically detectable ascites, tumor involving >50% of the liver), it is most suited to identify advanced disease carrying a poor prognosis but lacks the discriminatory ability needed to stratify patients with early and intermediate stage.

Cancer of the Liver Italian Program Scoring System

The CLIP score was derived from a retrospective analysis of 435 Italian patients with HCC between 1990 and 1992 [12]. At multivariate analysis, the independent predictive factors of survival were Child–Pugh stage, tumor morphology, AFP, and portal vein thrombosis. These parameters have been integrated into a simple linear

Table 8.3 Okuda staging system [11]

Parameters	Points 0	1
Tumor size	<50% of liver	>50% of liver
Ascites	No	Yes
Albumin (g/dl)	≥3	<3
Bilirubin (mg/dl)	<3	≥3

Okuda Stage I: 0 point, Okuda Stage II: 1–2 points, and Okuda Stage III: 3–4 points
Modified from Okuda et al. [11] (with permission)

Table 8.4 CLIP staging system [12]

Parameters	Scores 0	1	2
Child–pugh score	A	B	C
Tumor morphology	Uninodular and extension ≤50%	Multinodular and extension ≤50%	Massive or extension >50%
AFP (ng/ml)	<400	≥400	
Portal vein thrombosis	No	Yes	

Reproduced from [12] (with permission)

scoring system (Table 8.4) [12]. The CLIP system has been prospectively validated [42, 45, 46]. The 2-year survival rates for a CLIP score of 0, 1, 2, 3, and 4–6 were 65%, 45%, 17%, 12%, and 0%, respectively [45]. The CLIP system has been validated in various patient populations [37, 42, 43, 45–49], although the survival rate in an Asian population was different from the original experience [37]. It has been shown to have a better discriminatory ability than the Okuda and TNM systems, particularly in patients undergoing nonsurgical treatments. The main shortcoming of the CLIP system is the limited discriminatory ability of the early stages (scores 1–3) [15, 41, 43, 50–53]. Therefore, it is limited in its ability to assess patients undergoing curative therapies, such as resection or transplantation. The CLIP system is accepted by the American Hepato-Pancreato-BIliary Association (AHPBA) and the AJCC consensus group as a staging of choice because it is easily applicable to all patients and has been prospectively validated [32].

There have been attempts at modifying the CLIP score by replacing the AFP component with the more sensitive protein induced by vitamin K absence or antagonist II (PIVKA-II). The modified score had an improved prognostic prediction in patients who underwent hepatic resection [54, 55]. Modification of the CLIP system by replacing Child–Pugh score with the Model for End-Stage Liver Disease (MELD) may improve its ability to predict outcomes in patients undergoing locoregional therapy for HCC [56]. Recently, a combination of CLIP score and the baseline plasma vascular endothelial growth factor (V-CLIP) or performance status (CLIP + PS) has been noted to be a good prognostic predictor in those with advanced HCC and in palliative settings [57, 58].

Table 8.5 The Groupe d'Etude et de Traitement du Carcinome Hépatocellulaire (GRETCH) scoring system

Parameters	Points			
	0	1	2	3
Karnofsky index	≥80%			<80%
Bilirubin (μg/l)	<50			≥50
Alkaline phosphatase (ULN)	<2		≥2	
AFP (μmol/l)	<35		≥35	
Portal vein obstruction	No	Yes		

Risk group: low (A)—score 0, intermediate (B)—score 1–5, and high (C)—score ≥6
Reproduced from Chevret et al. [13] (with permission)
ULN upper limit of normal range

Group d'Etude et de Traitement du Carcinome Hépatocellulaire Scoring System

The Group d'Etude et de Traitement du Carcinome Hépatocellulaire (GRETCH) scoring system is a clinical scoring system that accounts for tumor characteristics, liver function, and performance status. It was introduced in 1999 by GRETCH investigators (Table 8.5). They conducted a prospective study of 761 patients with HCC, used five prognostic variables (Karnofsky index, serum bilirubin, alkaline phosphatase, AFP, and ultrasonographic evidence of portal vein obstruction), and stratified patients into three risk groups: The 1-year survival rates were 72–79% for low risk, 31–34% for intermediate risk, and 4–7% for high-risk group [13]. Subsequent evaluations have shown that it has a limited prognostic capability compared to other models, particularly in patients in early HCC [40, 43, 53].

Japanese Integrated System

Kudo et al. [15] proposed the Japanese integrated system (JIS) system in 2003 by incorporating the Child–Pugh score into the TNM staging based on the LCSGJ criteria (Table 8.6). In a retrospective analysis of 722 patients treated for HCC, the authors reported significant differences in survival curves for nearly all JIS scores (0–5) [15]. The JIS system has been validated by several reports and confirmed to be a good predictor of prognosis [52, 59, 60].

Modification of the conventional JIS score by replacing Child–Pugh score with either liver disease severity classification by LCSGJ [61–63] or MELD [64] has improved predictive ability compared with the original system. Kitai et al. proposed the bm-JIS score by adding HCC-specific biomarkers, including AFP, Lens culinaris agglutinin-reactive three fraction of AFP (AFP-L3), and des-gamma-carboxy prothrombin (DCP), to the c-JIS score. Both bm-JIS and AFP-combined c-JIS have demonstrated a better predictor of prognosis than c-JIS, especially in early disease [65–67].

Table 8.6 Variables included in JIS [15], CUPI [68], Tokyo [71], ALCPS [72], SLiDe [73], BALAD [75], and TIS scoring systems [76]

Staging system	Tumor stage	Liver function	Global health status	Tumor marker
c-JIS	TNM by LCSGJ	CP score	No	No
bm-JIS	TNM by LCSGJ	CP score	No	AFP, AFP-L3, DCP
CUPI	TNM by AJCC	Ascites, bilirubin, ALP	Presence of symptoms	AFP
Tokyo	Tumor size, number of tumors	Albumin, bilirubin	No	No
ALCPS	Tumor size, portal vein thrombosis, lung metastases	CP score, Ascites, bilirubin, ALP	Abdominal pain, weight loss, serum urea	AFP
SLiDe	TNM by LCSGJ	Ascites, albumin, bilirubin, $ICGR_{15}$, PT	No	DCP
BALAD	No	Albumin, bilirubin	No	AFP, AFP-L3, DCP
TIS	Total tumor volume	CP score	No	AFP

CP Child–Pugh, *ALP* alkaline phosphatase, *PT* prothrombin time, $ICGR_{15}$ indocyanine green retention rate at 15 min

It is important to note that evidence supporting the superior performance of the JIS system is retrospective and is based exclusively on studies evaluating patients from Japan. Studies conducted on Western populations have drawn a different conclusion [40, 43].

Other Staging Systems

The Chinese University Prognostic Index (CUPI) was developed from a cohort of 926 patients in Hong Kong (Table 8.6) [68]. As expected, the majority of patients (79%) had hepatitis B, in contrast to most other staging systems which have been derived in a population where hepatitis C and/or alcoholic cirrhosis predominate [68]. It has been shown to be more accurate than TNM, CLIP, and Okuda staging systems in prognosis stratification in patients with advanced disease. These observations have been prospectively validated in subsequent multicenter studies [49, 69, 70].

The Tokyo scoring system is a simple system which provides good prediction of prognosis for Japanese patients with HCC undergoing percutaneous ablation [71]. The Advanced Liver Cancer Prognosis System (ALCPS) can predict 3-month survival in advanced HCC patients who are not candidates for locoregional therapy [72]. The SLiDe (S, stage; Li, liver damage; De, DCP) score can be a good predictor of prognosis for patient who had undergone hepatic resection [73, 74]. The BALAD score, a novel scoring system based on serum markers (bilirubin, albumin, AFP-L3, AFP, and DCP), can predict patient outcomes with discriminative ability [75]. However, it demonstrated lesser performance characteristics than that of the system which combines both biomarkers and tumor stage in subsequent validation [65]. Recently, Taipei Integrated

Scoring (TIS) system has been introduced following a single center retrospective analysis of 2,030 HCC patients in Taiwan [76]. This study suggested that the TIS model can provide a better prognostic ability than currently used staging systems (Table 8.6).

Barcelona Clinic of Liver Cancer Staging System

BCLC system is a clinical staging model comprised of four components that are based on the anatomic extent of the tumor, Child–Pugh score, the presence portal hypertension, and the Eastern Cooperative Oncology Group (ECOG) performance status (Table 8.7 and Fig. 8.1) [8, 14, 77]. It was developed, based on a combination of data, from several independent studies representing various disease stage and treatment modalities and was introduced in 1999 by Llovet et al. [8, 14]. This classification has been externally validated [40, 50, 78, 79] and is endorsed by the American Association for the Study of Liver Diseases (AASLD) and the European Association for the Study of the Liver (EASL) [16]. Several large comparison studies demonstrated that the BCLC system offered the best discrimination of HCC prognosis, especially in patients with early and intermediate stage HCC [40, 41, 43, 80]. Thus, it has been used in many major prospective clinical trials of HCC therapy to define and stratify the population to be studied [81–83]. The major advantage of the BCLC staging system is that it links staging with a potential treatment algorithm and with an estimation of life expectancy that is based on published experiences (Fig. 8.1).

In the BCLC system, patients are stratified into five categories: (1) Very early stage (Stage 0) is defined as a single ≤2 cm HCC in well-compensated liver disease and without portal hypertension. These tumors are usually detected incidentally or as part of a surveillance program. Patients at this stage can be treated by resection with very high likelihood of cure. Five-year survival rate exceeds 90% after resection [8, 84, 85]. (2) Early stage (Stage A) consists of physically well patients with single-lesion HCC or with up to three nodules <3 cm, and preserved liver function (Child–Pugh A and B). These patients are likely to benefit from radical therapies such as resection, liver transplantation, or percutaneous ablation with possibility of long-term cure. The choice of treatment depends on portal pressure, liver reserve, local expertise, and organ availability. Long-term survival in these patients is reported to be in the range of 50–75% over 5 years [86]. (3) Intermediate stage (Stage B) is in asymptomatic patients with single large HCC and those with multifocal HCC who have preserved liver function and do not have vascular invasion or extrahepatic spread. These patients are likely to benefit from palliative therapy such as chemoembolization. Expected median survival is 8–15 months without treatment, whereas treatment with chemoembolization improves outcome to a median survival of 17–21 months and with a 2-year survival rate of 31–63% [81, 87–89]. (4) Advanced stage (Stage C) includes symptomatic patients who have limited performance status (ECOG performance scale 1–2) and/or aggressive tumor with vascular invasion or extrahepatic spread. These patients have short life expectancy, with median survival of 5–10 months and 20–35% survival at 1 year,

Table 8.7 Performance scales [77]

Eastern Cooperative Oncology Group (ECOG) performance scale

Performance status	Definition
0	Fully active; no performance restriction
1	Restricted in physically strenuous activity but ambulatory and able to carry out work of a light or sedentary nature, e.g., light house work, office work
2	Ambulatory and capable of all self-care but unable to carry out any work activities. Up and about >50% of waking hours
3	Capable of only limited self-care, confined to bed or chair >50% of waking hours
4	Completely disabled. Cannot carry on any self-care. Totally confined to bed or chair
5	Death

Karnofsky performance scale

Rating	Definitions
100	Normal no complaints; no evidence of disease
90	Able to carry on normal activity; minor signs or symptoms of disease
80	Normal activity with effort; some signs or symptoms of disease
70	Cares for self; unable to carry on normal activity or to do active work
60	Requires occasional assistance but is able to care for most of his personal needs
50	Requires considerable assistance and frequent medical care
40	Disabled; requires special care and assistance
30	Severely disabled; hospital admission is indicated although death not imminent
20	Very sick; hospital admission necessary; active supportive treatment necessary
10	Moribund; fatal processes progressing rapidly
0	Dead

Able to carry on normal activity and to work; no special care needed
Unable to work; able to live at home and care for most personal needs; varying amount of assistance needed
Unable to care for self; requires equivalent of institutional or hospital care; disease may be progressing rapidly

Modified from Oken et al. [77]

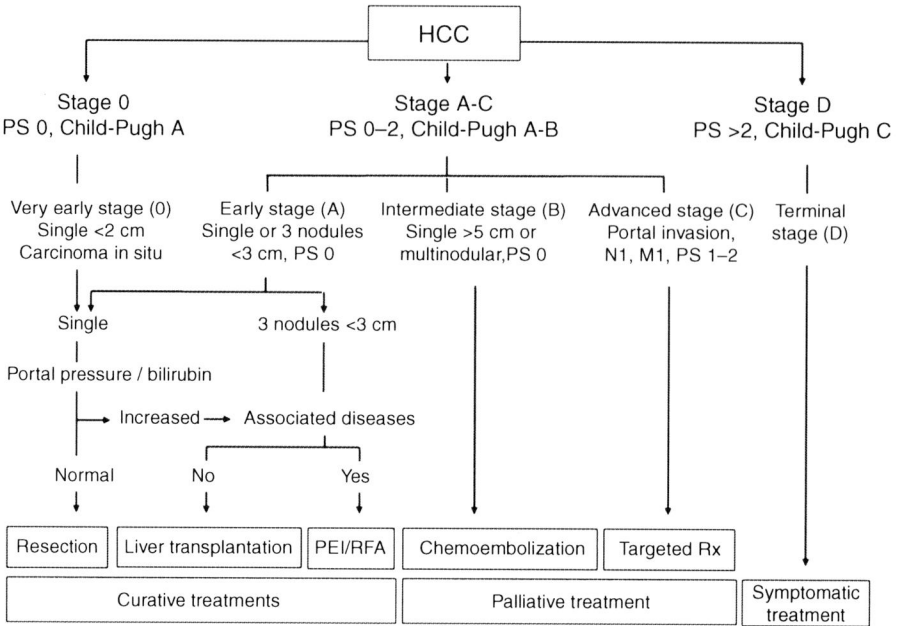

Fig. 8.1 Barcelona Clinic of Liver Cancer (BCLC) staging system [8, 14]. Reproduced from Forner et al. [8]. *HCC* hepatocellular carcinoma, *PS* performance status, *PEI* percutaneous ethanol injection, *RFA* radiofrequency ablation

and are candidates for systemic therapy [81–83]. (5) Terminal stage (Stage D) applies to patients with severe impairment of liver function (Child–Pugh C) and/or performance status. Their median survival is <3 months and symptom management is recommended.

One of the limitations of the BCLC system is that it does not take into consideration expanded tumor size criteria that allow curative therapy through liver transplantation in some BCLC stage B tumors [90]. It is also obvious that some patients with Child C cirrhosis and small tumors can undergo liver transplantation with good results. There are also difficulties associated with the implementation of a universal treatment algorithm. Differences in local expertise, as well as potential differences in tumor behavior in different populations, may lead to different outcomes [49, 52, 53, 60].

Conclusion

Hepatocellular carcinoma (HCC) is a heterogeneous tumor in terms of its biological behavior. The prediction of prognosis and the decision of a particular therapeutic approach are complex because the underlying liver function affects outcomes. A precise staging of HCC should define the prognosis as well as determine therapeutic options with the greatest survival potential. It has to integrate the prognostic parameters in various categories that include tumor stage, underlying liver function, global health status, and also efficacy of treatment. Although there is no universally adopted HCC staging system, most evidence points toward the BCLC as the staging system that most accurately defines prognosis and relates to an evidence-based therapeutic approach. A guideline for surveillance and management of HCC has also been developed by The National Comprehensive Cancer Network (NCCN) [91]. This NCCN guideline stratifies HCC patients similar to BCLC and is also well accepted by the oncology community [91]. Despite some limitations, the CLIP system is easily applicable and is useful for the prognostic prediction of HCC, particularly in patients who have intermediate and advanced disease. The TNM staging can be applied for early HCC patients undergoing resection or transplantation, or can be used as a part of any newer staging model. The CUPI staging may be utilized in patients who had advanced HCC with underlying chronic hepatitis B. In light of the recent advancements, biomarkers of HCC are being investigated extensively [92]. The future challenge is to identify the biomarkers which define the biological characteristic and the microenvironment of HCC and then integrate them into the clinical staging in order to provide the best prognostic prediction and to determine the most appropriate treatment for patients with HCC.

References

1. Bosch FX, Ribes J, Diaz M, Cleries R. Primary liver cancer: worldwide incidence and trends. Gastroenterology. 2004;127(5 Suppl 1):S5–16.
2. Sherman M, Peltekian KM, Lee C. Screening for hepatocellular carcinoma in chronic carriers of hepatitis B virus: incidence and prevalence of hepatocellular carcinoma in a North American urban population. Hepatology. 1995;22(2):432–8.
3. Manno M, Camma C, Schepis F, et al. Natural history of chronic HBV carriers in northern Italy: morbidity and mortality after 30 years. Gastroenterology. 2004;127(3):756–63.
4. Chen CJ, Yang HI, Su J, et al. Risk of hepatocellular carcinoma across a biological gradient of serum hepatitis B virus DNA level. J Am Med Assoc. 2006;295(1):65–73.
5. Survival and stage of liver and intrahepatic bile duct cancers. http://seer.cancer.gov/statfacts/html/livibd.html#survival. Accessed 28 Feb 2011.
6. Yamamoto J, Iwatsuki S, Kosuge T, et al. Should hepatomas be treated with hepatic resection or transplantation? Cancer. 1999;86(7):1151–8.
7. Llovet JM, Fuster J, Bruix J. Intention-to-treat analysis of surgical treatment for early hepatocellular carcinoma: resection versus transplantation. Hepatology. 1999;30(6):1434–40.
8. Forner A, Reig ME, de Lope CR, Bruix J. Current strategy for staging and treatment: the BCLC update and future prospects. Semin Liver Dis. 2010;30(1):61–74.
9. Edge SB, Compton CC. The American Joint Committee on Cancer: the 7th edition of the AJCC cancer staging manual and the future of TNM. Ann Surg Oncol. 2010;17(6):1471–4.
10. Christensen E, Schlichting P, Fauerholdt L, et al. Prognostic value of Child–Turcotte criteria in medically treated cirrhosis. Hepatology. 1984;4(3):430–5.
11. Okuda K, Ohtsuki T, Obata H, et al. Natural history of hepatocellular carcinoma and prognosis in relation to treatment. Study of 850 patients. Cancer. 1985;56(4):918–28.
12. The Cancer of the Liver Italian Program (CLIP) Investigators. A new prognostic system for hepatocellular carcinoma: a retrospective study of 435 patients. Hepatology. 1998;28(3):751–5.

13. Chevret S, Trinchet JC, Mathieu D, Rached AA, Beaugrand M, Chastang C. A new prognostic classification for predicting survival in patients with hepatocellular carcinoma. Groupe d'Etude et de Traitement du Carcinome Hepatocellulaire. J Hepatol. 1999;31(1):133–41.

14. Llovet JM, Bru C, Bruix J. Prognosis of hepatocellular carcinoma: the BCLC staging classification. Semin Liver Dis. 1999;19(3):329–38.

15. Kudo M, Chung H, Osaki Y. Prognostic staging system for hepatocellular carcinoma (CLIP score): its value and limitations, and a proposal for a new staging system, the Japan Integrated Staging Score (JIS score). J Gastroenterol. 2003;38(3):207–15.

16. European Association For The Study Of The Liver, European Organisation For Research And Treatment Of Cancer. EASL-EORTC Clinical Practice Guidelines: Management of hepatocellular carcinoma. J Hepatol. 2012;56(4):908–43.

17. Tandon P, Garcia-Tsao G. Prognostic indicators in hepatocellular carcinoma: a systematic review of 72 studies. Liver Int. 2009;29(4):502–10.

18. Vauthey JN, Klimstra D, Franceschi D, et al. Factors affecting long-term outcome after hepatic resection for hepatocellular carcinoma. Am J Surg. 1995;169(1):28–34. discussion 34–25.

19. Lauwers GY, Terris B, Balis UJ, et al. Prognostic histologic indicators of curatively resected hepatocellular carcinomas: a multi-institutional analysis of 425 patients with definition of a histologic prognostic index. Am J Surg Pathol. 2002;26(1):25–34.

20. Ikai I, Yamaoka Y, Yamamoto Y, et al. Surgical intervention for patients with stage IV-A hepatocellular carcinoma without lymph node metastasis: proposal as a standard therapy. Ann Surg. 1998;227(3):433–9.

21. Vauthey JN, Lauwers GY, Esnaola NF, et al. Simplified staging for hepatocellular carcinoma. J Clin Oncol. 2002;20(6):1527–36.

22. Nzeako UC, Goodman ZD, Ishak KG. Hepatocellular carcinoma in cirrhotic and noncirrhotic livers. A clinico-histopathologic study of 804 North American patients. Am J Clin Pathol. 1996;105(1):65–75.

23. Poon RT, Fan ST. Evaluation of the new AJCC/UICC staging system for hepatocellular carcinoma after hepatic resection in Chinese patients. Surg Oncol Clin N Am. 2003;12(1):35–50. viii.

24. Wu CC, Cheng SB, Ho WM, Chen JT, Liu TJ, P'Eng FK. Liver resection for hepatocellular carcinoma in patients with cirrhosis. Br J Surg. 2005;92(3):348–55.

25. Varotti G, Ramacciato G, Ercolani G, et al. Comparison between the fifth and sixth editions of the AJCC/UICC TNM staging systems for hepatocellular carcinoma: multicentric study on 393 cirrhotic resected patients. Eur J Surg Oncol. 2005;31(7):760–7.

26. Ramacciato G, Mercantini P, Cautero N, et al. Prognostic evaluation of the new American Joint Committee on Cancer/International Union Against Cancer staging system for hepatocellular carcinoma: analysis of 112 cirrhotic patients resected for hepatocellular carcinoma. Ann Surg Oncol. 2005;12(4):289–97.

27. Lei HJ, Chau GY, Lui WY, et al. Prognostic value and clinical relevance of the 6th Edition 2002 American Joint Committee on Cancer staging system in patients with resectable hepatocellular carcinoma. J Am Coll Surg. 2006;203(4):426–35.

28. Kee KM, Wang JH, Lee CM, et al. Validation of clinical AJCC/UICC TNM staging system for hepatocellular carcinoma: analysis of 5,613 cases from a medical center in southern Taiwan. Int J Cancer. 2007;120(12):2650–5.

29. Vauthey JN, Ribero D, Abdalla EK, et al. Outcomes of liver transplantation in 490 patients with hepatocellular carcinoma: validation of a uniform staging after surgical treatment. J Am Coll Surg. 2007;204(5):1016–27. discussion 1027–1018.

30. Choi SB, Lee JG, Kim KS, et al. The prognosis and survival analysis according to seven staging systems of hepatocellular carcinoma following curative resection. Hepatogastroenterology. 2008;55(88):2140–5.

31. Vauthey JN, Lauwers GY. Prognostic factors after resection of hepatocellular carcinoma: are there landmarks in the wild forest? J Hepatol. 2003;38(2):237–9.

32. Henderson JM, Sherman M, Tavill A, Abecassis M, Chejfec G, Gramlich T. AHPBA/AJCC consensus conference on staging of hepatocellular carcinoma: consensus statement. HPB (Oxford). 2003;5(4):243–50.

33. Lu W, Dong J, Huang Z, Guo D, Liu Y, Shi S. Comparison of four current staging systems for Chinese patients with hepatocellular carcinoma undergoing curative resection: Okuda, CLIP, TNM and CUPI. J Gastroenterol Hepatol. 2008;23(12):1874–8.
34. Contreras CM, Vauthey JN. Staging systems: is there a surgical staging and a medical one? A surgeon's perspective. J Hepatobiliary Pancreat Sci. 2010;17(4):438–9.
35. Edge SB, Byrd DR, Compton CC, Fritz AG, Greene LF, Trotti A. AJCC (American Joint Committee on Cancer) cancer staging manual. 7th ed. New York: Springer; 2010.
36. Japan ISGo. General Rules for the Clinical and Pathological Study of Primary Liver Cancer 2nd English [corresponds to the 2000 4th Japanese edition.] ed. Tokyo: Kanehara; 2003.
37. Ueno S, Tanabe G, Nuruki K, et al. Prognostic performance of the new classification of primary liver cancer of Japan (4th edition) for patients with hepatocellular carcinoma: a validation analysis. Hepatol Res. 2002;24(4):395–403.
38. Makuuchi M, Belghiti J, Belli G, et al. IHPBA concordant classification of primary liver cancer: working group report. J Hepatobiliary Pancreat Surg. 2003;10(1):26–30.
39. Minagawa M, Ikai I, Matsuyama Y, Yamaoka Y, Makuuchi M. Staging of hepatocellular carcinoma: assessment of the Japanese TNM and AJCC/UICC TNM systems in a cohort of 13,772 patients in Japan. Ann Surg. 2007;245(6):909–22.
40. Cillo U, Bassanello M, Vitale A, et al. The critical issue of hepatocellular carcinoma prognostic classification: which is the best tool available? J Hepatol. 2004;40(1):124–31.
41. Grieco A, Pompili M, Caminiti G, et al. Prognostic factors for survival in patients with early-intermediate hepatocellular carcinoma undergoing non-surgical therapy: comparison of Okuda, CLIP, and BCLC staging systems in a single Italian centre. Gut. 2005;54(3):411–8.
42. Levy I, Sherman M. Staging of hepatocellular carcinoma: assessment of the CLIP, Okuda, and Child–Pugh staging systems in a cohort of 257 patients in Toronto. Gut. 2002;50(6):881–5.
43. Marrero JA, Fontana RJ, Barrat A, et al. Prognosis of hepatocellular carcinoma: comparison of 7 staging systems in an American cohort. Hepatology. 2005;41(4):707–16.
44. Rabe C, Lenz M, Schmitz V, et al. An independent evaluation of modern prognostic scores in a central European cohort of 120 patients with hepatocellular carcinoma. Eur J Gastroenterol Hepatol. 2003;15(12):1305–15.
45. The Cancer of the Liver Italian Program (CLIP) Investigators. Prospective validation of the CLIP score: a new prognostic system for patients with cirrhosis and hepatocellular carcinoma. Hepatology. 2000;31(4):840–5.
46. Ueno S, Tanabe G, Sako K, et al. Discrimination value of the new western prognostic system (CLIP score) for hepatocellular carcinoma in 662 Japanese patients. Cancer of the Liver Italian Program. Hepatology. 2001;34(3):529–34.
47. Farinati F, Rinaldi M, Gianni S, Naccarato R. How should patients with hepatocellular carcinoma be staged? Validation of a new prognostic system. Cancer. 2000;89(11):2266–73.
48. Siddique I, El-Naga HA, Memon A, Thalib L, Hasan F, Al-Nakib B. CLIP score as a prognostic indicator for hepatocellular carcinoma: experience with patients in the Middle East. Eur J Gastroenterol Hepatol. 2004;16(7):675–80.
49. Huitzil-Melendez FD, Capanu M, O'Reilly EM, et al. Advanced hepatocellular carcinoma: which staging systems best predict prognosis? J Clin Oncol. 2010;28(17):2889–95.
50. Marrero JA. Staging systems for hepatocellular carcinoma: should we all use the BCLC system? J Hepatol. 2006;44(4):630–2.
51. Pons F, Varela M, Llovet JM. Staging systems in hepatocellular carcinoma. HPB (Oxford). 2005;7(1):35–41.
52. Toyoda H, Kumada T, Kiriyama S, et al. Comparison of the usefulness of three staging systems for hepatocellular carcinoma (CLIP, BCLC, and JIS) in Japan. Am J Gastroenterol. 2005;100(8):1764–71.
53. Camma C, Di Marco V, Cabibbo G, et al. Survival of patients with hepatocellular carcinoma in cirrhosis: a comparison of BCLC, CLIP and GRETCH staging systems. Aliment Pharmacol Ther. 2008;28(1):62–75.
54. Nanashima A, Morino S, Yamaguchi H, et al. Modified CLIP using PIVKA-II for evaluating prognosis after hepatectomy for hepatocellular carcinoma. Eur J Surg Oncol. 2003;29(9):735–42.

55. Nanashima A, Omagari K, Tobinaga S, et al. Comparative study of survival of patients with hepatocellular carcinoma predicted by different staging systems using multivariate analysis. Eur J Surg Oncol. 2005;31(8):882–90.
56. Huo TI, Huang YH, Lin HC, et al. Proposal of a modified Cancer of the Liver Italian Program staging system based on the model for end-stage liver disease for patients with hepatocellular carcinoma undergoing loco-regional therapy. Am J Gastroenterol. 2006;101(5):975–82.
57. Kaseb AO, Hassan MM, Lin E, et al. V-CLIP: Integrating plasma vascular endothelial growth factor into a new scoring system to stratify patients with advanced hepatocellular carcinoma for clinical trials. Cancer. 2011;117(11):2478–88.
58. Tournoux-Facon C, Paoletti X, Barbare JC, et al. Development and validation of a new prognostic score of death for patients with hepatocellular carcinoma in palliative setting. J Hepatol. 2011;54(1):108–14.
59. Kudo M, Chung H, Haji S, et al. Validation of a new prognostic staging system for hepatocellular carcinoma: the JIS score compared with the CLIP score. Hepatology. 2004;40(6):1396–405.
60. Chung H, Kudo M, Takahashi S, et al. Comparison of three current staging systems for hepatocellular carcinoma: Japan integrated staging score, new Barcelona Clinic Liver Cancer staging classification, and Tokyo score. J Gastroenterol Hepatol. 2008;23(3):445–52.
61. Ikai I, Takayasu K, Omata M, et al. A modified Japan Integrated Stage score for prognostic assessment in patients with hepatocellular carcinoma. J Gastroenterol. 2006;41(9):884–92.
62. Nanashima A, Sumida Y, Abo T, et al. Modified Japan integrated staging is currently the best available staging system for hepatocellular carcinoma patients who have undergone hepatectomy. J Gastroenterol. 2006;41(3):250–6.
63. Nanashima A, Sumida Y, Morino S, et al. The Japanese integrated staging score using liver damage grade for hepatocellular carcinoma in patients after hepatectomy. Eur J Surg Oncol. 2004;30(7):765 70.
64. Huo TI, Lin HC, Huang YH, et al. The model for end-stage liver disease-based Japan Integrated scoring system may have a better predictive ability for patients with hepatocellular carcinoma undergoing locoregional therapy. Cancer. 2006;107(1):141–8.
65. Kitai S, Kudo M, Minami Y, et al. Validation of a new prognostic staging system for hepatocellular carcinoma: a comparison of the biomarker-combined Japan integrated staging score, the conventional Japan integrated staging score and the BALAD score. Oncology. 2008;75 Suppl 1:83–90.
66. Kitai S, Kudo M, Minami Y, et al. A new prognostic staging system for hepatocellular carcinoma: value of the biomarker combined Japan integrated staging score. Intervirology. 2008;51 Suppl 1:86–94.
67. Yen YH, Changchien CS, Wang JH, et al. A modified TNM-based Japan Integrated Score combined with AFP level may serve as a better staging system for early-stage predominant hepatocellular carcinoma patients. Dig Liver Dis. 2009;41(6):431–41.
68. Leung TW, Tang AM, Zee B, et al. Construction of the Chinese University prognostic Index for hepatocellular carcinoma and comparison with the TNM staging system, the Okuda staging system, and the cancer of the liver Italian Program staging system: a study based on 926 patients. Cancer. 2002;94(6):1760–9.
69. Leung TW, Mo F, Leow CK, et al. Multicenter validation of the Chinese University Prognostic Index (CUPI) of hepatocellular carcinoma (HCC). Proc Am Soc Clin Oncol. 2003;22:1040A.
70. Chan SL, Mo FK, Johnson PJ, et al. Prospective validation of the Chinese University Prognostic Index and comparison with other staging systems for hepatocellular carcinoma in an Asian population. J Gastroenterol Hepatol. 2011;26(2):340–7.
71. Tateishi R, Yoshida H, Shiina S, et al. Proposal of a new prognostic model for hepatocellular carcinoma: an analysis of 403 patients. Gut. 2005;54(3):419–25.
72. Yau T, Yao TJ, Chan P, Ng K, Fan ST, Poon RT. A new prognostic score system in patients with advanced hepatocellular carcinoma not amendable to locoregional therapy: implication for patient selection in systemic therapy trials. Cancer. 2008;113(10):2742–51.
73. Omagari K, Honda S, Kadokawa Y, et al. Preliminary analysis of a newly proposed prognostic scoring system (SLiDe score) for hepatocellular carcinoma. J Gastroenterol Hepatol. 2004;19(7):805–11.

74. Nanashima A, Omagari K, Sumida Y, et al. Evaluation of new prognostic staging systems (SLiDe score) for hepatocellular carcinoma patients who underwent hepatectomy. Hepatogastroenterology. 2009;56(93):1137–40.
75. Toyoda H, Kumada T, Osaki Y, et al. Staging hepatocellular carcinoma by a novel scoring system (BALAD score) based on serum markers. Clin Gastroenterol Hepatol. 2006;4(12):1528–36.
76. Hsu CY, Huang YH, Hsia CY, et al. A new prognostic model for hepatocellular carcinoma based on total tumor volume: the Taipei integrated scoring system. J Hepatol. 2010;53(1):108–17.
77. Oken MM, Creech RH, Tormey DC, et al. Toxicity and response criteria of the Eastern Cooperative Oncology Group. Am J Clin Oncol. 1982;5(6):649–55.
78. Cillo U, Vitale A, Grigoletto F, et al. Prospective validation of the Barcelona Clinic Liver Cancer staging system. J Hepatol. 2006;44(4):723–31.
79. Vitale A, Saracino E, Boccagni P, et al. Validation of the BCLC prognostic system in surgical hepatocellular cancer patients. Transplant Proc. 2009;41(4):1260–3.
80. Guglielmi A, Ruzzenente A, Pachera S, et al. Comparison of seven staging systems in cirrhotic patients with hepatocellular carcinoma in a cohort of patients who underwent radiofrequency ablation with complete response. Am J Gastroenterol. 2008;103(3):597–604.
81. Beaugrand M, Sala M, Degos F, et al. Treatment of advanced hepatolcellular carcinoma by seocalcitol (a vit D analogue): an International randomized double-blind placebo-controlled study in 747 patients. J Hepatol. 2005;42 Suppl 2:17A.
82. Cheng AL, Kang YK, Chen Z, et al. Efficacy and safety of sorafenib in patients in the Asia-Pacific region with advanced hepatocellular carcinoma: a phase III randomised, double-blind, placebo-controlled trial. Lancet Oncol. 2009;10(1):25–34.
83. Llovet JM, Ricci S, Mazzaferro V, et al. Sorafenib in advanced hepatocellular carcinoma. N Engl J Med. 2008;359(4):378–90.
84. Takayama T, Makuuchi M, Hasegawa K. Single HCC smaller than 2 cm: surgery or ablation?: surgeon's perspective. J Hepatobiliary Pancreat Sci. 2010;17(4):422–4.
85. Takayama T, Makuuchi M, Hirohashi S, et al. Early hepatocellular carcinoma as an entity with a high rate of surgical cure. Hepatology. 1998;28(5):1241–6.
86. Bruix J, Llovet JM. Prognostic prediction and treatment strategy in hepatocellular carcinoma. Hepatology. 2002;35(3):519–24.
87. Llovet JM, Bruix J. Systematic review of randomized trials for unresectable hepatocellular carcinoma: Chemoembolization improves survival. Hepatology. 2003;37(2):429–42.
88. Llovet JM, Real MI, Montana X, et al. Arterial embolisation or chemoembolisation versus symptomatic treatment in patients with unresectable hepatocellular carcinoma: a randomised controlled trial. Lancet. 2002;359(9319):1734–9.
89. Lo CM, Ngan H, Tso WK, et al. Randomized controlled trial of transarterial lipiodol chemoembolization for unresectable hepatocellular carcinoma. Hepatology. 2002;35(5):1164–71.
90. Yao FY, Ferrell L, Bass NM, et al. Liver transplantation for hepatocellular carcinoma: expansion of the tumor size limits does not adversely impact survival. Hepatology. 2001;33(6):1394–403.
91. National Comprehensive Cancer Network (NCCN) Guidelines Version 2.2011 Hepatocellular Carcinoma. http://www.nccn.org/professionals/physician_gls/f_guidelines.asp. Accessed 7 July 2011.
92. Meier V, Ramadori G. Clinical staging of hepatocellular carcinoma. Dig Dis. 2009;27(2):131–41.

Chapter 9
Liver Anatomy and Function in the Planning of Hepatic Interventions

Nicholas N. Nissen and Alagappan Annamalai

Introduction

The patient with newly diagnosed hepatic tumor faces the unique dilemma of having more cytoreductive treatment options available to them than any other type of solid organ cancer. As a simple example, a patient with well-compensated cirrhosis and a small tumor may be a candidate for any one of the options of hepatic resection, chemical or thermal ablation, or hepatic arterial therapy. Add to this the choice of an open versus laparoscopic versus percutaneous procedure, and the wide array of devices and hepatic artery infusates available, and the patient may have ten or more viable treatment options. Making sense of these options and in turn selecting the most appropriate treatment for an individual patient require a working knowledge of liver anatomy and function and require the practitioner to recognize the constraints of each modality. In this chapter, we will focus on liver anatomy and function as it pertains to decision-making in the treatment of hepatic tumors. We will focus first on how anatomy and function pertain to hepatic resection and later expand this to be applicable to decision-making regarding local and regional therapies.

N.N. Nissen, MD (✉)
Department of Surgery, Comprehensive Transplant Center, Cedars-Sinai Medical Center,
Los Angeles, CA 90048, USA

Center for Liver Diseases and Transplantation, 8635W 3rd Street, Suite 590W,
Los Angeles, CA 90048, USA
e-mail: Nicholas.nissen@cshs.org

A. Annamalai, MD
Department of Surgery, Comprehensive Transplant Center, Cedars-Sinai Medical Center,
Los Angeles, CA 90048, USA

N. Reau and F.F. Poordad (eds.), *Primary Liver Cancer: Surveillance, Diagnosis and Treatment*, Clinical Gastroenterology, DOI 10.1007/978-1-61779-863-4_9,
© Springer Science+Business Media New York 2012

Basics of Hepatic Anatomy

Most descriptions of liver anatomy are based on the classic descriptions of segmental and lobar anatomy from two different researchers Couinaud [1] and Healey [2], roughly 50 years ago (Fig. 9.1). The nomenclature embraced over the decades varied between surgeons and between centers, making comparative descriptions of treatments and outcomes difficult. In 1998, the International HepatoPancreaticoBiliary Association (IHPBA) convened an expert panel to come to consensus on an accurate, useful, and widely applicable terminology to describe liver anatomy and liver resections, which was subsequently accepted by the IHPBA in Brisbane, Australia [3]. The IHPBA terminology, sometimes called the Brisbane classification, has become widely accepted in the literature, but terms such as hepatic lobectomy and trisegmentectomy, which are not ideal descriptors, are still utilized in many circles.

The IHPBA paradigm recognizes right and left hemilivers (no longer called lobes), with two sections making up each hemiliver and two segments making up each section (except left medial section, consisting of only segment 4). The vascular watershed areas which artificially separate the liver are termed interhemispheric or intersectional planes. The terms lobe, lobectomy, trisegmentectomy, and Cantle's line are no longer favored [3, 4].

This segmental/sectional description has allowed fairly consistent terminology when describing "anatomic" hepatic resections (Table 9.1). *Anatomic* resections are those in which lobar or sectoral boundaries are followed, often utilizing division of

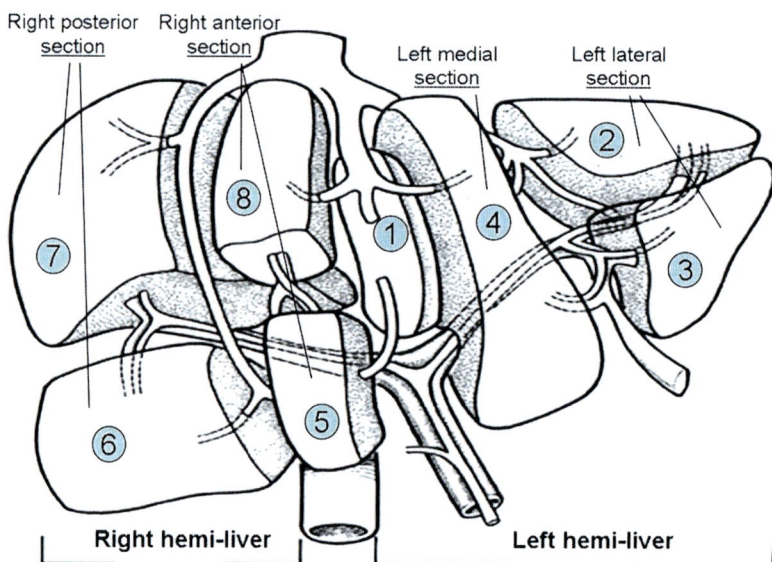

Fig. 9.1 Drawing showing hepatic terminology by IHPBA consensus (see text for details). Segments are numbered individually, and the four anatomic liver sections are noted

Table 9.1 IHPBA terminology of common liver resections

Resection type	Segments of liver removed
Left lateral sectionectomy or bisegmentectomy	2, 3
Left hemihepatectomy or left hepatectomy	2–4 (+/−1)
Left trisectionectomy or extended left hemihepatectomy	2–5, 8(+/−1)
Right hemihepatectomy or right hepatectomy	5–8
Right trisectionectomy or extended right hemihepatectomy	4–8

the vascular structures at or near the hilum of the liver. This expression, while not precise, implies both a method of dissection and a magnitude of resection encompassing at least two segments. In contrast, *nonanatomic* hepatic resections are those which do not follow a strict hemispheric (previously lobar) or sectoral plane and instead aim to simply remove the target lesion with an appropriate margin of normal liver. Resections involving a single segment usually are not called anatomic resections, but this distinction is arbitrary.

A precise understanding of anatomic detail is most critical when planning liver resections, in which the residual liver must maintain adequate function to allow full hepatic and overall recovery. In the simplest terms, the surgeon must ensure that at the end of a procedure, four key principles are met: (1) adequate volume of liver remaining, (2) adequate vascular inflow and outflow of liver remnant, (3) adequate biliary drainage, and (4) adequate functional hepatic reserve to tolerate the stress associated with recovery. Standard liver resections (Table 9.1) are crafted so that the planned liver remnant has independent portal, biliary, and hepatic vein integrity, and these factors rarely need to be considered independently. More complex scenarios, such as those in which lesions occupy the middle segments of the liver or involve central portal structures, or those in which prior interventions have already compromised some of the liver, require more detailed planning. An example of this process is presented in Fig. 9.2.

Assessment of Liver Volume

A key aspect of planning a successful hepatic resection is the determination of liver volume. Important measurements include total liver volume (TLV), tumor volume (TV), and residual liver volume (RLV). The term future liver remnant (FLR) is similar to RLV, but FLR is often used when discussing methods to increase hepatic volume such as preoperative portal vein embolization. Total liver volume (TLV, Table 9.2) is the volume of the entire native liver and can be either calculated from cross-sectional imaging or estimated using body surface area or body mass. TV refers to the volume of tumor in the liver and is an important concept to recognize, since this is considered nonfunctional parenchyma and should be removed from TLV when estimating the effect of resection of normal parenchyma. Since most tumors are roughly spherical, this can be estimated by the formula $TV = r^3\pi(4/3)$, where r is

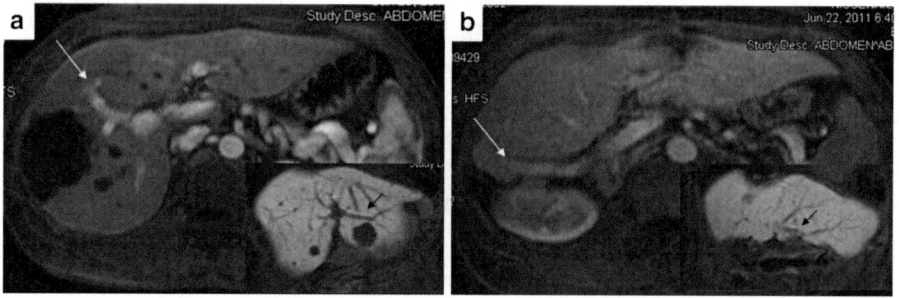

Fig. 9.2 Treatment of bilobar hepatic tumors. (**a**) Preoperative MRI shows large mass in posterior right liver on axial view, with left-sided lesion seen on coronal imaging (*inset*). In order to preserve parenchyma, the portal structures to the anterior section of the right lobe (*white arrow*) are preserved and posterior right sectionectomy is performed. Wedge resection of segment 3 mass is performed to preserve portal structures to left lateral section (*black arrow*). (**b**) Postoperative MRI showing preservation of the right anterior section and left lateral section

Table 9.2 Common acronyms

TLV	Total liver volume	Estimate or direct measurement of volume of entire liver
FLR	Future liver remnant	Portion of liver that will remain after surgical resection of diseased liver
RLV	Residual liver volume	Volume of liver that will remain after surgical resection
TV	Tumor volume	Amount of tumor that is planned for removal during liver resection (does not include surrounding normal liver)
DLH	Degree of liver hypertrophy	Change in RLV or FLR measured before and after preoperative PVE
PPVE	Preoperative portal vein embolization	Deliberate occlusion of the portal vein of planned resection area in order to induce hypertrophy of FLR
DRGBWR	Donor graft to recipient graft body weight ratio	Ratio of the weight of liver used in liver transplant to the weight of the recipient

maximal radius of the tumor in cm. FLR or RLV refers to the amount of liver that will remain after resection. FLR is an acronym often used to discuss the planned volume before and after portal vein embolization, but for consistency in this chapter, we will generally refer to this as RLV. TV and RLV, because they will vary with the type of planned resection, must be calculated using cross-sectional imaging. Of note, for a straightforward hemihepatectomy (or lobectomy) in a healthy liver, calculating liver volumes is usually not necessary unless there is an unusually small-appearing remnant lobe. In larger resections or those performed on patients with underlying liver dysfunction, calculating liver volumes in advance should be routine.

Table 9.3 Formulas for calculating liver mass and liver resection

TLV by body mass[a]	TLV (cc) = 18.5 (cc/kg) × body mass (kg) + 191 (cc)
TLV by body surface area[a]	TLV (cc) = 1,280 (cc/m²) × body surface area (m²) − 700 (cc)
Residual liver volume index (goal for safe resection is >0.5%)	RLV index = residual liver volume (cc) divided by body mass (kg) (×100%) (×1 kg/1,000 cc)
Residual liver volume ratio (goal for safe resection is >30%)	RLV ratio = residual liver volume (cc)/(TLV−TV) (cc) × 100%

[a]Vauthey et al. [5, 10]

TLV total liver volume, *TV* tumor volume, *RLV* residual liver volume

TLV can be estimated or calculated by several methods. In broad terms, TLV is around 2% of the total body mass and the right lobe (segments 5–8) makes up ~55–65% of the TLV. When more precise information is required, as is often the case, TLV can be estimated by slightly more detailed formulas listed in Table 9.3. These formulas are based on large series of patients and may be subject to some geographic or age bias [5]. Weight-based formulas may slightly overestimate TLV in older patients, and there may also be mild variations across nationality, as TLV measured in a large Japanese study showed liver volumes averaging ~300 cm³ less than in Western patients after correcting for body mass [5, 6]. Several commercially available programs can also be used to calculate liver volumes from cross-sectional imaging studies by summing slice volumes or the designated zone identified by the user. Calculation of TLV can also be performed "by hand" by manually outlining the liver on each slice of a CT or MRI scan to find a slice area and then summing this across the entire liver by multiplying each slice area by slice thickness. The assistance of a friendly radiologist in this tedious endeavor is invaluable.

Once TLV, TV, and RLV are calculated, a few simple calculations can be used to predict the risk of postresection hepatic failure (Table 9.3). The first of these formulas is the RLV to body weight ratio, or RLV index, which is simply RLV (in g) divided by body mass. Minimal acceptable RLV index has been reported as 0.5%, as patients with lower RLV index have increased risk of postresection liver failure and death [7]. The second useful formula is the RLV to TLV ratio, which is simply RLV divided by TLV−TV. In general, RLV/TLV ratio of 0.3 (or 30%) is considered safe in the presence of normal parenchyma, while ratios as low as 20% may be acceptable in select cases [8–10].

Remarkably, there continues to be some inconsistency in how liver volumes are expressed and how surgical decisions are made. In general, formulas which include TLV and TV may be less reliable in cases with multiple tumors or segments of dysfunctional parenchyma such as in the case of biliary obstruction because the planned FLR may be functionally more important than the area of planned resection, making the calculation of RLV/TLV ratio less valid. Our practice is to measure RLV directly with cross-sectional imaging and to calculate TLV based on body mass, and to then calculate RLV index with a goal of >0.5%.

Live donor liver transplantation is accompanied by an extra measure of complexity, in that both the resected portion of liver and the liver remnant must be of sufficient size and quality to thrive. In planning this procedure, the donor should have an RLV index of at least 0.7% to minimize risk of hepatic failure and the recipient should receive a graft of appropriate mass to provide a *donor graft to recipient body weight ratio* of at least 0.8%. Smaller grafts have been reported to function in live donor liver transplantation, but as the size of the partial graft decreases, the risk of graft failure and graft dysfunction increases. This scenario, often termed small-for-size syndrome, includes the constellation of hyperbilirubinemia, synthetic dysfunction, and ascites in the absence of other causes of graft failure [11].

Assessment of Liver Function

When considering a patient for hepatic intervention, the assessment of liver function and reserve should begin with clinical and laboratory assessment. Liver function can be considered in three broad categories: synthesis and metabolism, detoxification, and portal homeostasis, which are reflected in the analysis of serum albumin, prothrombin time, and serum bilirubin and the assessment of any evidence of portal hypertension or portosystemic shunting. Portal hypertension should be suspected in any patient with low or low-normal platelet count or any clinical or radiographic evidence of ascites, encephalopathy, or varices. In some cases with borderline features, such as the patient with lower-than-expected platelet count or radiographic features suggesting portal hypertension or cirrhosis, measurement of the hepatic vein to portal vein gradient can be easily accomplished by a transjugular approach and can be combined with transjugular liver biopsy to assess hepatic histology. The finding of portal hypertension in turn should cause the surgeon to limit the resection size or consider nonsurgical treatment options.

A concise description of hepatic reserve remains elusive, but for purposes of planning hepatic intervention, it refers to the capacity of the liver to recover from an insult and to restore the patient to normal performance and liver function. Ideally, the patient's hepatic reserve would return to normal as well, but in clinical practice this is rare, and the sum total of prior hepatic interventions always has to be considered in planning. Numerous clinical, biochemical, and imaging modalities have been utilized to determine hepatic functional reserve and are considered here.

Clinical Assessment of Hepatic Reserve

The most widely utilized clinical measures of hepatic reserve include the Child–Turcotte–Pugh (CTP) score, the model of end-stage liver disease score (MELD), and the Barcelona Center for Liver Cancer score (BCLC). Each of these has different origin and utility. The Child–Pugh classification (Table 9.4), sometimes referred to as the Child–Turcotte–Pugh score, is a tool used to help classify the severity of liver disease and to assess the prognosis of chronic liver disease.

Table 9.4 Child–Turcotte–Pugh classification and survival

Clinical factor	1 point	2 points	3 points
Albumin (g %)	>3.5	3–3.5	<3.0
Bilirubin (mg %)	<2.0	2.0–3.0	>3.0
Ascites	None	Controlled	Refractory
Encephalopathy	Absent	Minimal	Advanced
INR	<1.7	1.7–2.3	>2.3
Class	A	B	C
Points	5–6	7–9	10–15
1-year survival (%)	100	80	60
2-year survival (%)	85	60	35

CTP scoring was first reported as a predictor of death after surgical portacaval shunting, but over several decades, this quickly became the system by which patients with cirrhosis were classified for purposes ranging from determining risk of surgical intervention to determining organ allocation in liver transplantation. While CTP scoring has the apparent advantage that it is largely a physiologic and intuitive scoring system, it has the disadvantage of being subjective and poorly reproducible. The "Child's class," as it is often referred, provides a relatively simple broad categorization of hepatic reserve and function and is probably most valuable in risk stratification of nonhepatic interventions. For example, the mortality risk of umbilical hernia repair in a cirrhotic patient can be estimated as roughly 5%, 20%, or 50% for Child's A, B, or C class, respectively.

Model for end-stage liver disease (MELD) is an objective measure of liver disease-related mortality that is based on an easily reproducible logarithmic calculation composed of three laboratory values: creatinine, bilirubin, and international normalized ratio (INR) [12]. It has been validated as a prognostic index in patients with cirrhosis [13, 14]. Each single-point increment in the MELD score increases perioperative risk, suggesting a certain amount of precision in its ability to predict mortality [15, 16]. In the past, it had been suggested that MELD score had a poor predictive value in terms of postoperative morbidity and mortality after hepatic resection [17, 18]. The majority of those studies did not differentiate between resections with or without underlying cirrhosis [18–20]. Recently, it has been suggested that there is a 1% increase in mortality for each one-point increase in MELD from 5 to 20 and 2% increase with MELD scores >20 after any surgery [21]. MELD scores of ≤7, 8–11, and 12–15 have mortality rates of 5.7%, 10.3%, and 25.4%, respectively, with an almost linear risk of death beyond a MELD of 8 [20]. Overall, it has been shown that mortality rates are as high as 25% after hepatic resection in patients with cirrhosis [22]. Risk stratification utilizing MELD score in cirrhotic patients has yielded death rates of 29% when the score is ≥9 and 0% with score ≤8 [23]. In addition to predicting mortality, MELD has the potential to predict morbidity after liver resection [15]. MELD scores of <9, 9–10, and >10% are associated with liver failure 0%, 3.6%, and 37.5% of the time, respectively [24]. On the other hand, MELD score fails to predict outcomes in noncirrhotic patients who undergo hepatic resection for hepatocellular carcinoma. In summary, MELD is useful to stratify patients into low- and high-risk resection groups just as is seen with CTP scoring, as those with MELD >8 do very poorly with liver resection. The real value of MELD in treating liver cancer, however, is likely to be in the stratification and management of patients who are not candidates for resection but are considering other potentially hepatotoxic therapies.

The Barcelona Clinic Liver Cancer (BCLC), Cancer of the Liver Italian Program (CLIP), Japan Integrated Scoring (JIS) system, tumor-node-metastasis (TNM), and Tokyo score are all systems developed to prognosticate and treat hepatocellular cancer [25]. The only externally validated system is the BCLC classification. The BCLC staging system is not a scoring system but rather a staging classification that was derived from results of multiple studies identifying various prognostic indicators for HCC. It was developed from a cohort of studies and randomized clinical trials [26, 27]. The BCLC classification system uses multiple variables including tumor stage, liver functional status, physical status, and cancer-related symptoms. Based on these variables, prognostic stages can be determined, from very early (Stage 0) and early (Stage A) to terminal (Stage D). These stages are then linked to treatment options to create a management algorithm. Hepatic resection for HCC is only advised with a BCLC Stage 0 (carcinoma in situ, HCC <2 cm) and early stage A1 (single lesion and well-preserved liver function with normal liver function and <10 mmHg hepatic venous pressure gradient) [18, 26, 27].

Biochemical and Nuclear Imaging Assessment of Liver Function

In addition to volumetric analysis and clinical risk stratification, a tremendous amount of research has been performed on identifying a useful functional assessment of liver function that goes beyond common laboratory analysis. These tests are most useful in patients with some degree of underlying hepatic dysfunction or fibrosis or in those with marginal FLR volume in whom portal vein embolization might be considered. The best tests to assess preoperative hepatic function should be noninvasive, rapid, reproducible, and relatively easy to perform.

Many currently utilized quantitative liver function tests were developed based on the understanding that the liver cytochrome p450 system sequentially metabolized certain foreign compounds yielding a detectable metabolite. The most widely used metabolite is indocyanine green (ICG) which is a tricarbocyanine dye entirely metabolized by the liver. After binding to albumin and alpha-1 lipoproteins, it is actively transported into liver cells. Serum sampling of ICG after 15 min is generally accepted as a single useful measure for determining hepatic parenchymal function. ICG retention is not only affected by parenchymal function, but it is also substantially influenced by hepatic blood flow. Impaired hepatic function is suggested by 15% or more retention of ICG within the plasma after 15 min from the injection. Patients with higher degree of 15-min ICG retention have been reported to have poor outcomes after major liver resections [28, 29]. ICG clearance may be affected by hepatic blood flow and is decreased after portal vein embolization as reported by Wayakabashi et al. Interestingly, in this report, mortality rates did not correlate with changes in ICG clearance after portal vein embolization. Despite a possible limitation in the assessment of patients undergoing preoperative portal vein embolization (PPVE), ICG clearance remains the most widely reported and utilized functional test for assessment of risk during hepatic resection.

Nuclear imaging, utilizing single-photon emission computed tomography (SPECT), is another method to assess hepatic functional reserve. 99m-Tc is a radio-label attached to synthetic proteins such as galactosyl glycoalbumin which bind to hepatic receptors. SPECT imaging is not only able to provide volumetric and ana-tomic assessment of the liver but also provides a functional assessment of the liver's ability to clear the radiolabeled glycoproteins [16, 25, 26]. Stadalnik et al. demon-strated the correlation of glycoprotein clearance with the Child's score, the amin-opyrine breath test, and ICG retention [30]. A summary of the Japanese experience with a similar glycoprotein analog showed clear evidence correlating hepatic func-tion with the index of cirrhosis, whereas a similar correlation between ICG retention and cirrhosis was not elucidated. Hwang et al. revealed that SPECT images could predict the quantity of functional receptors remaining after hepatic resection [31]. Multiple studies have combined SPECT imaging with portal vein embolization. After portal vein embolization, there has been a trend suggesting an increase in receptor numbers but on an uncertain timetable. Kubo et al. demonstrated a shift in receptor numbers to the contralateral lobe after portal vein embolization as hyper-plasia ensued [32]. Kokudo et al. elaborated on receptor recovery after hepatic resection by showing that an initial decline in receptor concentration in the first several weeks was followed by an increase in receptor number up to 150 days postresection [33]. The use of SPECT imaging as a guide to resection remains rela-tively limited in clinical practice, but there may be an increased role for this modal-ity as the trend toward increased sequential hepatic interventions continues.

The LiMAx test is a recently described test which can be used both preopera-tively and postoperatively to predict liver failure. This test involves the intravenous administration of C-13-methacetin which is metabolized in a manner dependent on liver function to C-13-CO2, which is in turn easily measured by breath analysis. When given on the day after hepatic resection, the LiMAx test correlates with the risk of death from hepatic failure [34].

Postoperative Liver Failure

The diagnosis of liver failure after hepatic resection (posthepatectomy liver failure, or PHLF) is made if there is evidence of significant synthetic dysfunction, hyper-bilirubinemia, encephalopathy, or portal hypertension during the recovery period. Several criteria have been developed to diagnose postresection liver failure, but these are largely useful in the standardization of reporting across centers, since there are limited treatments available in the present day to the patient who carries this diagnosis. In its most ominous form, postresection liver failure has similarities to fulminant hepatic failure or the syndrome of primary nonfunction after liver transplant. This severe form is rarely amenable to salvage liver transplant because of issue of underlying malignancy and the multisystem organ failure these patients often encounter, although extracorporeal liver support may hold some promise as a bridge to recovery. The vast majority of PHLF is more subtle and until recently was subject to variable degrees of reporting and diagnostic bias. Recent efforts to standardize the definition and diagnosis of postoperative liver failure are promising. Most patients diagnosed with PHLF will recover, but the impact on future ability to tolerate treatments is greatly diminished.

The International Study Group of Liver Surgery (ILSGLS) has proposed a definition of PHLF as increased INR or bilirubin on or after postoperative day 5, with grading of severity based on the impact to a patients' clinical management [35]. Two other useful scoring systems include postoperative MELD score and the 50/50 criteria. The first of these has been described previously and is appealing because it includes kidney function and as such may reflect a trend toward multiorgan dysfunction. The 50/50 criteria is similar to the ILSGLS criteria in that it considers PHLF present if bilirubin is >50 µl/l or prothrombin time index is <50% of the normal on postoperative day 5 after liver resection [36].

The relative value of these three PHLF scoring systems in predicting outcome and mortality has been reported, and there remains some debate on the ideal reporting system. The MELD score, because it is routinely followed in patients with chronic liver disease, has the added benefit that it is used by interventional radiologists and other specialties to follow liver function before and after treatment, and as such may allow a delta MELD comparison across treatments.

The diagnosis of liver failure after nonsurgical hepatic treatments has not been well defined to date. In general, any significant increase in bilirubin, prothrombin time, or severity of encephalopathy or ascites should be considered as indicative of hepatic compromise. Since these modalities are often palliative, data are often reported as time to disease progression and time to death. However, as competing modalities arise, refinement in classification of liver failure after nonsurgical treatments will become increasingly important.

Planning a Hepatic Resection

The decisions surrounding liver resection are centered around a risk/benefit analysis. The risk of major hepatic resection includes both perioperative events such as liver failure and bleeding but also the risk related to loss of healthy parenchyma and the potential risks of future hepatic interventions. The benefit should be measured in improvement of symptoms or disease, prevention of cancer (as in the case of hepatic adenoma), or durable treatment of malignancy.

Risk assessment in planning a liver resection includes several factors, including liver volume, liver function, tumor location, and patient comorbidities. Analysis of liver volume and function is described above. Tumor size and location are important in planning because this determines the amount of diseased and healthy bystander liver that will be removed and also predicts blood loss and determines the surgical approach. Finally, the importance of considering patient reserve is paramount, and efforts to take this assessment beyond the traditional "eyeball test" are ongoing.

In cases involving a single liver tumor, the decision for the surgeon largely boils down to whether to perform anatomic or nonanatomic resection (defined above). The decision-making in these cases is not easily amenable to algorithms, but several key factors should always be considered: (1) can adequate margin be obtained with nonanatomic resection, (2) is there likelihood of requiring future interventions on the remnant liver, (3) if nonanatomic resection is performed, does the area of liver preserved have independent biliary and vascular integrity so that it is likely to show significant hypertrophy and be functionally significant, (4) is nonanatomic resection safe with respect to vascular control and risk of bile leak? If these factors favor nonanatomic resection, then this approach should be considered. As a general approach, however, single tumors in segments 2 and 3 are often treated with anatomic left lateral sectionectomy (formerly left lateral segmentectomy), which removes relatively little liver mass, is anatomically favorable, and often can be performed laparoscopically. In contrast, lesions in segments 4–8 are often treated with nonanatomic resection to maximize parenchymal preservation and future therapeutic potential options.

When dealing with multifocal tumors, the surgical decision-making increases in complexity, but the fundamental issues remain unchanged. When planning resection, the same four questions are addressed, with the caveat that multifocality implies that recurrence is more likely and there may be even greater incentive to spare as much parenchyma as possible. The risk of bile leak, however, increases with the number of discrete resection beds, and if the majority of tumors are in a sector or lobe, then it may be safer to consider anatomic sectionectomy or hemihepatectomy rather than subject the patient to multiple unilateral segmental resections. In some cases, the safest approach may be to combine hepatic resection and ablation, typically using resection for formal removal of large tumors or tumor clusters, and ablation to treat smaller discrete lesions that might create excessive risk if resected. If the decision is made for incomplete treatment at the time of surgery, it may be beneficial to address the most difficult lesions or those requiring the most portal dissection at the first setting when the tissue planes are most favorable.

Special Circumstances

Preoperative Portal Vein Embolization

In patients with an estimated RLV that is too small to allow safe attempt at hepatic resection, preoperative embolization of the portal vein contralateral to the hepatic remanent can be performed in an attempt to induce RLV (or FLR) hypertrophy.

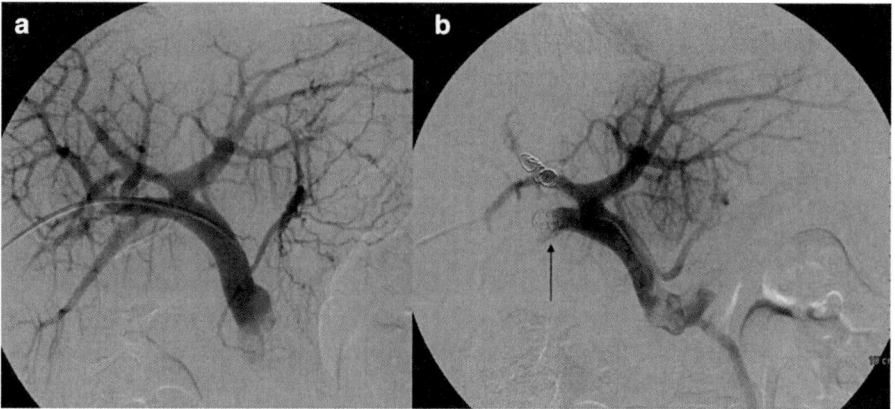

Fig. 9.3 Portal vein embolization. (**a**) Percutaneous portogram showing normal portal venogram in a patient with multifocal tumors in right hemiliver and segment 4. (**b**) Completion venogram after coils have been placed in the right portal vein and the segment 4 portal vein branch in an effort to induce hypertrophy of the left lateral section (see Fig. 9.4)

The premise of PVE is that preemptive hypertrophy lowers the risk of postoperative liver failure by either increased hepatocyte mass or lower risk of portal hyperperfusion. Several reports on PPVE have demonstrated increase in RLV of 20–40%, even in livers with fibrosis or cirrhosis. The exact mechanism by which PPVE induces hypertrophy is unknown, but presumably, it is related to the same mechanisms in play after a large liver resection. Physiologically, however, the stimulus for hypertrophy is less dramatic after PVE than after resection, as patients rarely develop hypophosphatemia or synthetic dysfunction after embolization.

The approach to PVE involves first measuring RLV (or FLR) directly by calculating the volume of the planned liver remnant from cross-sectional imaging, followed by an estimate of RLV index or RLV/TLV ratio. PPVE should be considered if the RLV index is 0.5% or the RLV/TLV ratio is <30% in the setting of an otherwise healthy liver remnant, or <0.7% or 40%, respectively in the patient with fibrosis or abnormal liver function [37]. Embolization is performed either by percutaneous or transjugular approach, with the degree of embolization tailored to the planned future resection (Figs. 9.3 and 9.4). PPVE is generally well tolerated, with side effects ranging from fevers and cholangitis to more severe events such as thrombosis of the RLV portal vein. There is also an obligate waiting time to allow RLV hypertrophy, which may carry additional risk in some cases.

Recent reports have demonstrated the moderate but predictable effectiveness in PVE both in achieving liver hypertrophy and in accomplishing surgical resection with low morbidity. In a fairly early Japanese study of PPVE, 43 patients were analyzed and found to have hypertrophic ratio of 1.4 in healthy livers and 1.2 in chronically diseased livers, where hypertrophic ratio was defined as the RLV after PVE/RLV before PVE. Interestingly, portal hemodynamics after PPVE were maintained after liver resection, questioning whether portal vascular capacitance increases

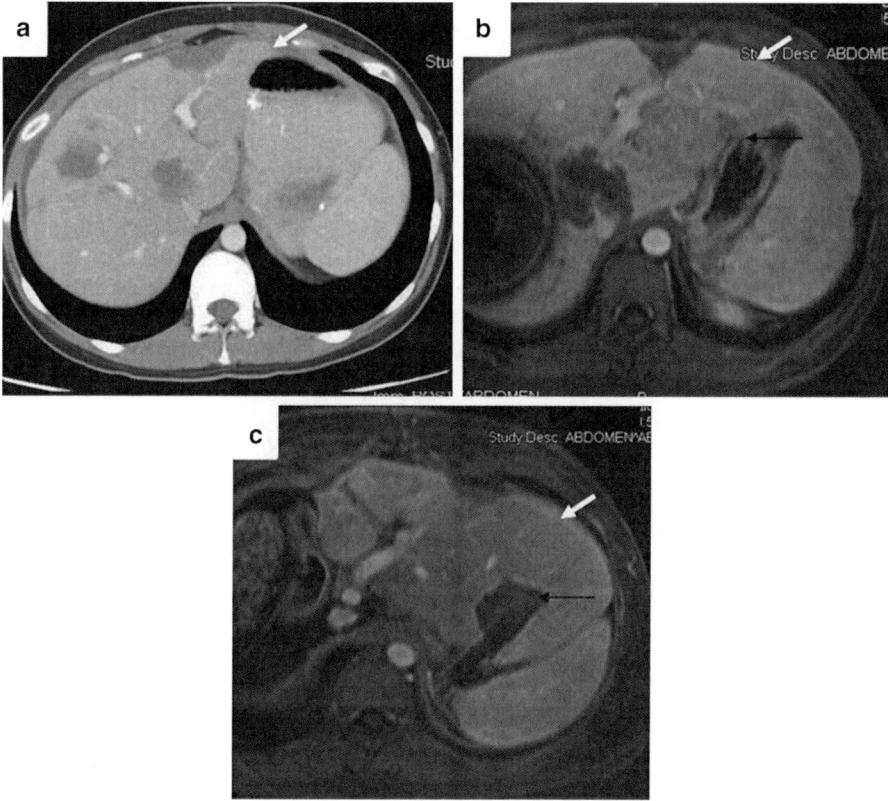

Fig. 9.4 Use of preoperative portal vein embolization in liver resection. (**a**) The patient shown in Fig. 9.3 has multiple colorectal metastases in the right lobe of the liver and in segment 4. There is a very small remnant of relatively uninvolved liver in the left lateral section (*white arrow*). (**b**) Four weeks after portal vein embolization, the left lateral section has increased markedly in size (*white arrow*), allowing right trisectionectomy and simultaneous ablation of a small focus of tumor in the left lobe (*black arrow*). (**c**) Postoperative MRI showing successful right trisectionectomy and ablated mass (*black arrow*)

substantially with PPVE. Liver failure was more common in patients with higher portal pressures or lower hypertrophic ratios [38]. A more recent series reporting the degree of liver hypertrophy using several methods of measuring TLV found a mean increase in FLR% (previously termed RLV ratio in this report) of 0.27%, with patients on average increasing RLV ratio from 0.58% to 0.85%. Mathematically, this represents an increase of 47% in the volume of the planned liver remnant [37]. Of patients undergoing PVE, ~25% of patients ultimately do not go on to hepatic resection, either due to tumor progression or inadequate hypertrophy [37, 39]. In those undergoing resection, however, posthepatectomy liver failure and mortality rates are low. Interestingly, liver function as measured by scintigraphy may increase to a greater extent in the RLV than the volume change, suggesting a benefit that goes beyond simply increased hepatocyte mass [39].

Staged Hepatic Treatments

An approach to multifocal tumors with some similarities to PPVE is the principle of using two or more planned hepatic resections separated by a period of time to allow for a period of recovery and hypertrophy between interventions. This approach is especially practical in the setting of bilobar tumors, in which portal vein embolization is not favored because of the risk of loss of otherwise healthy parenchyma or when intraoperative findings prevent the full resection of all lesions. For example, if a patient with multiple hepatic tumors is found at surgery to have a greater degree of steatosis or chemotherapy effects than anticipated, the surgeon may opt to limit the current resection with plans to return at a later date. An example of this is demonstrated in Fig. 9.5.

In addition to considering a later surgical intervention, it is becoming commonplace to use ablative or hepatic arterial therapies in combination with resection to treat the multifocal tumor patient. The timing of interventions in these patients is very dependent on the bias, experience, and expertise of the patients' care team, and for that reason, these decisions are perhaps best made by multidisciplinary institutional planning teams. Factors to consider include: (1) optimizing hepatic reserve when undertaking interventions likely to involve significant risk of liver failure, for example, perform resection of large or central mass up front before risking compromise of residual liver with hepatic arterial therapy (Fig. 9.6); (2) optimizing access to percutaneous ablation, for example, preferentially remove or otherwise treat lesions not amenable to a percutaneous route; and (3) optimizing access to treatment by hepatic arterial therapy, for example, preferentially remove or ablate lesions on one side of liver if remainder of lesions could be treated with unilateral or unisegmental hepatic artery therapy.

Functional and Anatomic Approach to Ablation

The number of treatments available now for ablation of hepatic tumors continues to increase. At the present time, the primary modalities in use include chemical ablation with alcohol or similar injectates; cryoablation, which refers to freezing tissue to cause cell death; or radiofrequency ablation and microwave ablation, which cause tumor necrosis through tissue heating. The most common technique in the US is thermal ablation. Irreversible electroporation is another modality with the purported capacity to destroy tumors while leaving collagen lined structures such as large blood vessels and bile ducts intact, but at this time, the data are not sufficient to support its widespread application.

The decision on whether to use an ablative modality and which one to employ is multifactorial. General principles to consider include: (1) likelihood of local recurrence after ablation, (2) likelihood of remote recurrence after ablation, (3) morbidity of ablation compared to resection or other treatments, (4) options available for treatment failure, and (5) goals of treatment.

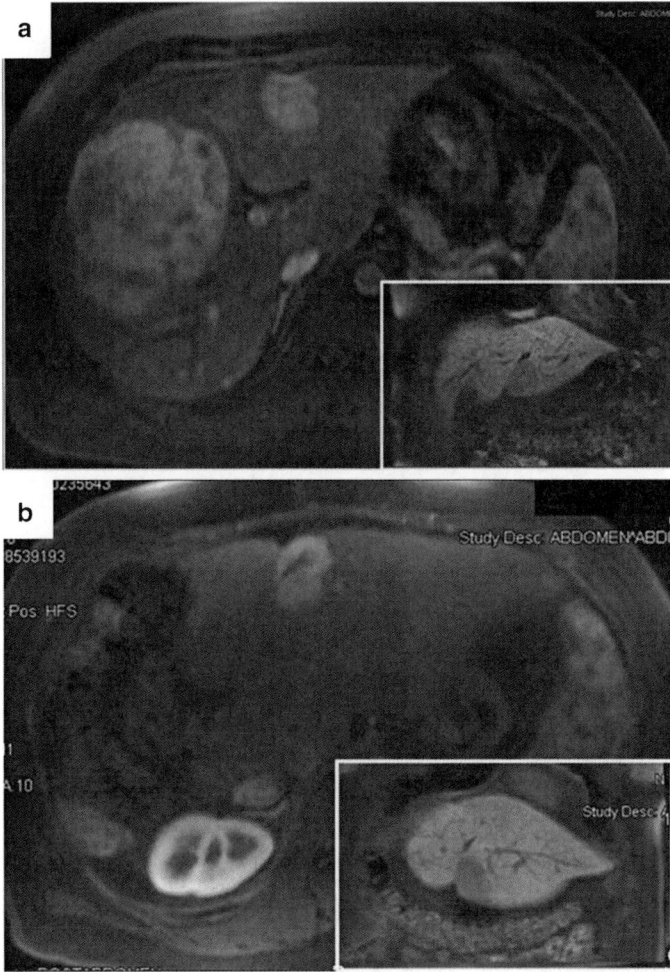

Fig. 9.5 Staged hepatic resections. (**a**) Patient with bilateral masses suspicious for adenoma (left-sided mass seen in *inset* on coronal section). Combined resection of both masses was not possible due to fatty liver and inadequate liver volume. Right hemihepatectomy performed with finding of benign adenoma and therefore planned to undergo repeat hepatic resection after liver recovery. (**b**) Three months after right hemihepatectomy, liver hypertrophy is sufficient to allow repeat laparotomy and resection of remaining left-sided lesion

The use of ablation in the treatment of hepatocellular carcinoma (HCC) exemplifies the complexities of these decisions. The patient with a unifocal HCC and otherwise well-compensated cirrhosis may be a candidate for either resection or ablation based on liver parameters. The perceived value of ablation is that in the presence of high-risk hepatic recurrence, the morbidity of the treatment should be kept low to offset risks of repeated surgical intervention. Randomized trials as to which modality is ideal are limited, but several reports suggest that ablation and

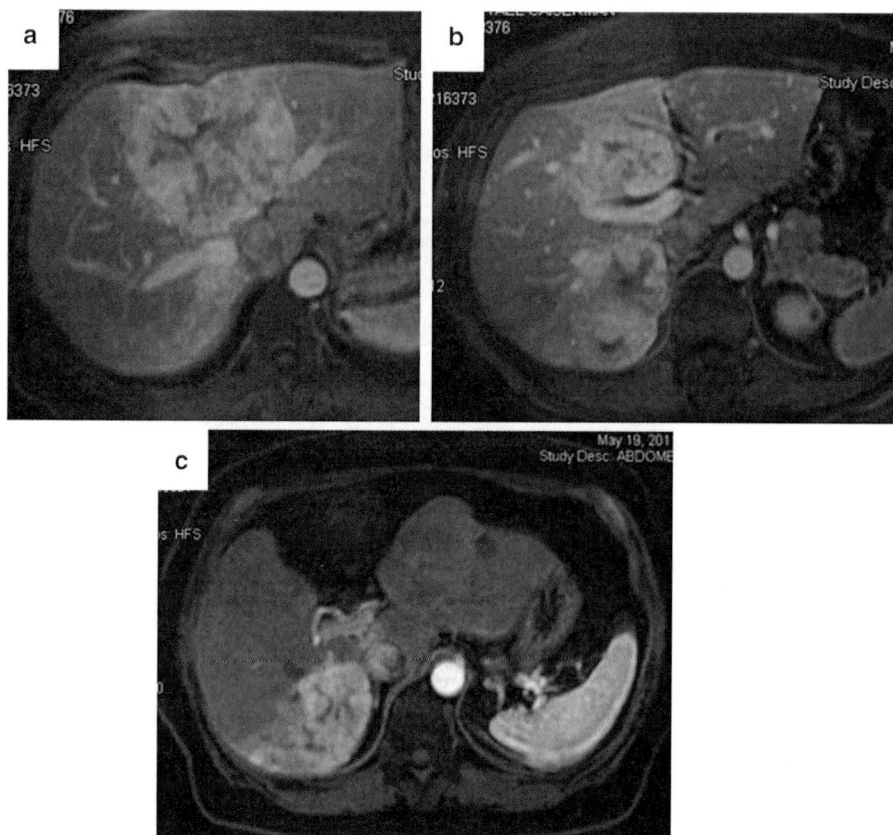

Fig. 9.6 Management of central hepatic lesion. (**a**) Hypervascular tumor (neuroendocrine carcinoma) located central in the liver in immediate proximity to hepatic veins. (**b**) Same tumor in proximity to central portal structures. The location makes ablation risky due to possible injury to underlying biliary structures. Hepatic arterial therapy is an option, but due to bilateral arterial supply, complete necrosis is unlikely. Surgical resection can be undertaken but is planned to spare maximal parenchyma in right and left to allow future treatment options. (**c**) After resection of the central mass, residual posterior right-sided tumor can be treated by direct ablation or hepatic arterial therapy

resection are largely equivalent for treatment of HCC ≤3 cm [40, 41]. More recent data from a study analyzing resection versus ablation in HCC meeting Milan criteria (1 lesion ≤5 cm; 2 or 3 lesions ≤3 cm) demonstrated superiority of resection over ablation in overall and subgroup analysis [42] both in recurrence rates and overall survival. This is further complicated by the transplant guidelines for HCC in the USA, which only provide for expedited transplant in a patient who has undergone ablation but provide no advantage for those undergoing resection. In the scenario of planned transplant, ablation is thought of as a bridging modality, and a slightly increased risk of local recurrence is accepted because of the planned whole-organ replacement.

The anatomical and functional constraints facing the planned ablation are slightly different than those present in planning surgical resection. The benefits of ablation include generally less loss of parenchyma, lower risk of bile leak and bleeding, and, if performed percutaneously, less morbidity from surgical incisions. The unique risks include unintended injury to surrounding viscera, unanticipated vascular or biliary injury, and a higher risk of local treatment failure. Radiofrequency ablation is well known to be less effective in tumors close to large vessels that can act as a heat sink, which in turn will lead to higher local treatment failure. Microwave ablation is less susceptible to heat sink effect but requires greater caution because of rapid and large ablation zones it can create.

Planning an ablation should proceed very similar to planning resection, in that the patient should be assessed to ensure adequate hepatic volume and function. Child's class A or MELD <15 patients are generally good candidates for tumors up to 3 cm in size and in some cases up to 5 cm in size. Treatment of larger lesions carries not only the risk of excessive local tissue damage from overlapping treatment beds but also the risk of compromising uninvolved liver peripheral to the treated tumor. These factors should be considered in volumetric planning of ablation.

The ablative treatment of tumors close to the central biliary structures warrants special consideration. In most cases, an unintended thermal injury to the central hepatic ducts completely outweighs the benefit of ablative treatment because of subsequent morbidity from biliary obstruction, cholangitis, and liver failure. Piecemeal ablation may be an option in these cases, whereby small-zone ablations are performed over a longer staged interval to assess the response over time. Another option is to place a biliary catheter to allow cooling of the bile ducts during active tumor heating. Finally, central lesions in close proximity to bile ducts may be better treated with hepatic arterial therapy to avoid any risk of thermal spread or with surgical resection during which the central structures can be deliberately preserved (see Fig. 9.6).

Functional and Anatomic Approach to Hepatic Arterial Therapy

Hepatic arterial therapies are based on the premise that certain tumors are primarily fed by hepatic arterial flow and that treatment by means of the hepatic artery selectively targets these lesions while causing relatively little damage to surrounding hepatic parenchyma. The normal parenchyma is thought to be protected by the property of dual blood flow from the portal vein. This premise is most well studied in highly hypervascular tumors such as neuroendocrine carcinomas and hepatocellular carcinomas, and in some cases, even simple hepatic artery embolization to induce tumor hypoxia can be effective. More commonly, chemotherapy either eluted onto microparticles or in a slurry of Ethiodol is infused in order to effect tumor necrosis by both hypoxia and cytotoxicity from the chemotherapy. Recently, infusion of yttrium-rich beads into the hepatic artery circulation has shown tremendous

Table 9.5 Selection criteria for hepatic therapy

Factor	SIRT	Hepatic artery chemoembolization	Radiofrequency ablation	Microwave ablation
Serum bilirubin	2 mg/dl	3 mg/dl	1.5 mg/dl[a]	1.5 mg/dl[a]
Ascites	Contraindicated	Increased risk of liver failure	Increased risk of bleeding, tumor seeding, and liver failure[a]	Increased risk of bleeding, tumor seeding, and liver failure[a]
Proximity to major blood vessels	Minimal effect	Minimal effect	May cause heat sink, higher local recurrence rate	Minimal effect
Proximity to major bile ducts	Minimal effect	Minimal effect	May cause biliary injury (consider intraductal cooling techniques)	May cause biliary injury
Prior hepatic radiation	Cannot exceed maximal hepatic dose	No direct effect	No direct effect	No direct effect
Prior hepatic chemoembolization	May limit arterial access to tumor or cause uneven distribution of treatment	Minimal effect	Minimal direct effect	Minimal direct effect
Portal vein thrombosis	May be tolerated if unilateral; selective use if main portal vein thrombosis	Relative contraindication	Minimal direct effect	Minimal direct effect

[a]Treatment risk increased in Child's B cirrhosis
SIRT selective internal radiation therapy

efficacy in several tumor types (SIRT, or selective internal radiation therapy). This approach is unique among the hepatic arterial therapies in that it can be performed in a high-dose segmental approach that leads to planned segmental or sectional atrophy along with tumor destruction. This "radiation segmentectomy" approach does not rely on tumor avidity or hypervascularity but rather on the premises of Couinaud and Healey that the hepatic arteries accurately and reliably supply certain segments of the liver.

Preoperative planning in the setting of planned hepatic arterial therapy must factor hepatic reserve, patient reserve, and goals of therapy. In general, most hepatic arterial therapies are considered palliative and not curative, although long-standing treatment responses are well described in many tumor types. In the case of HCC, most patients will ultimately die of underlying liver disease and not the cancer, and for that reason, the use of hepatic-based therapy must be judicious. A recent large study analyzing hepatic artery chemoembolization in HCC with ascites found that posttreatment liver failure occurred in 17% of patients and that 94% of these patients died within the next year. Risk factors for liver failure in this study included CTP class B and history of gastrointestinal bleeding [43]. In addition, poor performance status was independently associated with early death.

Guidelines for selecting patients for hepatic arterial therapies have been proposed, with the most recent reports focusing on SIRT [44, 45]. Some of these are listed in Table 9.5. Additional factors to be considered in an individual patient include the goals of therapy, the other options available to the patient, and, in transplant patients, the expected wait time for transplantation. If we again use the example of the HCC patient, regional therapy may be used for palliation of symptoms, for purposes of bridging while on the wait list, or for downstaging a patient who is beyond transplant criteria. Almost no toxicity is acceptable in a patient being treated for symptom palliation, while the patient who is being bridged to transplant may tolerate a more aggressive approach because of the safety net offered by transplant. In contrast, the patient who requires downstaging may be accepting a risky intervention because of limited other options, but in fact, these patients are required to wait an additional 6 months or more after treatment prior to transplant, and therefore, hepatic therapies are often completed in stages, both to allow maximal hepatic recovery and to allow observation of biological behavior of the tumor.

Summary

The growing number of options available for the treatment of liver tumors has made the accurate assessment of liver anatomy and function more important than ever before. Consensus guidelines for selection of treatments and nomenclature are uncommon but are increasing in the last few years. The next decade is likely to be accompanied by greater use of computer-assisted imaging techniques, improved biochemical and imaging analysis of liver function reserve, and greater sophistication of ablative techniques. With the steady evolution of systemic therapies such as targeted biologic agents, the role of liver-directed cytoreductive therapy will need to be continually evaluated.

References

1. Couinaud CLeFoie. Etudes anatomiques et chirugicales. Paris: Masson & Cie; 1957.
2. Healey Jr JE, Schroy PC. Anatomy of the biliary ducts within the human liver; Analysis of the prevailing pattern of branchings and the major variations of the biliary ducts. Arch Surg. 1953;66:599–616.

3. Terminology Committee of the IHPBA. Terminology of liver anatomy and resections. HPB Surg. 2000;2:333–9.
4. Strasberg SM. Nomenclature of hepatic anatomy and resections: a review of the Brisbane 2000 system. J Hepatobiliary Pancreat Surg. 2005;12:351–5.
5. Vauthey JN, Abdalla EK, Doherty DA, et al. Body surface area and body weight predict total liver volume in western adults. Liver Transplant. 2002;8(3):233–40.
6. Urata K, Kawasaki S, Matsunami H, et al. Calculation of child and adult standard liver volume for liver transplantation. Hepatology. 1995;21:1317–21.
7. Truant S, Oberlin O, Sergent G, et al. Remnant liver volume to body weight ration >0.5%: a new cut-off to estimate postoperative risks after extended resection in noncirrhotic liver. J Am Coll Surg. 2007;204(1):22–33.
8. Shoup M, Gonen M, D'Angelica M, et al. Volumetric analysis predicts hepatic dysfunction in patients undergoing major liver resection. J Gastrointest Surg. 2003;7:325–30.
9. Yigitler C, Farges O, Kianmanesh R, et al. The small remnant liver after major liver resection: how common and how relevant? Liver Transplant. 2003;9:S18–25.
10. Vauthey JN, Chaoui A, Do KA, et al. Standardized measurement of the future liver remnant prior to extended liver resection: methodology and clinical associations. Surgery. 2000;127: 512–9.
11. Kiuchi T, Kasharah M, Uryuhara K, et al. Impact of graft size mismatching on graft prognosis in liver transplantation from living donors. Transplantation. 1999;67:321–7.
12. Malinchoc M, Kamath PS, Gordon FD, Peine CJ, Rank J, ter Borg PC. A model to predict poor survival in patients undergoing transjugular protosystemic shunts. Hepatology. 2000;31: 864–71.
13. Kamath PS, Wesner RH, Malinchoc M, et al. A model to predict survival in patients with end-stage liver disease. Hepatology. 2001;33:464–70.
14. Forman LM, Luccy MR. Predicting the prognosis of chronic liver disease: An evolution from the CHILD to MELD. Mayo end-stage liver disease. Hepatology. 2001;33:473–5.
15. Friedman LS. Surgery in the patient with liver disease. Trans Am Clin Climatol Assoc. 2010;121:192–205.
16. O'Leary JG, Friedman LS. Predicting surgical risk in patients with cirrhosis: from art to science. Gastroenterology. 2007;132(4):1609–11.
17. Schroeder RA, Marroquin CE, Bute BP, Khuri S, Henderson WG, Kuo PC. Predictive indices of morbidity and mortality after liver resection. Ann Surg. 2006;243:373–9.
18. Jarnagin W, et al. Surgical treatment of hepatocellular carcinoma: expert consensus statement. HPB. 2010;12:302–10.
19. Teh SH, Sheppard BC, Schwartz J, Orloff S. Model for end-stage liver disease score fails to predict perioperative outcome after hepatic resection for hepatocellular carcinoma in patients without cirrhosis. Am J Surg. 2008;195:697–701.
20. Teh SH, Nagorney DM, Stevens SR, et al. Risk factors for mortality after surgery in patients with cirrhosis. Gastroenterology. 2007;132:1261–9.
21. Northup PG, Wanamaker RC, Lee VD, Adams RB, Berg CL. Model for end-stage liver disease (MELD) predicts nontransplant surgical mortality in patients with cirrhosis. Ann Surg. 2005;242:244–51.
22. Mullin EJ, Metcalfe MS, Maddern GJ. How much liver resection is too much? Am J Surg. 2005;190:87–97.
23. Teh SH, Christein J, Donohue J, et al. Hepatic resection of hepatocellular carcinoma in patients with cirrhosis: model of end-stage disease (MELD) score predicts perioperative mortality. J Gastrointest Surg. 2005;9(9):1207–15.
24. Cucchetti A, Ercolani G, Vivarelli M, et al. Impact of model for end-stage liver disease (MELD) score on prognosis after hepatectomy for hepatocellular carcinoma on cirrhosis. Liver Transplant. 2006;12:966–71.
25. Tu R, Xia LP, Yu AL, Wu L. Assessment of hepatic functional reserve by cirrhosis grading and liver volume measurement using CT. World J Gastroenterol. 2007;13(29):3956–61.
26. Vauthey JN, Dixon E, Abdalla EK, et al. Pretreatment assessment of hepatocellular carcinoma: expert consensus statement. HPB (Oxford). 2010;12(5):289–99.

27. Torzilli G, et al. Hepatectomy for stage B and stage C hepatocellular carcinoma in the Barcelona Clinic Liver Cancer classification. Arch Surg. 2008;143(11):1082–90.
28. Schneider PD. Preoperative assessment of liver function. Surg Clin North Am. 2004;84: 355–73.
29. Tarantino G. Could quantitative liver function tests gain wide acceptance among hepatologists? World J Gastroenterol. 2009;15(28):3457–61.
30. Stadalnik RC, Vera DR. The evolution of (99m)Tc-NGA as a clinically useful receptor-binding radiopharmaceutical. Nucl Med Biol. 2001;28(5):499–503.
31. Hwang EH, Taki J, Shuke N, et al. Preoperative assessment of residual hepatic functional reserve using 99mTc-DTPA-galactosyl-human serum albumin dynamic SPECT. J Nucl Med. 1999;40(10):1644–51.
32. Kubo S, Shiomi S, Tanaka H, et al. Evaluation of the effect of portal vein embolization on liver function by (99m)tc-galactosyl human serum albumin scintigraphy. J Surg Res. 2001;107(1): 113–8.
33. Kokudo N, Vera DR, Koizumi M, et al. Recovery of hepatic asialoglycoprotein receptors after major hepatic resection. J Nucl Med. 1999;40(1):137–41.
34. Stockmann M, Lock JF, Malinowski M, Niehues SM, Seehofer D, Neuhaus P. The LiMAx test: a new liver function test for predicting postoperative outcome in liver surgery. HPB (Oxford). 2010;12(2):139–46.
35. Rahbari NN, Garden OJ, Padbury R, et al. Posthepatectomy liver failure: a definition and grading by the International Study Group of Liver Surgery (ISGLS). Surgery. 2011;149(5): 713–24.
36. Balzan S, Belghiti J, Farges O, et al. The "50–50 criteria" on postoperative day 5: an accurate predictor of liver failure and death after hepatectomy. Ann Surg. 2005;242(6):824–8.
37. Shah A, Goffette P, Hubert C, et al. Comparison of different methods to quantify future liver remnants after preoperative portal vein embolization to predict postoperative liver failure. Hepatogastroenterology. 2011;58(105):109–14.
38. Wakabayashi H, Ishimura K, Okano K, et al. Application of preoperative portal vein embolization before major hepatic resection in patients with normal or abnormal liver parenchyma. Surgery. 2002;131(1):26–33.
39. de Graaf W, van Lienden KP, van den Esschert JW, Bennink RJ, van Gulik TM. Increase in future remnant liver function after preoperative portal vein embolization. Br J Surg. 2011;98: 825–34.
40. Livraghi T, Meloni F, Di Stasi M, et al. Sustained complete response and complications rates after radiofrequency ablation of very early hepatocellular carcinoma in cirrhosis: Is resection still the treatment of choice? Hepatology. 2008;47(1):82–9.
41. Chen MS, Li JQ, Zheng Y, et al. A prospective randomized trial comparing percutaneous local ablative therapy and partial hepatectomy for small hepatocellular carcinoma. Ann Surg. 2006;243(3):321–8.
42. Huang J, Yan L, Cheng Z, et al. A randomized trial comparing radiofrequency ablation and surgical resection for HCC conforming to the Milan criteria. Ann Surg. 2010;252(6):903–12.
43. Hsin IF, Hsu CY, Huang HC, et al. Liver failure after transarterial chemoembolization for patients with hepatocellular carcinoma and ascites: incidence, risk factors, and prognostic prediction. J Clin Gastroenterol. 2011;45(6):556–62.
44. Lau WY, Kennedy AS, Kim YH, et al. Patient selection and activity planning guide for selective internal radiotherapy with yttrium-90 resin microspheres. Int J Radiat Oncol Biol Phys. 2010;80(4):1280.
45. Coldwell D, Sangro B, Wasan H, Salem R, Kennedy A. General selection criteria of patients for radioembolization of liver tumors: an international working group report. Am J Clin Oncol. 2011;34(3):337–41.

Chapter 10
Treatment of HCC: Resection, Local-Regional Therapy, Systemic Therapy, and Liver Transplantation

Nate Susnow, Talia B. Baker, and Laura Kulik

Introduction

The burden of hepatocellular carcinoma (HCC) worldwide has escalated to the sixth most common cancer worldwide [1]. Furthermore, it is now recognized as the third leading cause of cancer related mortality [1]. While orthotopic liver transplantation (OLT) offers the best chance for long-term survival, organ shortage limits its availability to all those in need, and the priority for OLT is dependent upon meeting the current selection criteria, Milan criteria [2]. There is a growing need for efficacious therapies for HCC. Treatment for HCC is dependent upon the degree of underlying liver dysfunction and tumor burden as the majority of such tumors occur in the background of cirrhosis. Therefore, any therapy for HCC should be performed in a manner to minimize the risk of mortality related to decompensated liver disease with appropriate patient selection. The Barcelona Clinic Liver Cancer Staging classification (BCLC) takes into account tumor characteristics, liver function, and the patient's performance status and pairs each BCLC stage with a recommended treatment modality [3] (Fig. 10.1). However, in clinical practice, adherence to the BCLC is not always absolute. This chapter will focus on the therapeutic options for HCC.

N. Susnow, MD
Division of Gastroenterology, University of Washington, Seattle, WA, USA

T.B. Baker, MD • L. Kulik, MD (✉)
Department of Transplantation Surgery, Feinberg School of Medicine,
Northwestern University, Chicago, IL, USA
e-mail: lkulik@nmff.org

N. Reau and F.F. Poordad (eds.), *Primary Liver Cancer: Surveillance, Diagnosis and Treatment*, Clinical Gastroenterology, DOI 10.1007/978-1-61779-863-4_10, © Springer Science+Business Media New York 2012

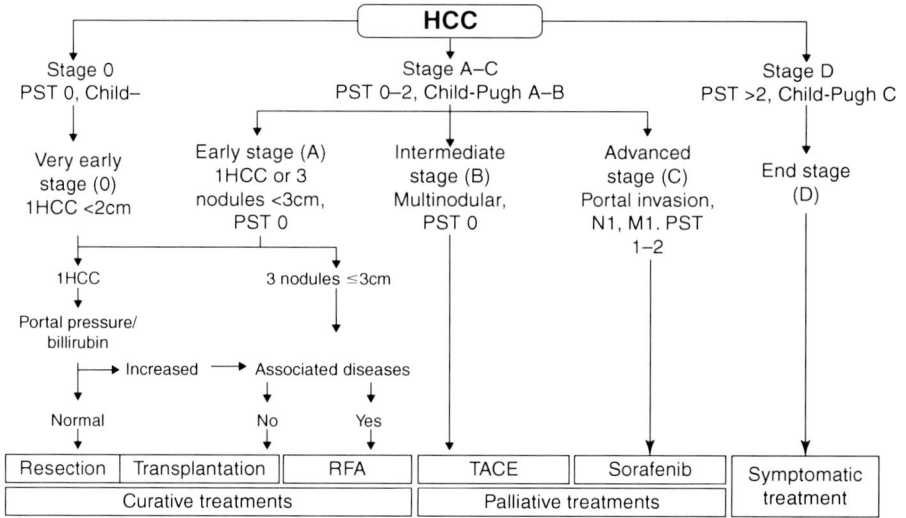

Fig. 10.1 The Barcelona Clinic Liver Cancer Staging classification (BCLC) differentiates patients based on size and number of tumors, severity of liver disease, and performance status. Based on the results of this staging, recommendations for treatment modalities are given

Early HCC: BCLC 0-A

The recognized potential curative therapies for hepatocellular carcinoma (HCC) include liver transplantation (OLT), resection, and radiofrequency ablation (RFA). These patients embody the BCLC A group.

RFA has been showed to be superior to other local ablative therapies due to its need for fewer treatment sessions, superior local tumor control, and higher overall survival rates in a meta-analysis [4, 5]. The comparison of RFA vs. resection has been limited to only a few RCTs; one reported no significant difference in overall or disease-free survival after a median follow-up of 2 years [6]. A more recent RCT comparing RFA to resection among patients meeting the Milan criteria showed a superior 5-year overall survival among those who underwent hepatic resection (76% vs. 55%) and significantly less recurrence at 5 years (42% vs. 63%) compared to RFA [7]. A large prospective nonrandomized trial of resection ($n = 2,857$) compared to RFA ($N = 3,022$) and PEI ($n = 1,306$) reported a significantly lower recurrence rate in those who underwent resection [8]. Overall survival was not significantly different between the groups; however, median follow-up was limited to 10.4 months. In very early HCC (BCLC 0), 5-year overall survival has been reported to be 68%, leading most authorities to agree that resection and RFA are equivalent in a solitary lesion less than 2 cm [9].

In lieu of RCTs, others have employed Markov models to simulate a large RCT and propensity score matching analysis to reduce the inevitable cofounding variables that influence the results of nonrandomized studies. Molinari et al. demonstrated with Markov modeling (simulating a 10,000 person RCT) that resection is superior in terms of less recurrence compared to RFA; however, in patients older than 75, RFA emerged as the preferred treatment modality due to less associated mortality [10]. With sensitivity analysis, operating on the assumption of an equal probability of performing RFA for recurrent HCC in either treatment arms, RFA became the preferred strategy for solitary HCC < 5 cm. The feasibility of repeat RFA for recurrent disease after initial RFA as a viable treatment option was recently reported by Rossi and colleagues with no procedure-related deaths in 1921 RFA sessions [11]. The authors reported a 5-year OS and disease-free survival of 40.1% and 38.0%, respectively, after repeated RFA for recurrent HCC in 577 patients. The risk of death associated with underlying liver disease was highlighted in a 40.3% mortality rate unrelated to HCC. Factors independently associated with survival were CP B, first recurrence <24 months post-RFA, and local or advanced recurrence.

A recent retrospective study examined overall survival and recurrence rates in 419 patients with HCC (≤5 cm, ≤3 lesions) treated with anatomic resection ($N = 229$) and RFA ($N = 190$) [12]. Those treated with resection had a significantly lower 5-year recurrence rate (43.9% vs. 79.5%; $p < 0.001$) and improved 5-year overall survival (79.3% vs. 67.4%; $p = 0.009$). Patients that received RFA were significantly more likely to be older, female, have lower platelets, lower AFP levels, smaller tumors, and be HCV positive. The authors used propensity analysis to match patients who underwent anatomic resection with those who had RFA in order to make the two groups more homogenous. After matching for baseline patient and tumor characteristics, overall survival was comparable between the two treatment strategies; however, HCC recurrence remained significantly higher in the RFA group. A subanalysis including only BCLC 0 showed equivalent overall survival (5 year: 84.6% resection; 77.8% RFA) and recurrence rates both before and after propensity score matching.

The optimal initial treatment for early HCC in patients with preserved liver function remains a subject of intense debate. Hepatic resection has always been and remains the primary treatment for HCC in patients with limited disease. The efficacy of partial hepatectomy depends on the ability to achieve a complete resection (R0) that leaves behind an adequate liver remnant. Like transplantation, disease extent is closely linked with outcomes after resection with the best results achieved in patients with solitary lesions. In addition, resection is largely limited to patients with either normal livers or Child–Pugh class A cirrhosis. Importantly, unlike transplantation, resection does not address the diseased precancerous liver remnant and therefore may be associated with a higher tumor recurrence rate. The 5-year tumor recurrence-free survival rate after resection of early HCC within the Milan criteria in Child A cirrhotic patients was 40–48% as compared to 60–80% after transplantation [13, 14]. The benefit of transplantation in terms of disease-free survival, however, is counteracted by long-term complications associated with transplant such as graft rejection, disease recurrence, and immunosuppression-related complications. These long-term transplant-related morbidities explain the similar overall 5-year survival rates of 60–70% after partial hepatectomy for early HCC as compared to studies of transplantation for similar lesions [15]. Furthermore, patients on the transplant waiting list have a significant risk of tumor progression and drop out, while liver resection may be immediately accessible. Dropout rates at 1 year of 25% have been reported in patients awaiting a deceased donor graft [16].

The severe shortage of donor organs leading to the risk of dropout due to tumor progression on the transplant waiting lists has encouraged the practice of primary liver resection for early HCC in carefully selected patients. EASL (European Association for Study of Liver) in 2001 and AASLD published guidelines for HCC treatment trying to define the role of each therapeutic option [17–19]. Well-defined indications for hepatectomy for HCC were reported. Patients with single lesions and preserved liver function without portal hypertension were considered optimal candidates. Notably, nodule size was not considered a limit to resection, but the authors emphasized that it was uncommon to resect tumors > 5 cm because of the high risk of vascular invasion.

As experience with liver resection for HCC grows and new surgical techniques emerge, most experienced liver transplant centers now offer resections to selected patients with more advanced disease than defined by the EASL/AASLD guidelines. In general, the Child–Pugh classification is reasonably effective in stratifying patient risk on the basis of underlying hepatic function and for selecting patients for resection. In most recent series, only patients with either normal hepatic parenchyma (noncirrhotic) or Child–Pugh class A cirrhosis are candidates for major resection. Carefully selected patients with Child–Pugh B liver disease and small peripheral tumors may be eligible for more limited resections. Strategies aimed at better identifying the subgroup of Child–Pugh class A patients at increased risk of hepatic decompensation associated with resection have been adopted including indocyanine green clearance test and the direct measurement of portal pressure as determined by the hepatic venous pressure gradient. Bruix et al. were able to use this later approach to identify a subgroup of Child–Pugh class A patients with subclinical portal hypertension who decompensated after hepatic resection [20].

Laparoscopic hepatic resection has also emerged as a growing option in the field of liver surgery for hepatocellular cancer. It is now established as a safe and effective alternative to open liver resection for HCC. A recent meta-analysis of laparoscopic vs. open liver resection for HCC indicated potentially favorable outcomes in terms of blood loss, blood transfusion requirements, postoperative morbidity, and length of hospital stay [21]. Concerning the oncological outcomes, there was no difference between groups in surgical margin, overall survival, and disease-free survival. There are currently no randomized controlled trials comparing laparoscopic vs. open liver resection in HCC.

The advent of living donor liver transplant (LDLT) has been another approach to decrease dropout by increasing organ availability to patients with HCC [22]. The use of LDLT is particularly relevant to patients exceeding the Milan criteria. The viable role of LDLT was demonstrated in a Japanese nationwide survey of LDLT that reported a 3-year survival of 60% in patients with tumors beyond the Milan criteria [23].

The outcome of HCC recurrence post-transplant and overall survival in patients undergoing LDLT compared with DDLT has not been fully elicited. The use of

LDLT to increase access to transplantation for patients with HCC requires careful consideration of the risk-to-benefit ratio of recurrent HCC post transplant with the goal of ensured safety to the donor. The Adult to Adult Living Donor Liver Transplantation (A2ALL) Study Cohort reported a significantly higher recurrence rate among the LDLT compared with DDLT recipients (17/56 vs. 0/31) [24]. The overall survival was similar between the two groups. Although in aggregate the LDLT patients had evidence of more advanced tumor (higher AFP, higher percent with vascular invasion, diameter of largest nodule), there were no significant differences in explant staging. The most notable findings were a 24% recurrence rate in the LDLT patients with early HCC and a lack of recurrence among the 13 DDLT patients with T3/T4 disease on explant.

Similarly, Lo et al. reported a significantly higher rate of recurrence in the LDLT patients compared with DDLT [25]. In both of these studies, the waiting times were significantly shorter in the LDLT group. It has been suggested that a shorter waiting period may not allow for the expression of a tumor's biologic behavior. Transplantation in patients with an unrecognized aggressive tumor may lead to increased HCC recurrence regardless of the explant stage [26]. A single center study reported significantly improved overall survival in the LDLT group compared to DDLT despite a significantly higher HCC recurrence rate among LDLT recipients [27]. Conversely, a multicenter study from Korea found no difference in HCC recurrence [28]. A2ALL more recently reported a significantly higher HCC recurrence rate in the LDLT compared to DDLT recipients in the MELD era with no difference in overall survival; however, after controlling for tumor characteristics, there was no longer a significant difference in HCC recurrence rates between the two groups [29]. Additional studies are needed to determine if an increased recurrence rate will offset an increased mortality on the waiting list for a DDLT.

Selection for Transplant Beyond the Milan Criteria

The Milan criteria continue to be the selection criteria utilized by UNOS to grant prioritization for OLT. There has been a growing debate that the Milan criteria are too stringent and that there is room for its expansion without significantly compromising post-transplant results. Response to liver-directed therapy may give insight into the biological behavior of tumors as reported by Otto et al. who reported that the lack of response to TACE while awaiting OLT was a significant predictor of posttransplant HCC recurrence regardless of Milan status [30]. Similarly, the UCSF group has demonstrated excellent posttransplant outcomes in patients that were successfully downstaged into the Milan criteria using various forms of liver-directed therapies [31]. Vitale and colleagues found a lack of response to liver-directed therapy to be the only independent predictor of dropout from the waiting list irrespective of tumor size [32]. The authors prioritized those with HCC for OLT, regardless of tumor size and number, in those without evidence of tumor response at 3 months (defined as stable, progressive, or untreated disease) post-liver-directed therapy and not fulfilling their institutions exclusionary criteria for OLT: evidence of macrovascular invasion, metastatic disease, and/or poorly differentiated HCC. All patients were restaged prior to receiving prioritization for transplant. Patients without response to therapy had a similar posttransplant survival compared to those who were not given prioritization for OLT based on a favorable response to therapy; however, the risk of HCC recurrence was noted to be higher in those with a lack of treatment response (13% vs. 2%; $p = 0.04$).

Intermediate HCC: BCLC B

Patients exceeding the Milan criteria without evidence of vascular invasion, metastasis, and/or tumor-related symptoms are considered intermediate HCC or BCLC B. The staple therapy has been TACE based on the results of RCT showing improved OS compared to supportive care.

TACE

Transarterial chemoembolization (TACE) is a regionally directed therapy for HCC. TACE as a therapy relies on the fact that HCC > 2 cm is a hypervascular tumor that is usually dependent on arterial blood supply, as opposed to surrounding normal hepatic parenchyma, which receives a dual blood supply from the hepatic artery and portal vein [33]. TACE results in improved survival in carefully selected patients but is felt to be inferior to surgical resection and RFA and is not considered a curative therapy of HCC [34, 35]. Arterial embolization without chemoembolization (bland embolization) has been used in patients deemed poor candidates for TACE, but there has been no demonstrated survival benefit with this technique [35, 36]. One of the two RCT that showed improved OS with TACE over supportive care included bland embolization; however, at the time of study termination, bland embolization had not reached a significant survival benefit survival compared to no therapy [36]. The goal of TACE is to extend overall survival, to bridge patients to liver transplant by preventing HCC expansion and subsequent removal from the transplant list (dropout), and in some centers to downstage patients so that transplant becomes a viable option.

   In this technique, the affected liver segment is accessed via hepatic artery angiography to identify the dense network of arterioles supplying the tumor (tumor blush). Chemotherapeutic agents used include various combinations of doxorubicin, cisplatin, mitomycin, and epirubicin. The most commonly used regimen is a three-drug regimen with doxorubicin, cisplatin, and mitomycin. The chemotherapeutic agent is often mixed in a 1:1 emulsion with lipiodol, a fat-soluble contrast agent that undergoes selective uptake into the tumor. Embolization is achieved with various approaches, most commonly via polyvinyl particles or gelatin foam administration, and rarely with coils, starch microspheres, and blood clot administration. Newer techniques include administration of chemotherapy and arterial embolization with drug-eluting beads (most data are for doxorubicin, size varies between 300 and 700 μm) which both obstruct tumor blood flow and allow local distribution of chemotherapeutics (see below). TACE may be reapplied as on demand based on tumor response or on a scheduled basis, usually every 6–8 weeks. There is no data regarding timing of treatment/retreatment, choice of chemotherapeutic agent, or choice of embolic agent.

The contraindications to TACE primarily relate to liver function and anatomy. The two primary side effects of TACE therapy are obstruction of arterial blood flow and damage to surrounding functional hepatic parenchyma. Patients who undergo TACE therapy are generally not candidates for more definitive therapies (resection, RFA), and decompensated liver disease is often present. TACE therapy invariably results in some loss of hepatic reserve, which may lead to hepatic decompensation. Therefore, TACE is avoided in patients with Child–Pugh C cirrhosis, significant encephalopathy, serum bilirubin >2 (as an indicator of significant liver dysfunction; however, studies have used up to a bilirubin of 5), or extensive tumor burden (>50% of liver). Bilobar and multifocal HCC are not absolute contraindications to therapy, but treatment to more than one liver lobe should not be performed simultaneously, in order to allow recovery from therapy to the first area treated before proceeding to another region. Thrombus in the main portal vein is considered a contraindication to TACE due to the fact that normal liver in the region being treated will be dependent on portal vein inflow after embolic occlusion of the arterial blood supply. If portal vein inflow is not present, then both tumor and nontumoral tissue will necrose following treatment, leading to further hepatic decompensation in cirrhotic patients. Branch portal vein thrombosis is no longer considered to be an absolute contraindication to therapy. An incompetent sphincter of Oddi (e.g., PSC with biliary stents in place) is a contraindication to TACE therapy. In this situation, the biliary tree may be colonized with bacteria, which may cause formation of a hepatic abscess in the treated area. Other relative contraindications include conditions where an arterial puncture is unsafe (platelet count < 50,000/mm^3, INR > 1.5), gastrointestinal bleeding, and renal failure.

Complications of TACE include worsening of liver disease, systemic effects of chemotherapy, and procedural complications. Postembolization syndrome (PES) is characterized by fever, abdominal pain, nausea, and vomiting. It is thought to result from symptoms of ischemia to the treated liver region. In early trials, PES affected up to 50% of patients and was felt to be a predictor of response [37]. The current rate of postembolization syndrome is thought to be lower, and in a 2009 study of 71 patients who underwent 98 procedures, the rate of postembolization syndrome was 32% on the first treatment and 23% following a second cycle of TACE [38]. Postembolization syndrome is treated supportively with hydration and analgesia. Antibiotics are not felt to be necessary. Although systemic delivery of chemotherapeutics is limited, patients may still develop bone marrow suppression and alopecia. In rare instances, tumor lysis syndromes may occur.

TACE is not considered to be definitive or curative therapy. The benefit of therapy is highly dependent on initial tumor burden, tumor biology, baseline hepatic function, and the initial response to therapy. In a metaanalysis, overall survival in patients undergoing TACE therapy was 20 months vs. 16 months for untreated controls [39]. However, due to the above factors, these numbers are unhelpful when predicting outcomes in individual patients. TACE therapy does continue to advance with regard to technical ability to selectively target tumor and in some cases treating patients with portal vein thrombus. A recent prospective study examined the difference in outcome between lobar TACE and selective/superselective TACE by examining the explants specimen at the time of liver transplant. Sixty-seven consecutive patients undergoing TACE for HCC prior to transplant were studied, of whom 53% underwent selective/superselective TACE. Superselective TACE demonstrated a superior degree of mean necrosis (75% vs. 53%) and also a significantly higher rate of complete necrosis (54% vs. 30%) [40]. Another recent study out of Seoul, Korea, examined the impact of TACE in patients with main portal vein invasion [41]. From 2003 to 2007, 125 patients presented with main PV invasion and without decompensated cirrhosis. Sixty-six percent were treated with TACE and showed significantly improved survival of 7.4 vs. 2.6 months. There were no procedure-related deaths. The study was limited by the fact that of those treated with TACE, 69% were Childs A, while in the supportive treatment group only 36% were Childs A. However, this study does appear to offer support to previous reports of selected patients with PVT (compensated and with good collateral circulation) being successfully treated with TACE [42–44].

Advancement in TACE has been the introduction of drug-eluting beads (DEBs). The beads vary in size (300–500 and 500–700 μm) and are loaded with doxorubicin. This form of delivery differs from conventional TACE in that the chemotherapeutic agent is slowly released with a prolonged dwell time of drug within the tumor and thereby enhances drug delivery to the tumor. Additionally, pharmacokinetic studies have demonstrated less systemic absorption of doxorubicin, leading to less toxicity associated with DEBs [45, 46]. A RCT of DEBs vs. TACE, PRECISION V, showed no significant difference in radiographic response (EASL) at 6 months post therapy; however, in a subanalysis of patients with more advanced disease (CP B, ECOG 1, bilobar disease, and recurrent disease), there was a significant improvement in response observed in those who received DEBs [47]. A retrospective trial of TACE ($N=26$) vs. DEBs ($N=45$) reported a significantly improved survival in patients treated with DEBs compared to TACE (median survival from time of initial treatment of 403 vs. 114 days; $p=0.01$) [48]. A sub-analysis of OS based on CP classification demonstrated that CP A–B had superior survival associated with DEBs therapy; however, survival was not different based on therapy in CP C patients. These results emphasize the associated mortality with advanced underlying liver disease and support the recommendation of avoiding any form of liver-directed therapy in those with CP C as the risk is likely to outweigh any potential benefit derived from an antitumor effect.

TARE

Radioembolization (TARE) has emerged as another form of transarterial therapy for unresectable HCC. Microspheres, coated with y-90, a pure beta emitter, are injected into the hepatic artery in a similar fashion to TACE. They are preferentially trapped

Table 10.1 TARE vs. TACE

	Lewandowski et al. [54] #: 43 vs. 35	Carr et al. [8] #: 99 vs. 691	Kooby et al.[c] [9] #: 27 vs. 44	Salem et al. [52] #: 123 vs. 122
Median OS (mo.)	35.7 vs. 18.7; $p=0.18$	11.5 vs. 8.5; $p=<.05^a$	6 vs. 6; $p=0.74$	20.5 vs. 17.4; $p=0.23$
Radiographic response	61 vs. 37; $p=0.12$	41 vs. 60[b]	11 vs. 6;	49 vs. 36;
WHO response (%)	58 vs. 31; $p=0.023$	N/A	$p=0.73^d$	$p=0.10$
T3 to T2 (%)			N/A	N/A
TTP (mo.)	33.3 vs. 12.8; $p=0.005$	N/A	N/A	13.1 vs. 8.4; $p=0.023$
Tolerability		N/A		
Median hospitalization (d)	0 vs. 2; $p<0.001$		1.7 vs. 5.0; $p=0.05$	0 vs. 1.8; $p<0.001$
Any complication (%)			44 vs. 70; $p=0.05$	
Hyperbilirubinemia (%)	Grade ¾: 26 vs. 7		>3 mg/dl: 4 vs. 16; $p=0.1$	

[a]OS between Y-90 and TACE became NS after adjusting for baseline bilirubin, presence of PVT, and baseline AFP level

[b]Single dose of TARE to lobe with dominant disease burden; 43% bilobar in TARE. TACE q 8–10 weeks

[c]Sir-Spheres (Y-90 resin-based beads FDA approved in the USA only for colorectal metastases, but in Europe for liver neoplasia)

[d]Radiographic response by RECIST at three mos

in the tumor capillary bed due to their small size of 30 μm. This enables higher doses of radiation to be delivered to exert a greater tumorcidial effect. At the same time, there is minimization of damage to the nontumorous tissue.

There are two forms of TARE that are commercially available: ThereaSphere® and Sir-Sphere® [49, 50]. They differ in some of their physical properties which are highlighted in Table 10.1.

TARE is mechanistically different from TACE in that it is microembolic (25–35 μm) and therefore has minimal postembolization syndrome. Absolute contraindications to TARE include an inability to embolize nontargets (to avoid inadvertent delivery of radiation to nontumorous tissue such as gallbladder, bowel, stomach) and a Technetium-99 macroaggregated albumin (MAA) scan (MAA) showing anticipated delivery of greater than 30 Gy with a single injection and/or a cumulative dose of >50 Gy to the lungs. Preparation for TARE does require a staging angiogram in order to rule out such a contraindication and to perform dosimetry calculations. Cross-sectional imaging with CT or MRI is used to determine the targeted liver mass which is converted into the volume of liver that will be exposed to radiation. The dose of radiation is calculated using the targeted liver mass and the calculated lung shunt. Radioembolization is generally performed 7–10 days after the staging angiogram. The patient is discharged 6 h later with no special radiation precautions.

Table 10.2 Ongoing trials

Agent/clinical trials identifier	Phase	Targeted population	Estimated N
Brivanib vs. sorafenib: BRISK FL NCT00858871	III	First line in advanced HCC	1,050
Brivanib vs. placebo: BRISK PS NCT00825955	III	Second line in Sor failure in advanced HCC	414
Brivanib vs. placebo: BRISK TA NCT00908752	III	Adjuvant Tx to TACE in unresectable HCC	870
Sorafenib + erlotinib vs. sorafenib: SEARCH NCT00901901	III	First line in advanced HCC	700
Sorafenib + doxorubicin vs. sorafenib: SoraDox NCT01272557	II	First line in advanced HCC	170
ABT-869 vs. sorafenib NCT01009593	III	First line in advanced HCC	900
BIBF-1120 vs. sorafenib NCT01004003	II	First line in advanced HCC	115
Sorafenib vs. placebo ECOG 1208 NCT01004978	III	In combination with TACE in unresectable HCC	400
Sorafenib vs. placebo: SPACE NCT00855218[a]	II	In combination with DEBs in intermediate HCC	307
Sorafenib vs. placebo: STORM NCT 00692770[a]	III	Adjuvant therapy in ablation or resection	1,115
Sorafenib + everolimus NCT00828594[a]	I/II	Advanced HCC	130

[a]Active but not recruiting

While there has been growing enthusiasm for TARE in HCC, it has been tempered by a lack of RCTS. There are currently no RCTs comparing TARE to any other form of liver-directed or systemic therapy. Hilgard and colleagues proposed the incorporation of TARE into their institutional treatment algorithm as a modification of the BCLC staging system based on a median OS of 16.4 months and time to progression of 10 months in a retrospective study of 108 patients with advanced HCC [51]. The results of this study independently corroborated the results reported by another retrospective study with 291 patients treated with TARE and validated the safety of TARE in HCC [52].

Until recently, the results with TARE have been limited to single center experiences. A multicenter experience among European centers with resin microspheres also showed efficacy of TARE with a median OS of 12.8 months among 325 patients with HCC [53].

The two clinical scenarios where TARE has been shown to be of particular interest are in patients with PVT and downstaging. Lewandowski et al. reported a retrospective analysis of patients with T3 disease that were treated with TACE compared to TARE. Those treated with TARE were more likely to be successfully downstaged into Milan criteria [54]. As stated above, there is concern regarding the safety of TACE in patients with PV invasion due to risk of ischemic hepatitis leading to liver failure. Unlike TACE, TARE is microembolic and therefore the patency of the hepatic artery is maintained. The safety of TARE has been reported in patients with the presence of PVT [51–53].

Various retrospective studies have shown similar overall survival between TARE and TACE and are highlighted in Table 10.2.

Advanced HCC: BCLC C

To date, sorafenib (400 bid) is the only systemic therapy that has demonstrated an overall survival benefit in patients with unresectable HCC. Sorafenib is a multikinase inhibitor with antiproliferative, antiangiogenic, and proapoptotic activities [55]. Two RCTs, which encompassed a patient population from the West (SHARP) and the East (Asia-Pacific), demonstrated a similar degree of survival benefit associated with sorafenib relative to placebo [56, 57].

There is a paucity of data of the safety and efficacy of sorafenib in patients with CP B cirrhosis (95% of the patients enrolled in the phase III trials were CP A). The competing risk of mortality associated with chronic liver disease is underscored by a decreased OS in those with more advanced liver disease. Inferior overall survival in CP B compared to CP A patients does not appear to be mediated by an inferior antitumor activity, suggested by a similar time to progression regardless of CP class in one retrospective study [58]. The same study reported an OS of 6.5 months in 23 CP B patients. In a small phase II trial, there was no significant difference in pharmacokinetics noted between CP A and CP B patients [59]. Additionally, GIDEON, a prospective observational trial of patients on sorafenib, recently reported no significant increase in drug-related adverse events in CP B patients [60]. Only a RCT with a placebo group will be able to determine if treatment of advanced HCC in CP B patients leads to a clinically meaningful improvement in survival. The benefit of therapy via prevention of tumor progression becomes less meaningful as liver function declines and has a greater role in determining patient survival. This is clearly evident in a report of ten CP C patients treated with sorafenib in whom the median OS was dismal at 1.5 months; therefore, it is not recommended [58].

The utility of continuing sorafenib after disease progression is not known. Currently, there are no approved alternative options for sorafenib treatment failure. Such patients could participate in a clinical trial whenever available. Until there are data to refute or support the role of sorafenib in this clinical context, treating physicians may consider continuation of sorafenib in a patient who is otherwise tolerating therapy.

A RCT of sorafenib (400 bid) vs. sunitinib (37.5 mg/day) conducted in the USA was discontinued due to observed toxicity associated with sunitinib. An earlier study of sunitinib in advanced HCC reported 10% of the deaths to be related to treatment despite using the lower dose of 37.5 mg/day rather than 50 mg/day, the dose for renal cell carcinoma [61]. Therefore, it does not appear that there will be a role for sunitinib in the treatment of HCC.

Brivanib, also a multikinase inhibitor (anti VEGFR-2 and fibroblast growth factor receptor 1), may be a contender for second-line therapy after sorafenib failure. An OS of 9.8 months and TTP of 5.5 months after initiation of brivanib in sorafenib failures have been reported [62]. This has led to a phase III RCT (BRISK PS) of brivanib (800 mg/day) vs. placebo as a second-line agent. A phase II, open-label study has reported a median survival of 10 months in patients with advanced HCC treated with brivanib as a first-line therapy [63]. A phase III RCT (BRISK FL) of brivanib vs. sorafenib as first-line therapy is ongoing.

The additive therapeutic effects of sorafenib in combination with a second targeted therapy are also being investigated. Improved efficacy compared to sorafenib alone and without limiting toxicity associated with combination therapy will need to be demonstrated in order to become the recognized standard of care for the intended population that the study is being conducted. A small phase II trial showed a significant increase in OS in patients treated with doxorubicin plus sorafenib with a median OS of 13.8 months compared to 6.5 months(less than placebo in SHARP) with doxorubicin alone [64]. While these results are quite encouraging, there was a noted increase in LV dysfunction: 19% in the combination group vs. 2% in doxorubicin alone. There is now an ongoing trial of sorafenib plus doxorubicin vs. sorafenib alone. This trial and other trials are listed in Table 10.2.

Sorafenib gained approval based on its safety and efficacy of RCTs that predominately were composed of BCLC C patients. It is approved with the broad indication of unresectable HCC. The role of sorafenib in other clinical settings such as in conjunction with TACE/DEBs or as adjuvant therapy post-RFA/resection is anticipated to be answered when the results of ongoing RCTs are reported (SPACE and STORM, respectively). Similarly, there is a RCT examining the safety/efficacy of brivanib vs. placebo with TACE. Such a therapeutic approach makes sense from a mechanistic standpoint as it is known that VEGF levels increase post TACE and resection; moreover, VEGF levels have been shown to be prognostic [65]. Disruption of the pro-angiogenesis signal induced by hypoxemia would be expected to have a positive effect; however, combination therapy cannot be recommended as standard of care unless the results of these trials support their use.

Terminal HCC (BCLC D)

The natural history of patients with decompensated liver disease, CPC and/or poor performance status have a median survival of 3 months. Therefore, no treatment other than supportive care is recommended in these patients.

Conclusion

The goal of therapy for HCC is tumor control while minimizing risk of hepatic decompensation. In order to attain this goal, patients need to be carefully selected based on tumor stage, liver function, and performance status, in terms of when therapy is appropriate and which therapy will provide the best potential outcome.

References

1. Ferlay J, Shin HR, Bray F, Forman D, Mathers C, et al. Estimates of worldwide burden of cancer in 2008: GLOBOCAN 2008. Int J Cancer. 2010;127(12):2893–917.
2. Mazzaferro V, Regalia E, Doci R, Andreola S, Pulvirenti A, et al. Liver transplantation for the treatment of small HCC in patients with cirrhosis. N Engl J Med. 1996;334:693–9.
3. Sala M, Forner A, Varela M, Bruix J. Prognostic prediction in patients with hepatocellular carcinoma. Semin Liver Dis. 2005;25(2):171–80.
4. Cho YK, Kim JK, Kim MY, Rhim H, Han JK. Systematic review of randomized trials for hepatocellular carcinoma treated with percutaneous ablation therapies. Hepatology. 2009;49: 453–9.
5. Orlando A, Leandro G, Olivo M, Andriulli A, Cottone M. Radiofrequency thermal ablation vs. percutaneous ethanol injection for small hepatocellular carcinoma in cirrhosis: meta-analysis of randomized controlled trials. Am J Gastroenterol. 2009;104(2):514–24.
6. Chen MS, Li JQ, Zheng Y, Guo RP, Liang HH, et al. Carcinoma. Ann Surg. 2006;243:321–8.
7. Huang J, Yan L, Cheng Z, Wu H, Du L, Wang J, Xu Y, Zeng Y, et al. A randomized trial comparing radiofrequency ablation and surgical resection for HCC conforming to the Milan criteria. Ann Surg. 2010;252(6):903–12.
8. Hasegawa K, Makuuchi M, Takayama T, Kokudo N, Arii S, et al. Surgical resection vs. percutaneous ablation for hepatocellular carcinoma: a preliminary report of the Japanese nationwide survey. J Hepatol. 2008;49:589–94.
9. Livraghi T, Meloni F, Di Stasi M, Rolle E, Solbiati L, et al. Sustained complete response and complications rates after radiofrequency ablation of very early hepatocellular carcinoma in cirrhosis: Is resection still the treatment of choice? Hepatology. 2008;47:82–9.
10. Molinari M, Helton S. Hepatic resection versus radiofrequency ablation for hepatocellular carcinoma in cirrhotic individuals not candidates for liver transplantation: a Markov model decision analysis. Am J Surg. 2009;198:396–06.
11. Rossi S, Ravetta V, Ghittoni G, Viera FT, et al. Repeated radiofrequency ablation for management of patients with cirrhosis with small hepatocellular carcinomas: a long-term cohort study. Hepatology. 2011;53:136–47.
12. Hung H-H, Chiou Yi-You, Hsia C-Y, Chien-Wei Su, Chou Yi-Hong, et al. Survival rates are comparable after radiofrequency ablation or surgery in patients with small hepatocellular carcinomas. Clin Gastroenterol Hepatol. 2011;9:79–86.
13. Bigourdan JM, Jaeck D, Meyer N, Meyer C, Oussoultzoglou E, et al. Small hepatocellular carcinoma in child A cirrhotic patients: hepatic resection vs transplantation. Liver Transplant. 2003;9:513–20.
14. Margarit C, Escartín A, Castells L, Vargas V, Allende E, et al. Resection for HCC is a good option in Child Turcotte Pugh class A patients with cirrhosis who are eligible for transplantation. Liver Transplant. 2005;11:1242–51.
15. Mazzaferro V, Regalia E, Doci R, Andreola S, Pulvirenti A, et al. Liver transplantation for the treatment of small HCC in patients with cirrhosis. N Engl J Med. 1996;334:693–9.
16. Yao FY, Bass NM, Nikolai B, Davern TJ, Kerlan R, et al. Liver transplantation for hepatocellular carcinoma: analysis of survival according to the intention-to-treat principle and dropout from the waiting list. Liver Transplant. 2002;8(10):873–83.
17. Bruix J, Sherman M, Llovet JM, Beaugrand M, Lencioni R, et al. Clinical management of hepatocellular carcinoma. Conclusions of the Barcelona-2000 EASL conference. European Association for the Study of the Liver. J Hepatol. 2001;35(3):421–30.
18. Bruix J, Sherman M. Management of HCC. AASLD practice guideline. Hepatology. 2005;42(5):1208–35.
19. Bruix et al. Management of HCC. AASLD practice guideline. Hepatology 2010.
20. Bruix J, Castells A, Bosch J, Feu F, Fuster J, et al. Gastro 1996;111:1018–22.
21. Zhou YM, Shao WY, Zhao YF, Xu DH, Li B. Meta-analysis of laparoscopic versus open resection for hepatocellular carcinoma. Dig Dis Sci. 2011;56(7):1937–43.

22. Lo CM, Fan ST, Liu CL, Chan SC, Wong J. The role and limitation of living donor liver transplantation for hepatocellular carcinoma. Liver Transplant. 2004;10(3):440–7.
23. Todo S, Furukawa H. Living donor liver transplantation for adult patients with hepatocellular carcinoma: experience in Japan. Ann Surg. 2004;240(3):451–61.
24. Fisher RA, Kulik LM, Freise CE, Lok AS, Shearon TH, et al. Hepatocellular carcinoma recurrence and death following living and deceased donor liver transplantation. Am J Transplant. 2007;7(6):1601–8.
25. Lo CM, Fan ST, Liu CL, Chan SC, Ng IO, et al. Living donor versus deceased donor liver transplantation for early irresectable hepatocellular carcinoma. Br J Surg. 2007;94(1):78–86.
26. Kulik L, Abecassis M. Living donor liver transplantation for hepatocellular carcinoma. Gastroenterology. 2004;127(5 Suppl 1):S277–82.
27. Vakili K, Pomposelli JJ, Cheah YL, Akoad M, Lewis WD, et al. Living donor liver transplantation for hepatocellular carcinoma: Increased recurrence but improved survival. Liver Transplant. 2009;15(12):1861–6.
28. Hwang S, Lee SG, Joh JW, Suh KS, Kim DG. Liver transplantation for adult patients with hepatocellular carcinoma in Korea: comparison between cadaveric donor and living donor liver transplantations. Liver Transplant. 2005;11(10):1265–72.
29. Kulik L, Fisher R, Lok A, Del Rodrigo, Freise C et al. HCC Recurrence and Survival in Living Donor Liver Transplant (LDLT) Compared to Deceased Donor Liver Transplant (DDLT): Results of the Adult to Adult Living Donor Liver Transplantation (A2ALL) Cohort Study. American Association for the Study of Liver Disease; 2010.
30. Otto G, Herber S, Heise M, Lohse AW, Mönch C, et al. Response to transarterial chemoembolization as a biological selection criterion for liver transplantation in hepatocellular carcinoma. Liver Transplant. 2006;12(8):1260–7.
31. Yao FY, Hirose R, LaBerge JM, Davern 3rd TJ, Bass NM, et al. A prospective study on downstaging of hepatocellular carcinoma prior to liver transplantation. Liver Transplant. 2005;11(12):1505–14.
32. Vitale A, D'Amico F, Frigo AC, Grigoletto F, Brolese A, et al. Response to therapy as a criterion for awarding priority to patients with hepatocellular carcinoma awaiting liver transplantation. Ann Surg. 2010;17:2290–302.
33. Nakashima T, Kojiro M. Pathologic characteristics of hepatocellular carcinoma. Semin Liver Dis. 1986;6:259–66.
34. Arii S, Yamaoka Y, Futagawa S, Inoue K, Kobayashi K, et al. Results of surgical and nonsurgical treatment for small-sized hepatocellular carcinomas: a retrospective and nationwide survey in Japan. Hepatology. 2000;32:1224–9.
35. Llovet JM, Bruix J. Systematic review of randomized trials for unresectable hepatocellular carcinoma: Chemoembolization improves survival. Hepatology. 2003;37:429.
36. Llovet JM, Real MI, Montanya X, Planas R, Coll S, et al. Arterial embolization, chemoembolization versus symptomatic treatment in patients with unresectable hepatocellular carcinoma: a randomized controlled trial. Lancet. 2002;359:1734–9.
37. Castells A, Bruix J, Ayuso C, et al. Transarterial embolization for hepatocellular carcinoma. Antibiotic prophylaxis and clinical meaning of postembolization fever. J Hepatol. 1995;22: 410–15.
38. Rodolfo S, Marco B, Pasquale P, Michele B, Irene B, et al. Clinical impact of selective transarterial chemoembolization on hepatocellular carcinoma: A cohort study. World J Gastroenterol. 2009;15(15):1843–8.
39. Llovet JM, Bruix J. Systematic review of randomized trials for unresectable hepatocellular carcinoma: Chemoembolization improves survival. Hepatology. 2003;37:429.
40. Golfieri R, Cappelli A, Cucchetti A, Piscaglia F, Carpenzano M, et al. Efficacy of selective transarterial chemoembolization in obtaining tumor necrosis in small (<5 cm) hepatocellular carcinomas. Hepatology. 2011;53(5):1580–9.
41. Chung GE, Lee JH, Kim HY, Hwang SY, Kim JS, et al. Transarterial chemoembolization can be safely performed in patients with hepatocellular carcinoma invading the main portal vein and may improve the overall survival. Radiology. 2011;258(2):627–34.

42. Georgiades CS, Hong K, D'Angelo M, Geschwind JF. Safety and efficacy of transarterial chemoembolization in patients with unresectable hepatocellular carcinoma and portal vein thrombosis. J Vasc Interv Radiol. 2005;16(12):1653–9.
43. Kim KM, Kim JH, Park IS, Ko GY, Yoon HK, et al. Reappraisal of repeated transarterial chemoembolization in the treatment of hepatocellular carcinoma with portal vein invasion. J Gastroenterol Hepatol. 2009;24(5):806–14.
44. Lee HS, Kim JS, Choi IJ, Chung JW, Park JH, et al. The safety and efficacy of transcatheter arterial chemoembolization in the treatment of patients with hepatocellular carcinoma and main portal vein obstruction: a prospective controlled study. Cancer. 1997;79(11):2087–94.
45. Varela M, Real MI, Burrel M, Forner A, Sala M, et al. Chemoembolization of hepatocellular carcinoma with drug eluting beads: efficacy and doxorubicin pharmacokinetics. J Hepatol. 2007;46:474–8.
46. Poon RT, Tso WK, Pang RW, Ng KK, Woo R, et al. A phase I/II trial of chemoembolization for hepatocellular carcinoma using a novel intra-arterial drug-eluting bead. Clin Gastroenterol Hepatol. 2007;5(9):1100–8.
47. Lammer J, Malagari K, Vogl T, Pilleul F, Denys A, et al. Prospective randomized study of doxorubicin-eluting-bead embolization in the treatment of hepatocellular carcinoma: results of the PRECISION V study. Cardiovasc Intervent Radiol. 2010;33(1):41–52.
48. Dhanasekaran R, Kooby DA, Staley CA, Kauh JS, Khanna V, et al. Comparison of conventional transarterial chemoembolization (TACE) and chemoembolization with doxorubicin drug eluting beads (DEB) for unresectable hepatocelluar carcinoma (HCC). J Surg Onc. 2010;101:476–80.
49. Thereasphere yttrium-90 microspheres package insert. MDS Nordion, Kanata, Canada 2004. Available at http://www.mds.nordion.com/therasphere/documents/package_insert.
50. SIR-Spheres Yttrium -90 microspheres package insert [Sirtex Medical Web site] 2004. Available at:http//www.sirtex.com/usa/-datapage/549/SIR-Spheres-User-Manual2pdf.
51. Hilgard P, Hamami M, Fouly AE, Scherag A, Müller S, et al. Radioembolization with yttrium-90 glass microspheres in hepatocellular carcinoma: European experience on safety and long-term survival. Hepatology. 2010;52(5):1741–9.
52. Salem R, Lewandowski RJ, Mulcahy MF, Riaz A, Ryu RK, et al. Radioembolization for hepatocellular carcinoma using Yttrium-90 microspheres: a comprehensive report of long-term outcomes. Gastroenterology. 2010;138(1):52–64.
53. Sangro B, Carpanese L, Cianni R, Golfieri R, Gasparini D, et al. Survival after Yttrium-90 resin microsphere radioembolization of hepatocellular carcinoma across Barcelona clinic liver cancer stages: A European evaluation. Hepatology. 2011;54(3):868–78.
54. Lewandowski RJ, Kulik LM, Riaz A, Senthilnathan S, Mulcahy MF, et al. A comparative analysis of transarterial downstaging for hepatocellular carcinoma: chemoembolization versus radioembolization. Am J Transplant. 2009;9(8):1920–8.
55. Wilhelm SM, Carter C, Tang L, Wilkie D, McNabola A, et al. Angiogenesis. Cancer Res. 2004;64:7099–109.
56. Llovet JM, Ricci S, Mazzaferro V, Hilgard P, Gane E, et al. Sorafenib in advanced hepatocellular carcinoma. N Engl J Med. 2008;359(4):378–90.
57. Cheng AL, Kang YK, Chen Z, Tsao CJ, Qin S, et al. Efficacy and safety of sorafenib in patients in the Asia-Pacific region with advanced hepatocellular carcinoma: a phase III randomised, double-blind, placebo-controlled trial. Lancet Oncol. 2009;10(1):25–34.
58. Pinter M, Sieghart W, Graziadei I, Vogel W, Maieron A, et al. Sorafenib in unresectable hepatocellular carcinoma from mild to advanced stage liver cirrhosis. Oncologist. 2009;14:70–6.
59. Abou-Alfa GK, Schwartz L, Ricci S, Amadori D, Santoro A, et al. Phase II study of sorafenib in patients with advanced hepatocellular carcinoma. J Clin Oncol. 2006;24:4293–300.
60. Bronowicki JP, Marrero J, Lim H et al. Sorafenib treatment and safety profile in Childs Pugh B patients characterized in the first and term results of GI DEON (Global Investigation of therapeutic DEcisions and hepatocellular carcinoma and Of its treatment with sorafeNib) Eastern Western experiences (IMHCC 2011) 7th international meeting, 14–15 January 2011, Paris, France.

61. Faivre S, Raymond E, Boucher E, Douillard J, Lim HY, et al. Safety and efficacy of sunitinib in patients with advanced hepatocellular carcinoma: an open-label, multicentre, phase II study. Lancet Oncol. 2009;10(8):794–800.
62. Raoul JL, Finn RS, Kang YK, Park JW, Harris R, Coric V, Donica M, Walters I. An open-label phase II study of first- and second-line treatment with brivanib in patients with hepatocellular carcinoma (HCC). J Clin Oncol. 2009;27(15s). suppl; abstr 4577.
63. Park JW, Finn RS, Kim JS, Karwal M, Li RK, et al. Phase II, open-label study of brivanib as first-line therapy in patients with advanced hepatocellular carcinoma. Clin Cancer Res. 2011;17(7):1973–83.
64. Abou-Alfa GK, Johnson P, Knox JJ, Capanu M, Davidenko I, et al. Doxorubicin plus sorafenib vs. doxorubicin alone in patients with advanced hepatocellular carcinoma: a randomized trial. J Am Med Assoc. 2010;304(19):2154–60.
65. Sergio A, Cristofori C, Cardin R, Pivetta G, Ragazzi R, et al. Transcatheter arterial chemoembolization (TACE) in hepatocellular carcinoma (HCC): the role of angiogenesis and invasiveness. Am J Gastroenterol. 2008;103(4):914–21.

Chapter 11
Recurrence: Prevention and Management

Natasha Chandok and Paul Marotta

Abbreviations

AFP	Alfa-fetoprotein
CUS	Contrast ultrasound
CT	Computed tomography
DCP	Des-gamma carboxy prothrombin
DEBs	Drug-eluting beads
FL-HCC	Fibrolamellar-type hepatocellular carcinoma
FLR	Future liver remnant
HBV	Hepatitis B virus
HCV	Hepatitis C virus
HCC	Hepatocellular carcinoma
LDLT	Living donor liver transplantation
MELD	Model for end-stage liver disease
LT	Liver transplantation
PVT	Portal vein thrombosis
TTV	Total tumor volume
TACE	Transarterial chemoembolization
TAE	Transarterial embolization
US	Ultrasound
UCSF	University of California at San Francisco

N. Chandok, MD • P. Marotta, MD, FRCPC (✉)
Division of Gastroenterology, University of Western Ontario,
339 Windermere Road, London, ON N6A5A5, Canada
e-mail: Paul.Marotta@lhsc.on.ca

N. Reau and F.F. Poordad (eds.), *Primary Liver Cancer: Surveillance, Diagnosis and Treatment*, Clinical Gastroenterology, DOI 10.1007/978-1-61779-863-4_11,
© Springer Science+Business Media New York 2012

Introduction

Although hepatocellular carcinoma (HCC) is the sixth most common cancer worldwide, it is the third leading cause of cancer-related mortality, owing to its aggressive natural history. While therapeutic approaches to the optimal management of HCC continue to evolve, less is known on the ideal strategies for the prevention and management of recurrent HCC. With the increasing global burden of HCC due to epidemiologic trends such as an aging population and high prevalence rates of viral hepatitis, among other factors, recurrence of HCC after the initial application of curative surgical therapy is an emerging and poorly understood phenomenon.

The expanding arsenal of treatment modalities for HCC includes surgical resection, liver transplantation (LT), locoregional therapies, and systemic therapies. Novel approaches utilizing multimodality treatments offer further promise for select patients, but further studies are needed to the clarify the efficacy, safety, and cost-effectiveness of these approaches. In the setting of recurrent HCC, early recognition is vital to facilitating timely aggressive therapy and a favorable clinical outcome.

Too often, however, recurrent HCC portents a worse clinical prognosis as compared with primary HCC due to the higher prevalence of advanced, poorly differentiated HCC, multifocal tumor, and lymphovascular involvement. Moreover, immunosuppression in the posttransplantation setting accelerates tumor proliferation. Optimal methods for surveillance for recurrent HCC and therapeutic approaches to management must be individualized, as factors such as tumor biology, patient functional status, hepatic reserve, health-care resources, and local expertise heavily weigh into treatment decisions and protocols for prevention.

Epidemiology and Risk Factors

This section will discuss the incidence of HCC and the known risk factors for recurrent HCC following LT and surgical resection, respectively.

Estimations on the rate of recurrent HCC following LT are derived from transplantation registries and publications on single-center experiences. Despite careful selection, HCC recurs in 8–20% of transplant recipients whose tumor stage prior to transplantation fulfilled widely accepted transplantation criteria.

The Milan criteria, the most widely used and best validated guide for hepatic transplantation for HCC, is associated with a 4-year recurrence-free survival of 92% [1]. An extension of the Milan criteria has been implemented by the University of California at San Francisco (UCSF) group. Outcome studies on the UCSF criteria reveal an acceptable recurrence rate of 11.4% at a mean of 8.1 months [2–22] following transplantation; this is noninferior to the recurrence rates from patients transplanted under Milan criteria [2]. The UCSF criteria have been validated by an independent transplant program, suggesting external validity [3]. There is some debate in the literature, however, as to whether patients within UCSF criteria but outside of Milan criteria may in fact have unacceptably higher rates of recurrence [4], but this finding is inconsistent. More recently, criteria from the University of

Alberta, established after combining HCC transplant data from the Denver and Toronto transplant programs, suggest that a total tumor volume (TTV) of less than 115 cm^3 and an AFP <400 units/ml is a valid selection criterion as these characteristics predict a recurrence rate similar to the Milan criteria [5].

Risk factors for recurrence of HCC following LT are well described and are the basis for exclusionary criteria for LT for potential recipients with HCC. These risk factors include tumor size and number, bilobar spread of tumor, high AFP and des-gamma carboxy prothrombin (DCP) levels, poorly differentiated tumor, positive lymph nodes, and vascular invasion [6–8].

Data on recurrence rates of HCC following surgical resection rather than LT are less robust, and are largely derived from single-center experiences and population-based cancer registries. Data from HCC registries have notable limitations. For example, tumor misclassification could be present as HCC typically represents only 80% or so of primary liver cancers. Misclassification bias may be particularly problematic in Asian regions where cholangiocarcinoma related to infection with liver flukes is highly prevalent. Other limitations to studies estimating HCC recurrence after resection include selection bias, failure of authors to report disease-free survival, underreporting of cirrhosis, and lack of uniform criteria for resection, among other factors [3].

Risk factors for recurrence of HCC following surgical resection fit into two broad categories: tumor biology (differentiation, size, vascular involvement) and underlying liver disease. Chronic active viral hepatitis, presence of cirrhosis, and positive tumor margin are examples of such established risk factors. In the specific case of hepatitis B virus, high viral load and E-antigen positivity are also known risk factors for primary HCC based on epidemiologic data; by deduction, these factors would presumably also increase the risk of recurrent HCC in patients with chronic active hepatitis B [9].

Morris-Stiff et al. performed a systematic review of the medical literature from 1997 to 2006 to examine outcomes from surgical resection of HCC [10]. Their robust analysis of 28 series revealed significant reporting discrepancies. Only 12 of 28 publications, for example, reported disease-free survival [10]. The overall disease-free survivals at 1-, 3-, and 5-year intervals in their meta-analysis were 64%, 38%, and 27%, respectively [10]. The main cause of mortality was tumor recurrence, noted in a median of 54.5% of cases (27.3–73%) [10]. Perhaps, not surprising, Morris-Stiff et al. observed that 80–90% of recurrences are seen within the liver remnant following hepatic resection for HCC [10].

The high incidence of recurrent HCC after primary resection suggests the need to optimize surveillance strategies and to consider early and aggressive adjuvant therapy, whether it be reresection, LRT, or systemic treatments, in an attempt to improve the long-term survival.

For patients who have recurrent HCC after LT, even for those originally transplanted for early HCC within Milan criteria, recurrence is usually rapid, with median survival less than 1 year [11]. Patients with rapid recurrence clearly had metastatic disease that was not identified prior to LT. Understaging of HCC prior to LT, despite serial dynamic cross-sectional imaging in recipients, is not uncommon and occurs in at least 25% of recipients once the explant is carefully examined [12]. Standard agents for immunosuppression following LT, including calcineurin inhibitors (cyclosporine and tacrolimus), have been shown in vivo to accelerate oncogenesis and are likely strongly contributory to the accelerated natural history of HCC in the post-transplantation course [13, 14]. Although the majority of patients with HCC recurrence after LT have an unfavorable outcome due to advanced stage of the tumor at the time of recognition, some patients have an acceptable prognosis if they are promptly diagnosed at an early stage and aggressively treated.

In summary, recurrence of HCC following LT for tumors that fulfilled Milan criteria is approximately 10%, and recurrence after surgical resection occurs in more than 50% of cases within 5 years based on the published literature. The comparison of recurrence rates of HCC between LT and resection is difficult due to selection bias, as patient with advanced HCC do not undergo LT. There are numerous risk factors for recurrence both after LT and surgical resection; these risk factors primarily involve tumor characteristics and the presence of cirrhosis. While a 10% recurrence rate of HCC after LT is generally acceptable, expansion of the Milan criteria should not be undertaken without rigorous validation to ensure that patients without HCC on the waiting list do not receive an unjust survival disadvantage compared to patients with extended-criteria HCC.

Clinical Manifestations

In clinical practice, there are two general patterns for recurrence of HCC: early recurrence due to microsatellite metastasis in remnant liver after primary resection and late recurrence that presents with the development of a second primary HCC lesion. Although recurrence typically occurs within the liver, several reports reveal a myriad of extrahepatic sites of recurrence. The most common sites of recurrence include lung, bone, brain, adrenal gland, bladder, skin, and lymph nodes [15]. Symptoms of recurrence are variable and depend upon the baseline functional status and underlying liver function of the patient and of course the location and stage of the tumor(s). Symptoms commonly include fatigue, anorexia, weight loss, abdominal pain, and jaundice. Occasionally, patients may experience new-onset or worsened ascites due to tumor invasion of the portal vein. HCC is also associated with numerous paraneoplastic syndromes that occur at varying frequencies, including hypoglycemia, thrombocytosis, hypercholesterolemia, and hypercalcemia.

Treatment

Validated staging systems are important in predicting prognosis and guiding therapy for primary HCC. Although currently established HCC staging systems were not designed to guide treatment decisions for recurrent HCC, they can provide a foundation upon which to derive an aggressive, patient-centered treatment strategy.

Staging systems that are effective combine both liver function and tumor parameters. The Barcelona Clinic Liver Cancer (BCLC) staging system, devised from prospective cohort and randomized controlled studies, is arguably the best validated and most endorsed HCC staging system.

There is no high-level evidence or even global consensus on the optimal approach to the management of HCC recurrence. Clearly, the treatment options and outcomes are affected by many variables, including liver function, performance status, and tumor stage. Given the complexity involved in management decisions and the lack of clear evidence to support a uniform treatment algorithm, a multidisciplinary approach to develop an individualized treatment plan is both essential and strongly advised by multisociety expert panels [16]. Other considerations may also include local expertise and cost. For instance, in Japan where there is a low availability of cadaveric donors and a reported low mortality rate following resection, cadaveric LT may be a less feasible option than resection for local patients with recurrent HCC [17].

While recognizing that a universal algorithm may have impracticalities such as limitations on generalizability across different patient populations in different health systems, current evidence would support surgical resection for early recurrent hepatic solitary tumors in patients with preserved liver function. Also, primary resection of metastatic deposits, specifically lung metastases, should be aggressively managed with resection where appropriate [18, 19]. Otherwise, recurrence within the liver should be treated with LRT depending on the size, location, functional status of the liver and the patient, and local expertise. Systemic therapy (chemotherapy) should also be considered for select patients.

Several published surgical series on outcomes of surgical resection for recurrent HCC report favorable results in carefully selected subjects. For example, in a study of 231 patients who developed recurrent HCC, Nagano et al. found that repeat resection is the treatment of choice for recurrent HCC in patients with preserved liver function and without portal invasion at the first resection if recurrence developed more than 1.5 years since the initial surgery [17]. The extended timing of recurrence is likely a reflection of adequate surgical margins during the original resection.

There is also evidence to support resection after LT. Resection should be pursued if recurrence of HCC in the hepatic allograft is solitary as there is a predicted survival benefit. The repeat surgery may be complicated, however, due to the formation of adhesions after prior hepatectomy. Where available, laparoscopic reintervention (hepatic resection or radiofrequency ablation) and adhesionolysis should be considered as this approach may be safer with respect to blood loss and injury to viscera and in turn result in a speedier recovery for patients. Belli et al. reported on 15 patients who had laparoscopic reintervention for HCC after LT; the overall mortality was 0%, and morbidity was 26.6% [20]. Although this case series is small, and there is limited published data in the literature, laparoscopic reintervention may be a worthy option for further exploration given its proven benefits and efficacy for other types of surgeries.

Due to the high prevalence of HCC (the peak point prevalence is likely to occur in the decade 2015–2020), in combination with the extending life expectancy among many populations, older patients are increasingly being evaluated for management of both primary HCC and recurrent HCC. In a study of 121 curative repeat hepate-ctomies, Tsujita et al. found no significant difference in the incidence of postopera-tive complications or in the duration of postoperative hospital stay in patients more than 75 years of age versus younger patients [21]. Furthermore, the authors noted a similar 3-year disease-free survival in both groups [21]. These data suggest that older patients with adequate functional status should be considered for repeat resec-tion if clinically warranted.

Although published series by and large demonstrate better survival of patients treated by resection than other modalities of care such as locoregional therapy, there is case-selection bias in publications, and with retrospective data, it is impossible to distinguish between the role of surgery versus the influence of favorable tumor biol-ogy and patient biology to explain the difference in survival. Nevertheless, in expe-rienced hands, liver resection is safe and associated with improved survival in select patients, including post-LT recipients with recurrent HCC.

Because recurrent HCC after LT almost always represents metastatic disease, either from the original tumor or from an HCC tumor that was not detected prior to transplantation, retransplantation for recurrent HCC should not be performed. LT would generally only be considered in the rare LT recipient with de novo HCC, and management of such patients would fit conceptually in the validated framework of the Milan or UCSF criteria.

However, LT for early recurrent HCC following surgical resection in a patient with no prior liver transplant is a potentially curative treatment worthy of careful consideration because it removes both the tumor and the underlying cirrhotic state. Given worldwide organ shortages, LT is usually restricted only to patients with an expected 5-year posttransplant survival of >50%, and many programs hold that patients transplanted for HCC should have similar 5-year survival to patients trans-planted for benign disease (i.e., 70%). As such, candidates for LT for recurrent HCC following resection should fulfill criteria such as Milan or UCSF. HCC is account-ing for an increasingly higher proportion of LT, and hence, the ideal approach to handle recurrence of HCC is fraught with ethical challenges.

A number of locoregional therapies are available for adjunctive treatment for recurrent HCC in selected candidates. Unfortunately, there is virtually no literature that examines criteria for selecting the ideal locoregional therapy in the post-transplant patient and for recurrent HCC in general. While the role of locoregional therapies has not been clarified for recurrent HCC through trials, these modalities are utilized in much the same way as for primary HCC when LT or repeat resection is contraindicated.

Isolated hepatic recurrences after LT are the pattern of recurrence most suitable for locoregional treatment when surgical resection cannot be performed. One obvi-ous benefit in the posttransplant setting is that the liver is usually noncirrhotic, par-ticularly in the initial 2 years after LT when the majority of recurrences occur. Furthermore, locoregional therapies spare patients the inherent technical challenges of surgical resection after LT if it cannot be safely performed. As recurrent HCC in LT recipients is by definition metastatic, locoregional therapy offers no "curative" solution, but it is possible that with locoregional therapy and/or adjustments in the recipient's immunosuppression regimen, patients can have an extended survival. Numerous therapies fall under the umbrella of locoregional therapies and include transarterial embolization (TAE), transarterial chemoembolization (TACE), radioembolization (RE), and drug-eluding bead transarterial chemoembolization (DEB-TACE), among others.

TAE and TACE are the most widely used treatment modalities for intermediate HCC. A meta-analysis failed to show superiority of TACE over TAE [22], but nevertheless, many centers preferentially utilize TACE as some published studies showed its improved efficacy over bland embolization. TACE is the standard of care for patients with adequate liver function, and large or multifocal tumor recurrence without portal venous involvement or extrahepatic spread. Two randomized controlled trials have shown a significant survival advantage with TACE versus placebo [23, 24]. Treatment with TAE is also associated with a significantly higher 2-year survival rate than in control groups [25]. The degree of benefit from TACE varies, and both TACE and TAE are associated with potentially serious adverse events such as postembolization syndrome (right upper quadrant pain, nausea, fever, and elevation in liver enzymes typically lasting 3–4 days) and hepatic decompensation, necessitating careful patient selection. The optimal frequency of TACE has not been determined through prospective trials for both primary HCC and recurrent disease. At our center, we typically perform TACE at 8–12-week intervals.

There is also a lack of consensus on the use and type of chemotherapeutic agent for embolization, and there is discordance in the literature on the optimal embolic particle. However, the safety of TACE after LT has been demonstrated to some degree. For example, Shin et al. reported no complications in a series of 28 patients with recurrence of HCC after live-donor LT [26]. Concerns about the added risk of biliary ischemia in the post-transplantation hepatic allograft have not been supported by available evidence.

DEB-TACE is another promising modality that may be considered, although its precise role in the management of HCC and recurrent HCC requires much clarification. DEBs are beads containing chemotherapeutic agents (e.g., doxorubicin). DEB-TACE provides a method of delivering chemotherapy that reportedly enhances tumor drug delivery and reduces systemic absorption of the chemotherapeutic agent(s), thereby theoretically improving safety and patient tolerability. In a trial by Lammer et al., TACE showed no superiority over DEB-TACE, but among patients with Child-Pugh status B, impaired functional status, bilobar disease, and recurrent HCC, there was a significant increase in the objective response (as measured by the standardized sized-based criteria of the European Association for the Study of the Liver) to DEB-TACE compared to TACE [27]. There is also exciting evidence suggesting fewer recurrences of HCC with DEB-TACE [28], and improved tolerability with fewer liver toxicities [27], but clearly, those conclusions are premature in the absence of more substantial data. Further trials are needed to objectively assess DEB-TACE, including insight into the role of combination treatments such as DEB-TACE with sorafenib.

RE is an emerging novel treatment now also available for consideration in patients with recurrent HCC. Caution needs to be exercised, however, as there are no randomized trials on RE to guide management decisions in patients with primary HCC, let alone recurrent disease. RE involves a catheter-based delivery of yttrium-90 embedded microspheres into the hepatic artery, for eventual release into the tumor. Once administered, the yttrium microspheres emit high-energy, low-penetration radiation to the tumor, causing localized necrosis. An advantage to RE is that it might be an effective locoregional therapy for patients with portal vein thrombosis (PVT) for whom TAE/TACE is not suitable. Kulik et al. reported on 108 patients with unresectable HCC with and without PVT; response rates by the criteria of the European Association for the Study of the Liver (EASL) were an impressive 70%, with a favorable toxicity profile, although liver-related adverse events were higher in patients with cirrhosis and main PVT [29]. Clearly, more studies are needed to establish the safety and efficacy of locoregional therapies in patients with recurrent HCC.

For failed locoregional therapy, sorafenib is the standard of care. Sorafenib is a targeted agent with a proven survival benefit as monotherapy in patients who do not qualify for surgical resection or locoregional therapy. Sorafenib blocks tumor cell proliferation and angiogenesis by inhibiting the activity of vascular endothelial growth factor receptors 1, 2, and 3 and platelet-derived growth factor receptor beta, Raf-1, and beta Raf. The side effects of sorafenib are numerous, including diarrhea (6%), weight loss, hand–foot reaction (~10.7%), hypophosphatemia, and fatigue (3.4%), among others.

Nevertheless, for patients with advanced HCC, sorafenib is a reasonable option for consideration. In a randomized placebo-controlled trial, sorafenib was associated with a 31% relative lower risk of death than placebo in patients with advanced HCC and Child A cirrhosis [30]. In this trial, there was a significant difference in the survival time between the treatment groups in favor of sorafenib (median survival 10.7 months versus 7.9 months) [30]. In a second randomized controlled trial on sorafenib from the Asia-Pacific region, an absolute survival benefit for sorafenib was also demonstrated (6.5 months versus 4.2 months in the placebo arm) [31]. The survival benefit in the Asia-Pacific study was felt to be less impressive as subjects had a relatively poorer functional status, and a greater proportion of patients had distant metastases [31].

Based on current available evidence, systemic therapy other than sorafenib has a limited role in recurrent HCC. There is no compelling evidence from prospective studies that there is a survival benefit with single-agent systemic chemotherapeutic (e.g., doxorubicin) administration.

Most extrahepatic recurrence of HCC is associated with an unfavorable prognosis and limits therapeutic options for management. Bone metastases, in particular, are strongly associated with an especially poor survival. Symptomatic patients can, however, be palliated with radiation and/or zoledronic acid. Locoregional therapies are generally not pursued for extrahepatic recurrence given the dismal survival of such patients and the lack of evidence to extend survival. Pulmonary metastases, however, should be aggressively treated by resection as previously mentioned.

Published case series, such as that by Bates et al., suggest that survival after resection of pulmonary metastases is similar to patients with HCC who underwent liver resection alone [19].

Fibrolamellar HCC (FL-HCC) is a rare variant of HCC with distinct clinical and pathologic features and as such warrants a specialized approach to management of recurrence. Recurrence of FL-HCC usually presents as a well-circumscribed hepatic or extrahepatic mass or masses characterized by well-differentiated polygonal hepatic cells with eosinophilic and granual cytoplasm surrounded by thick, fibrous stroma arranged in bands. Given that FL-HCC typically occurs in young patients without underlying hepatitis or cirrhosis, criteria for both resection and LT are far more liberal than normal variant HCC, although there is no uniform consensus. Most surgical series report a significantly better survival after resection of FL-HCC than normal variant HCC (1-, 5-, and 10-year disease-free survival 97.6%, 66.2%, and 47.4%, respectively) [32]. However, FL-HCC frequently recurs after complete resection (20–60%), and recurrence is often 5 or more years from the time of the original surgery. For patients with unresectable FL-HCC, survival is only 12 months. It is thus our opinion and experience that after initial hepatic resection of FL-HCC, there are virtually no size criteria of recurrence within the liver that should preclude LT as a salvage therapy, and patients with FL-HCC have the distinction of impressive long-term survival with aggressive surgical management, including liver transplantation for disease recurrence.

Surveillance After Liver Transplantation

Following transplantation, recipients may benefit from a surveillance protocol to monitor for HCC recurrence. Many transplantation centers routinely conduct annual or biannual CT scans of the liver and thorax for this purpose, particularly in patients who were transplanted outside of Milan criteria (after review of the explant). In light of the fact that recurrent HCC manifests outside of the liver 40% of the time, solely imaging the liver for surveillance would not always be useful to accomplish early detection. Presently, the most effective imaging modality or the frequency of such for postoperative surveillance has not been established. Furthermore, the cost-effectiveness of routine surveillance has been challenged, and only surveillance for patients possessing risk factors for recurrence has been proposed by some experts [33].

Using histologic characteristics of the tumor from careful study of the liver explant, a risk stratification for recurrence can be used. Vascular invasion, size of tumor, number of lesions, differentiation, and the presence of microsatellites can be used to generate an HCC recurrence score. A novel scoring system based on these tumor characteristics in an individual patient can help stratify surveillance strategies according to the estimated recurrence risk [30].

Serial surveillance measurement of tumor markers may also play a role in timely diagnosis of recurrent HCC. In a study by Yamashiki et al., 100 patients with HCC who underwent living donor LT were followed prospectively with monthly to bimonthly tumor markers (alpha fetoprotein and des-γ carboxy prothrombin) and yearly CT scan of the abdomen [34]. The authors determined that in all nine cases of HCC recurrence among 82 subjects who fulfilled Milan criteria prior to transplantation, rise in tumor marker levels after LT was the first indication of recurrence [34]. Other tumor markers or variations, such as the L3 fractionation of AFP, may also play a role in surveillance, but further studies are needed.

To date, prospective studies are lacking to show that surveillance translates into improved survival for recurrent HCC. That being said, there is no doubt that patients with recurrent HCC at early stages have better chances of extended survival than patients whose tumor is advanced at the time of diagnosis.

Prevention

Recurrence of HCC, be it following resection or transplantation, can be ameliorated but unfortunately not avoided in all patients with a history of HCC due to unmodifiable factors pertaining to tumor biology and patient characteristics. Integral to minimizing the probability of recurrence of HCC is the application of evidence-based criteria to guide decisions regarding resection versus transplantation eluded to earlier in the chapter. Adherence to evidence-based transplantation criteria such as the Milan criteria, for instance, should be the standard of care for assessing potential transplant recipients. Given that recurrent HCC following transplantation is more aggressive and decreases survival, early detection, and preferably prevention, is of paramount importance.

One possible strategy to lower the risk of recurrence of HCC following LT is the use of sirolimus in lieu of calcineurin inhibitors such as tacrolimus or cyclosporine. Sirolimus is an mTOR inhibitor with potent immunosuppressive properties and has also been shown in preclinical studies to have antiproliferative effects in vitro. However, the cumulative experience with sirolimus-based immunosuppression is limited [35], and the potential benefit of reducing the probability for HCC recurrence must be weighed against possible risks such as adverse drug effects and suboptimal immunosuppression with graft dysfunction, for example. Based on a study that utilized the Scientific Registry of Transplant Recipients (SRTR) and included 2,491 adult recipients for isolated LT for HCC and 12,167 for non-HCC diagnoses between March 2002 and March 2009, sirolimus-based maintenance immunosuppression regimens were associated with improved survival after LT for HCC [36]. For this reason, many liver transplant centers use a sirolimus-based immunosuppressive regimen in patients at high risk for recurrent HCC, or with known recurrence. Registry data such as that in SRTR may have selection bias and hence should be reviewed with healthy skepticism in the absence of pending prospective, randomized trials. The SILVER study, an ongoing prospective randomized open-label trial comparing sirolimus versus mTOR-inhibitor-free immunosuppression in patients undergoing LT for HCC, will shed more light on the utility of this strategy.

Everolimus is another immunosuppressive agent of interest in the management of patients with recurrent HCC or at risk for recurrent HCC. While everolimus may have a role for prophylaxis against recurrent HCC [37], there is presently insufficient evidence upon which to make formal recommendations.

Other agents serving as antitumor adjuvant therapy may be a future consideration for prevention of recurrent HCC. The rationale behind antitumor therapy administered early after LT or at the time of surgery is to eliminate micrometastases and thus reduce the risk for recurrence. At the present time, there is only sparse data in this area. To date, a variety of agents in varying regimens and populations have been examined, with no conclusive evidence to support its routine use. One compelling controlled trial by Xu et al. found that licartin was associated with a 30% absolute risk reduction in HCC recurrence [38], but larger studies are warranted before definitely recommendations can be made.

Conclusion

This chapter reviewed the available evidence to support a management approach for recurrent HCC, an emerging and poorly understood phenomenon. Unfortunately, high-quality prospective data to guide clinical decision-making in this area are lacking. That being said, the indications for surgical resection and LT are fairly established. Furthermore, a variety of treatment modalities, including locoregional therapy and systemic therapy, can be employed, each with indications, as well as potential risks and benefits. In the absence of sufficient data studying optimal strategies for the management HCC recurrence, clinical decision-making often relies on extrapolation of existing data on primary HCC. Given the complexity in managing recurrent HCC, a multidisciplinary and algorithmic approach that reflects local resources and expertise will help individual centers navigate through the myriad of treatment options.

References

1. Yen TC, et al. Hypercalcemia and parathyroid hormone-related protein in hepatocellular carcinoma. Liver. 1993;13(6):311–5.
2. Yao FY, et al. Liver transplantation for hepatocellular carcinoma: expansion of the tumor size limits does not adversely impact survival. Hepatology. 2001;33(6):1394–403.
3. Sotiropoulos GC, et al. Liver transplantation for hepatocellular carcinoma in patients beyond the Milan but within the UCSF criteria. Eur J Med Res. 2006;11(11):467–70.
4. Ju MK, et al. UCSF criteria by pre-transplant radiologic study cannot assure similar post-transplant results of hepatocellular carcinoma within Milan criteria. Hepatogastroenterology. 2010;57(101):819–25.
5. Toso C, et al. Total tumor volume predicts risk of recurrence following liver transplantation in patients with hepatocellular carcinoma. Liver Transplant. 2008;14(8):1107–15.
6. Kimura H, et al. Prognostic factors in resected hepatocellular carcinomas and therapeutic value of transcatheter arterial embolization for recurrences. Int Surg. 1998;83(2):146–9.

7. Ouchi K, et al. Recurrence of hepatocellular carcinoma in the liver remnant after hepatic resection. Am J Surg. 1993;166(3):270–3.
8. Zendejas-Ruiz I, et al, Recurrent hepatocellular carcinoma in liver transplant recipients with hepatitis C. J Gastrointest Cancer. 2010 [Epub ahead of print].
9. Chen CJ, Yang HI, Iloeje UH. Hepatitis B virus DNA levels and outcomes in chronic hepatitis B. Hepatology. 2009;49(5 Suppl):S72–84.
10. Morris-Stiff G, et al. Surgical management of hepatocellular carcinoma: is the jury still out? Surg Oncol. 2009;18(4):298–321.
11. Hollebecque A, et al. Natural history and therapeutic management of recurrent hepatocellular carcinoma after liver transplantation. Gastroenterol Clin Biol. 2009;33(5):361–9.
12. Shah SA, et al. Accuracy of staging as a predictor for recurrence after liver transplantation for hepatocellular carcinoma. Transplantation. 2006;81(12):1633–9.
13. Hojo M, et al. Cyclosporine induces cancer progression by a cell-autonomous mechanism. Nature. 1999;397(6719):530–4.
14. Schumacher G, et al. Sirolimus inhibits growth of human hepatoma cells in contrast to tacrolimus which promotes cell growth. Transplant Proc. 2002;34(5):1392–3.
15. Yang Y, et al. Patterns and clinicopathologic features of extrahepatic recurrence of hepatocellular carcinoma after curative resection. Surgery. 2007;141(2):196–202.
16. Bruix J, Sherman M. Management of hepatocellular carcinoma. Hepatology. 2005;42(5): 1208–36.
17. Nagano Y, et al. Efficacy of repeat hepatic resection for recurrent hepatocellular carcinomas. ANZ J Surg. 2009;79(10):729–33.
18. Bates MJ, et al. Pulmonary resection of metastatic hepatocellular carcinoma after liver transplantation. Ann Thorac Surg. 2008;85(2):412–5.
19. Koide N, et al. Surgical treatment of pulmonary metastasis from hepatocellular carcinoma. Hepatogastroenterology. 2007;54(73):152–6.
20. Belli G, et al. Laparoscopic redo surgery for recurrent hepatocellular carcinoma in cirrhotic patients: feasibility, safety, and results. Surg Endosc. 2009;23(8):1807–11.
21. Tsujita E, et al. Outcome of repeat hepatectomy in patients with hepatocellular carcinoma aged 75 years and older. Surgery. 2010;147(5):696–703.
22. Marelli L, et al. Transarterial therapy for hepatocellular carcinoma: which technique is more effective? A systematic review of cohort and randomized studies. Cardiovasc Intervent Radiol. 2007;30(1):6–25.
23. Llovet JM, et al. Arterial embolisation or chemoembolisation versus symptomatic treatment in patients with unresectable hepatocellular carcinoma: a randomised controlled trial. Lancet. 2002;359(9319):1734–9.
24. Lo CM, et al. Randomized controlled trial of transarterial lipiodol chemoembolization for unresectable hepatocellular carcinoma. Hepatology. 2002;35(5):1164–71.
25. Llovet JM, Bruix J. Systematic review of randomized trials for unresectable hepatocellular carcinoma: Chemoembolization improves survival. Hepatology. 2003;37(2):429–42.
26. Shin WY, et al. Prognostic factors affecting survival after recurrence in adult living donor liver transplantation for hepatocellular carcinoma. Liver Transplant. 2010;16(5):678–84.
27. Lammer J, et al. Prospective randomized study of doxorubicin-eluting-bead embolization in the treatment of hepatocellular carcinoma: results of the PRECISION V study. Cardiovasc Intervent Radiol. 2010;33(1):41–52.
28. Malagari K, et al. Safety Profile of Sequential Transcatheter Chemoembolization with DC Bead(): Results of 237 Hepatocellular Carcinoma (HCC) Patients. Cardiovasc Intervent Radiol. 2010;34(4):774–85.
29. Kulik LM, et al. Safety and efficacy of 90Y radiotherapy for hepatocellular carcinoma with and without portal vein thrombosis. Hepatology. 2008;47(1):71–81.
30. Parfitt JR, et al. Recurrent hepatocellular carcinoma after transplantation: use of a pathological score on explanted livers to predict recurrence. Liver Transplant. 2007;13(4):543–51.
31. Cheng AL, et al. Efficacy and safety of sorafenib in patients in the Asia-Pacific region with advanced hepatocellular carcinoma: a phase III randomised, double-blind, placebo-controlled trial. Lancet Oncol. 2009;10(1):25–34.

32. Pinna AD, et al. Treatment of fibrolamellar hepatoma with subtotal hepatectomy or transplantation. Hepatology. 1997;26(4):877–83.
33. Ladabaum U, et al. Cost-effectiveness of screening for recurrent hepatocellular carcinoma after liver transplantation. Clin Transplant. 2011;25(2):283–91.
34. Yamashiki N, et al. Postoperative surveillance with monthly serum tumor markers after living-donor liver transplantation for hepatocellular carcinoma. Hepatol Res. 2010;40(4):278–86.
35. Campsen J, et al. Sirolimus and liver transplantation: clinical implications for hepatocellular carcinoma. Expert Opin Pharmacother. 2007;8(9):1275–82.
36. Toso C, et al. Sirolimus-based immunosuppression is associated with increased survival after liver transplantation for hepatocellular carcinoma. Hepatology. 2010;51(4):1237–43.
37. Bilbao I, et al. Indications and management of everolimus after liver transplantation. Transplant Proc. 2009;41(6):2172–6.
38. Xu J, et al. A randomized controlled trial of Licartin for preventing hepatoma recurrence after liver transplantation. Hepatology. 2007;45(2):269–76.

Chapter 12
The Impact of Treating Chronic Liver Diseases on Hepatocellular Carcinoma Prevention

Narayan Dharel and Daryl T. Lau

Etiology of Hepatocellular Carcinoma

Hepatocellular carcinoma (HCC) is the third most common cause of cancer death worldwide [1]. Chronic hepatitis B virus (HBV) infection is the single most important etiology that accounts for more than 52% of all the HCC cases globally [2]. Chronic hepatitis C virus (HCV) infection accounts for another 20–30%. Together, HBV and HCV cause approximately 80–85% of all HCC cases worldwide [3–6]. Another 10% of HCC can be attributed to alcohol and nonalcoholic steatohepatitis (NASH) [7–9]. Hereditary hemochromatosis (HH), autoimmune liver diseases, alpha-1 antitrypsin deficiency, Wilson's disease, glycogen storage disease, porphyria, tyrosinemia, etc., contribute to the remaining 5–10% (Fig. 12.1a) [10, 11].

In the United States, and in other Western countries and Japan, chronic hepatitis C is the leading cause of HCC. HCV infection accounts for about 50% of all HCC in the United States. Another 15–20% can be attributed to chronic HBV infection [12]. Alcohol abuse (>50–70 g/day for >10 years) used to be an important cause of HCC but is declining to about 10% in the recent years. NASH, in contrast, has an increase in incidence and is recognized as an emerging cause of cryptogenic cirrhosis and HCC [3, 13] (Fig. 12.1b).

All etiologies of chronic liver diseases can lead to progressive liver damage ultimately resulting in advanced fibrosis and cirrhosis. Cirrhosis is the single most important risk factor for HCC and is present in about 80% of patients with HCC, regardless of underlying liver disease [7, 8, 10]. The average annual risk of HCC among cirrhotics is between 1% and 6%. The risk of HCC in cirrhotic patients with HBV infection is about 2.5% per year [14], and the incidences among cirrhotic patients with HCV infection range between 1.3% and 6.7% per year [15].

N. Dharel, MD • D.T. Lau, MD, MSc, MPH (✉)
Liver Center, Division of Gastroenterology, Department of Medicine,
Beth Israel Deaconess Medical Center, Harvard Medical School, Boston, MA, USA
e-mail: dlau@bidmc.harvard.edu

N. Reau and F.F. Poordad (eds.), *Primary Liver Cancer: Surveillance, Diagnosis and Treatment*, Clinical Gastroenterology, DOI 10.1007/978-1-61779-863-4_12,
© Springer Science+Business Media New York 2012

Fig. 12.1 (**a**) Causes of HCC in the world. (**b**) Causes of HCC in the United States

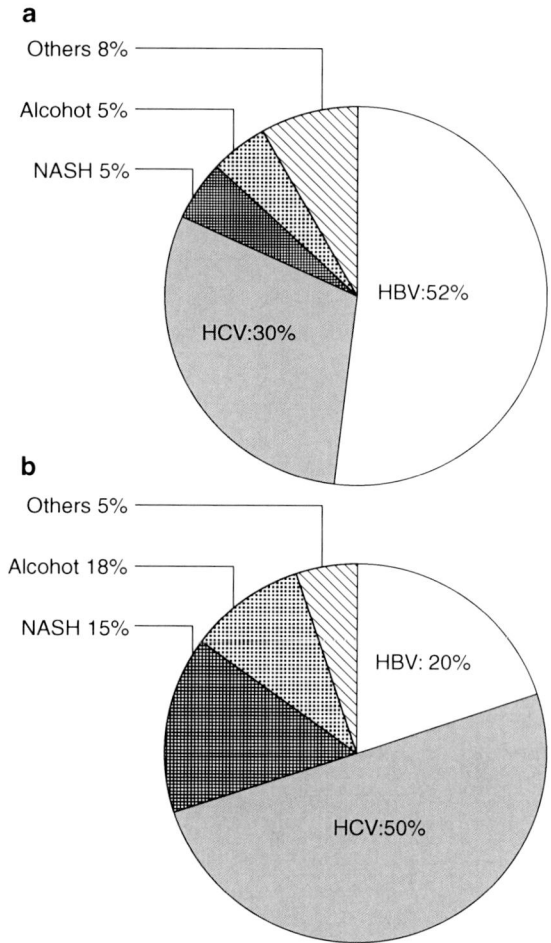

The presence of cirrhosis, however, is not always the prerequisite for HCC development. Almost 40% of HBV patients with HCC do not have documented cirrhosis [16]. Aflatoxin B is a potent hepatocarcinogen. High levels of dietary exposure to this toxin can greatly increase the risk of HCC among patients with chronic hepatitis B [17]. Drinking water contaminated by blue-green algae and microcystins in some regions of China also contributes to the risk of HCC [18]. There are reports that HCC can also occur without established cirrhosis in patients with chronic hepatitis C, NASH, as well as HH [19–22]. Apart from cirrhosis, increasing age, long disease duration, male sex, and presence of cocarcinogens such as tobacco, alcohol, and dietary iron are risk factors for malignant transformation in chronic liver disease [23].

In this chapter, we focus the discussion on the major etiologies of HCC including HBV, HCV, NASH, and hereditary hemochromatosis and whether treating these liver conditions can modify their associated HCC risk.

Prevention of HCC

HCC is associated with over 90% fatality rates and is one of the least curable malignancies [24]. It is a significant concern that the rate of HCC associated mortality has increased by about 40% over the period of 1990–2004, whereas the overall cancer deaths have declined by about 18% during this same period [6]. HCC is unique in the sense that 90% of the cases have discernible underlying etiologies that are either preventable or amenable to treatment. Prevention is the most effective strategy in reducing the morbidity and mortality from HCC. Preventing HCC entails both primary prevention such as HBV vaccination program and secondary prevention by surveillance, early detection, and treatment.

Yang and coworkers conducted a randomized controlled trial on more than 18,000 patients with chronic HBV infection and evaluated the survival benefit of HCC surveillance in China [25]. They reported an overall improved survival with 31% reduction in mortality secondary to HCC among patients who underwent 6-month HCC surveillance with abdominal ultrasound and AFP compared to those who did not undergo surveillance. Regular HCC surveillance among high-risk patients is therefore recommended by the AASLD practice guideline [26].

Prevention of HBV-Related HCC

Primary Prevention with HBV Vaccination

HBV infection is effectively preventable by vaccine. A vaccine that protects against HBV infection was invented in 1982 and is now one of the most commonly used vaccines. The primary focus of preventing HBV-related HCC, therefore, should aim at enhancing effective and timely vaccination of newborn, infants, and other high-risk individuals. Universal HBsAg vaccination with incorporation of HBsAg vaccine in the national vaccination programs has dramatically reduced the prevalence of HBV infection and carriers, with a concomitant decrease in the incidence of HCC in the vaccine-impacted populations [27]. HBsAg carriage among those aged below 20 years has fallen dramatically in countries like Korea, China, Thailand, Singapore, and Taiwan where universal vaccination programs have been in place since 1984 or soon after [27]. In fact, HBV vaccine is also a cancer-preventing vaccine. Taiwan has already demonstrated this with convincing epidemiological data showing that the annual incidence of childhood HCC has decreased from 0.52 to 0.13/100,000 children within 10 years of introducing the universal vaccination program [28]. Similarly, a reduction in the incidence of HCC was reported among Thai [29] and native Alaskan children [30] who received hepatitis B vaccination at birth. In addition to vaccination program, public health measures such as education and awareness, universal precautions, and screening of blood and blood products are also important process in arresting the transmission of HBV.

Secondary Prevention with Therapy

Vaccination is not helpful for the 350 million persons who are already chronically infected with HBV. Treating the HBV infection is another potential promising strategy for HCC prevention. Many prospective cohort studies have demonstrated that persistently high serum HBV DNA levels and presence of hepatitis B e antigen (HBeAg) are associated with an increased risk of cirrhosis and HCC [31–35]. Eradication of HBV would be the preferred strategy but is not usually possible, owing to the integration of viral cccDNA into the host cell DNA. Therapies are able to suppress HBV DNA replication and should theoretically reduce the risk of HCC. Interferon alpha (IFN-α) and five nucleoside and nucleotide inhibitors are currently approved by the Food and Drug Administration (FDA) for the treatment of chronic hepatitis B [36].

Interferon Alpha (IFN-α)

A randomized study in Taiwan by Lin et al. [37] provided evidence of HCC reduction with interferon therapy. The study was actually designed to examine long-term outcomes of IFN-treated patients with HBeAg-positive chronic hepatitis B after a cumulative and median follow-up period of 15 years and 6.8 years, respectively. The study showed significant benefit of IFN compared to no treatment in terms of HBeAg seroconversion (75% vs. 52%, $P=0.031$), HBsAg seroclearance (3.0% vs. 0.4%, $P=0.03$), cirrhosis (18% vs. 34%, $P=0.041$), and HCC development (2.7% vs. 13%, $P=0.011$). The cumulative incidence of HCC was significantly higher in the control group (20%) compared to the IFN-treated groups (<7%), with the benefits occurring after 72 months of post-treatment follow-up. This study also showed that IFN-treated patients who did not undergo HBeAg seroconversion had increased risk of HCC. One of the limitations of the study was the lack of adequately matched controls for it was originally designed to examine treatment outcomes of chronic hepatitis B.

Another small cohort study of Japanese patients with HBV-related cirrhosis showed that significantly fewer HCC development occurred in patients who achieved HBV DNA clearance with IFN treatment compared to those who failed to clear HBV DNA (6% vs. 34%, $P=0.026$) [38].

The effect of IFN in preventing HBV-related HCC has been evaluated in two meta-analyses. The first meta-analysis of 12 studies ($n=2,742$) compared IFN treatment with untreated controls. It included one randomized controlled trial, one case-control study, and ten cohort studies in the analysis (Table 12.1). Overall, the risk of HCC was reduced by 34% (relative risk 0.66, 95% CI 0.48–0.89) with IFN treatment [39]. Subgroup analyses showed that this benefit was significant in patients with early cirrhosis, but not among those without cirrhosis and was independent of virological response or the HBeAg status at baseline. In another more recent meta-analysis (11 studies; $n=2,082$), conventional IFN reduced the incidence of HCC in

Table 12.1 IFN versus placebo or no treatment in reducing HCC among patients with chronic hepatitis B

First author, year	Study type	N	Comment	HCC among treated n/N	HCC among untreated n/N	Odds ratio (95% CI)	Years of follow-up
Fattovich (1997) [62]	NRP	90	Cohort, 90 white patients	4/40	6/50	0.83 (0.25–2.75)	7.2
Benvegnu (1998) [65]	NRR	37	Retrospective cohort Child A cirrhosis	1/13	7/24	0.26 (0.04–1.92)	6.0
Brunetto (1998)	NRR	146	Retrospective cohort, Italy and Argentina	8/49	18/97	0.88 (0.41–1.88)	5.8
Ikeda (1998)	NRP	313	Prospective cohort, Japanese patients	10/94	51/219	0.46 (0.24–0.86)	7.0
Krogsgaard (1998)	NRR	308	Retrospective analysis of subgroups from three RCTs (EUROHEP)	2/210	1/98	0.93 (0.09–10.17)	4.7
DiMarco (1999)		302	Prospective cohort	2/109	6/193	0.59 (0.12–2.87)	7.8
Mazzella (1999)	RCT	61	RCT	1/33	2/31	0.47 (0.04–4.92)	7.2
Papatheodoridis (2001) [71]	NRP	404	Prospective cohort, Greece	17/209	15/195	1/06 (0.54–2.06)	6.0
Tangkijvanich (2001)	NRR	139	Retrospective cohort, Thai patients	2/67	9/72	0.24 (0.05–1.07)	5.0
Yuen (2011)	NRP	411	Prospective cohort	6/208	0/203	12.69 (0.72–223.79)	8.9
Truong (2005)	NRP	62	Prospective cohort	1/27	0/35	3.86 (0.16–91.12)	6.5
Lin (2007)	Case–control	466	Case–control, Taiwan	5/233	16/233	0.31 (0.12–0.84)	6.5
Total		2,742		59/1,292	131/1,450	0.66 (0.28–0.89)	

Adapted from Sung JJ et al., Aliment Pharmacol Ther 2008;28(9):1067–77
RCT randomized controlled trial, *NRR* nonrandomized retrospective, *NRP* nonrandomized prospective

patients with chronic hepatitis B by 41% compared with no treatment (95% CI 0.43–0.81) during the follow-up period of 4–7 years. The benefit of HCC risk reduction by IFN treatment was mainly among patients with sustained virological or biochemical response.

Even though these meta-analyses consistently demonstrate that IFN therapy is associated with reduced rates of HCC, most of the data were derived from retrospective or prospective cohort studies without matched controlled subjects. None of the studies evaluated the long-acting pegylated IFNs. The patient characteristics and clinical features that are correlated with reduced HCC rate from IFN treatment need to be better defined and evaluated.

Nucleos(t)ide Analogues

The oral antivirals are more potent than interferon in suppressing HBV replication [40]. Lamivudine is the first approved oral agent for chronic hepatitis B. Its long-term use is limited by high cumulative rate of drug-associated resistance [40, 41]. To date, most of the studies evaluating the role of antivirals in reducing disease progression and complications were generated from lamivudine therapy. Newer agents with better efficacy and resistance profile have been introduced into the practice more recently. It is yet to be determined if these newer agents will have protection against HCC development.

The key study that demonstrated efficacy of nucleoside analogues in preventing disease progression and perhaps reducing HCC risk was the Cirrhosis and Lamivudine Monotherapy (CALM) study [42]. This randomized controlled trial enrolled patients with biopsy-proven advanced fibrosis and cirrhosis with HBV DNA >140,000 IU/ml. The results conclusively showed that lamivudine was able to decrease the rates of hepatic decompensation in patients with advanced hepatic fibrosis. The benefit was greatest among those who did not develop lamivudine-associated resistance. This trial was terminated prematurely with median treatment duration of 32 months because of the significant benefit of lamivudine. The HCC rate was also lower in the lamivudine-treated patients; however, the difference in cancer rate was only approaching statistically significance. There have been debates that lamivudine would most likely show a reduction of HCC if the trial was allowed to continue for 5 years. Unfortunately, randomized controlled studies comparing antivirals to placebo in patients with advanced hepatitis B disease would no longer be considered ethical.

In a case-control study, Yuen et al. [43] compared 142 HBeAg-positive lamivudine-treated patients to 124 matched controls for a mean of 89 months and found that the controls developed HCC and/or cirrhosis at a significantly higher rate than lamivudine-treated patients ($P=0.03$). Similar to the CALM study, the presence of drug-associated resistance reduced the treatment benefits. Matsumoto et al. [44], in a retrospective study, compared 377 lamivudine-treated Japanese patients with controls matched for age of liver biopsy, gender, family history of HCC, stage of fibrosis, albumin levels, and platelet count. They found a significant reduction in

Table 12.2 Nucleos(t)ide analogues (NA) in the prevention of HCC among HBV patients

First author, year	Study type	N	HCC among treated n/N (%)	HCC among untreated n/N (%)	Odds ratio (95% CI)	Years of follow-up
Liaw (2004) [42]	RCT	651	17/436 (3.9)	16/215 (7.4)	0.49 (0.25–0.99)	2.7
Matsumoto (2005) [44]	NRR	754	4/377 (1.7)	50/377 (13.3)	0.02 (0.00–0.35)	2.7
Eun (2006)	RCT	222	5/111 (4.5)	36/111 (32.4)	0.14 (0.06–0.34)	4.4
Papatheodoridis (2005)	NRP	396	5/201 (2.49)	15/195 (7.69)	0.48 (0.16–1.40)	7.0
Yuen (2007) [43]	NRP	266	1/142 (0.7)	3/124 (2.41)	0.38 (0.28–0.97)	8.2
Total		2,289	37/1,267 (2.9)	120/1,022 (11.7)	0.66 (0.28–0.89)	

Adapted from Sung JJ et al., Aliment Pharmacol Ther 2008;28(9):1067–77

RCT randomized controlled trial, *NRR* nonrandomized retrospective, *NRP* nonrandomized prospective

HCC rate among the treatment group (0.4%/patient per year) compared to the controls (2.5%/ patient per year) ($P<0.001$). In another retrospective study, Di Marco et al. [45] confirmed that the loss of lamivudine response secondary to drug resistance was associated with higher risk of development of HCC, whereas patients who maintained a response to lamivudine were much less likely to develop progressive disease including HCC.

A meta-analysis of the impact of nucleoside analogues (mainly lamivudine) on HCC development included two randomized controlled trials, two cohort studies, and one case-control study (Table 12.2). The analysis showed an impressive 78% (RR 0.22, 95% CI 0.10–0.50) reduction in risk of HCC after treatment with nucleoside analogues compared to controls despite the heterogeneous study designs of the individual report [39]. A more recent systematic review on nucleos(t)ide-treated chronic HBV patients for at least 24 months included a total of 3,881 treated and 534 untreated patients in the analysis [46]. De novo HCC was diagnosed in 2.8% and 6.4% of treated and untreated patients, respectively, during a 46 (32–108)-month study period ($P=0.003$). Among the treated patients, cirrhosis, HBeAg negative at baseline, and failure to remain in virological remission were associated with an increased risk of HCC. In summary, medium-term continuous antiviral therapy significantly lowers but does not eliminate the risk of HCC.

Patients who have developed HCC and received treatment for HCC are at a particularly high risk for HCC recurrence. Antiviral therapies have been shown to reduce HCC recurrence in such patients as well. In a cohort study that included 157 patients treated for HBV-related HCC, 89 of them had undetectable serum HBV DNA and 68 were viremic; the 5-year cumulative HCC recurrence rate was significantly higher in the viremic group compared to the nonviremic group (73% vs. 55%; $P=0.043$) [47]. A smaller study on 72 patients undergoing HCC resection found that those with HBV DNA level >2,000 IU/ml had a significantly higher risk of HCC recurrence after tumor resection. The presence of viremia is the most significant correctable risk factor for HCC recurrence (odds ratio 22.3, 95% CI 3.3–151, $P = 0.001$) [48].

Despite the limitations of these studies, there is good evidence that prolonged suppression of HBV replication with nucleoside or nucleotide analogues can reduce the risk of HCC in patients with chronic hepatitis B. HCC risk also appears to decrease with limiting course of IFN therapy which may be attributable to its anti-proliferation property. The anticancer effect of nucleos(t)ide analogues and IFN appears to be most apparent among patients with significant hepatic fibrosis. Further prospective studies are necessary to determine the efficacy of prolonged therapy in reducing HCC risk among hepatitis B patients with less advanced liver disease using more potent antiviral therapy and pegylated interferon.

Prevention of HCV-Related HCC

Primary Prevention

Despite tremendous research, a reliable vaccine to prevent HCV infection is currently unavailable due to the high mutation rate of the HCV RNA. The key to the primary prevention is to prevent HCV transmission. Since HCV is predominantly a blood-borne pathogen [49], primary prevention is possible by adopting measures to avoid blood or blood product contaminations. Public health measures, such as education and awareness, universal precautions, screening of blood and blood products, use of disposable needles and supplies, and sterilization of all surgical instruments, have shown promising results in reducing the new HCV infections in many developed countries including the United States and should therefore be promoted [50]. Since the implementation of HCV screening programs for donated blood in 1992 in developed countries, the risk of HCV transmission from a blood transfusion is now less than 0.03% per unit transfused [51]. Other potential transmission routes of HCV include tattooing, body piercing, acupuncture, and cocaine snorting [49] which require specific preventive strategies. Efforts to prevent transmission should focus on education and identifying persons at increased risk of hepatitis C and providing them with counseling and testing. These preventive measures are especially important in developing and underdeveloped countries where resources for antiviral treatments are not readily available.

Secondary Prevention with Therapy

In chronic hepatitis C, the development of HCC is closely related to the disease duration and severity [52]. Eradication of HCV by interferon-based therapy has been shown to decrease the necroinflammatory process in the liver, reverse the hepatic fibrosis, delay the progression to cirrhosis, and reduce the risk of HCC [53–55]. In the absence of an effective vaccine for primary prevention, eradication of the virus by antiviral treatment is the most effective strategy to prevent or reduce risk of HCC in patients with chronic HCV infection.

There are numerous reports that demonstrate a reduction of HCC among patients with chronic hepatitis C who achieve sustained virological response (SVR) following interferon-based treatment. Most of these studies focused on patients with cirrhosis; however, reduction in HCC risk is significant even among patients with SVR without underlying cirrhosis [55–57]. One of the early evidence of the effects of therapy on HCC rate came from a small randomized controlled trial by Nishiguchi et al. [58] that included patients with compensated cirrhosis. In that study, 45 patients in each group were assigned to receive either IFN therapy or no treatment. HCC developed in 2 of 45 patients treated with IFN in 4.4 years of observation and 17 of 45 patients in the control arm in 5.5 years. The risk ratio of HCC development between treatment and no treatment was 0.067 (95% CI 0.009–0.530), indicating that the HCC rate was reduced by more than 90% with therapy. Subsequent long-term follow-up data on the same population with extended observation period to over 8 years showed that the risk ratio of HCC between the two groups was 0.256 (95% CI 0.125–0.522), a 75% risk reduction among the treatment group, suggesting a long-term protective effect [59]. The benefit was most evident among those who achieved SVR.

Similar encouraging outcomes have been replicated in several subsequent studies among patients with or without advanced fibrosis. Most of these early observations were from Japan and Europe based on retrospective or cohort study designs on patients who received a standard course of IFN with or without ribavirin for 6–12 months [58, 60–69] (Table 12.3). In a large prospective cohort study of 2,890 patients, Yoshida et al. [69] showed that HCC developed in 89/2,400 (3.7%) IFN-treated patients and 59/490 (12%) untreated patients during a mean follow-up period of 4.3 years. In multivariate analysis, IFN therapy was identified as an independent predictor of HCC-free survival. The adjusted risk ratio of HCC development for IFN treatment versus no treatment was 0.52 (95% CI 0.36–0.74), a 50% risk reduction with IFN therapy.

The protective effect of IFN has been further substantiated in at least three independent meta-analyses [70–72]. Singal et al. [70] performed a systematic review and meta-analysis of 20 studies with over 4,700 HCV cirrhotic patients treated with interferon alone or with ribavirin and compared the effect of treatment in HCC risk reduction. The overall HCC risk reduction was 53% (RR 0.43; 95% CI 0.33–0.56). Subgroup analysis of 14 studies that reported SVR rates demonstrated a 65% risk reduction among treated patients with SVR compared to nonresponders (NR) (risk ratio (RR) = 0.35; 95% CI 0.26–0.46). However, no benefit on HCC risk reduction was observed among nonresponders who continued maintenance IFN monotherapy (RR 0.58; 95% CI 0.33–1.03).

Morgan et al. [73] performed a prospective, long-term follow-up study of the HALT-C patients and evaluated the effect of achieving SVR with pegylated interferon and ribavirin treatment on death from any cause or liver transplantation and on liver-related morbidity and mortality including HCC. They found that patients who achieved SVR after pegylated interferon and ribavirin treatment had a significantly reduced risk of death from any cause/liver transplantation, and of liver-related morbidity and mortality, when compared with patients in the nonresponder (NR) group.

Table 12.3 IFN treatment in reducing HCC among patients with chronic hepatitis C

First author, year	Study type	N	IFN, dose, duration	HCC among treated n/N (%)	HCC among untreated n/N (%)	Odds ratio (95% CI)
Nishiguchi (1995) [58]	RP	90	6 MIU t.i.w. for 12–24 weeks	2/45 (4.4)	17/45 (37.8)	7.24 (2.64–19.81)
Mazella (1996) [60]	NRP	285	Mean dose, 3 MIU t.i.w for 6 (n=35) or 12 (n=158) months	5/193 (2.6)	9/92 (9.8)	4.64 (1.47–14.60)
Bruno (1997) [61]	NRP	163	6 MIU t.i.w. for 6 months	6/82 (7.3)	16/81 (19.7)	2.88 (1.18–7.06)
Fattovich (1997) [62]	NRR	129	Total dose 200 MIU for 166 patients	7/193 (3.6)	16/136 (11.8)	3.48 (1.96–8.22)
IHCSG, 1998	NRR	491	Median weekly dose, 9 MIU for median of 7 months	21/232 (9.0)	48/259 (11.8)	2.19 (1.32–3.64)
Imai 1998 [64]	NRR	52	Median total dose, 480 MIU in 6 months	8/32 (25.0)	7/20 (35.0)	1.61 (0.48–5.47)
Benvegnu (1998) [65]	NRR	152	3–6 MIU t.i.w. for 6–12 months	4/75 (5.3)	20/77 (26.0)	4.67 (1.96–11.15)
Serfaty (1998) [66]	NRP	103	3 MIU t.i.w. for a mean of 11 months	2/59 (3.3)	9/44 (20.4)	5.88 (1.67–20.69)
Valla (1999) [67]	NRR	81	3 MIU t.i.w. for 12 months	5/42 (11.9)	9/39 (23.1)	2.16 (0.69–6.80)
Yoshida (1999) [69]	NRR	337	Median total dose, 480 MIU in a median of 160 days	33/230 (14.3)	32/107 (29.9)	2.71 (1.52–4.84)
Okanoue (1999) [68]	NRR	95	6 MIU daily for 2 weeks, t.i.w. for 22–24 weeks	7/40 (17.5)	205/955 (21.5)	2.86 (1.19–6.89)
Total		2,178		100/1,223 (8.2)	205/955 (21.5)	3.02 (2.35–3.89)

Adapted from Papatheodoridis G.V., Aliment Pharmacol Ther 2001;15(5):689–98
RP randomized prospective, *NRR* nonrandomized retrospective, *NRP* nonrandomized prospective

Importantly, achieving SVR significantly reduced the risk of developing each component of liver-related morbidity and mortality (i.e., hepatic decompensation, HCC, and liver-related death or liver transplantation) when compared with NR patients. The incidence of HCC was much lower among those with SVR (1.4%; 2/140) compared to those with virological breakthrough/relapse (6.5%; 5/77) or nonresponders (9.1%; 28/309). While HCC incidence was significantly lower among treated patients with SVR, it did occur in two with SVR at least 4 years after achieving SVR. Both patients had evidence of cirrhosis in the resected liver. This underscores that HCC risk still exists even after achieving SVR, especially in patients with advanced fibrosis and cirrhosis. Patients with advanced hepatic fibrosis should have regular HCC surveillance even after achieving SVR.

While the benefits in preventing disease progression and reducing HCC risk were substantial for those with SVR after therapy, the benefits for those failed to achieve SVR, but had biochemical response with normalization of serum alanine aminotransferase (ALT), are not clear. In the HALT-C study [73], the risks of HCC, hepatic decompensation, and liver-related death or liver transplantation were lower among those with virological breakthrough/relapse compared to those without significant virological response (NR), but these differences did not reach statistical significance. Two large retrospective studies reported no difference in the incidence of HCC among nonresponders (NR) and untreated controls [74, 75], confirming the importance in achieving SVR. On the other hand, a recent meta-analysis of three randomized controlled trials and six cohort studies included over 3,200 patients. Miyake et al. [72] found that standard therapy with IFN reduced incidence of HCC even among treatment nonresponders.

Accordingly, there has been substantial interest in the potential role of prolonged maintenance IFN monotherapy in reducing the HCC risk among treatment nonresponders. The effects of long-term low-dose maintenance IFN among nonresponders were evaluated in at least three large, multicenter, randomized controlled trials, namely, HALT-C, COPILOT, and EPIC3 [76–78], with at least 3–4 years of follow-up. In the HALT-C trial [76], over 1,000 patients were randomized for a low-dose pegylated interferon (Peg-IFN) or no treatment and followed for 3.5 years. While the levels of ALT, HCV RNA, and histological grading were improved, there was no significant difference in the clinical events like death, HCC, or decompensate disease. The COPILOT study [77] prospectively compared low-dose Peg-IFN with colchicines among 555 HCV patients with advanced fibrosis who have failed prior antiviral therapy. It demonstrated that maintenance therapy with Peg-IFN was associated with improved disease-free survival only in a subset of patients with portal hypertension. Similarly, in the EPIC3 study [78] where prior nonresponders were randomized to low-dose maintenance Peg-IFN or no treatment, and followed for up to 5 years, there was no significant difference in time to first clinical event of hepatic complication in both study arms. In subgroup analysis, however, the time to first clinical event was significantly delayed by Peg-IFN maintenance therapy among patients with preexisting portal hypertension.

All of these trials failed to show clear benefit of maintenance IFN therapy in terms of HCC risk reduction. It is debatable whether the chemopreventive effect of

IFN would be apparent with longer follow-up observations. In fact, patients in the HALT-C study had extended observation for a median of 6.1 years, some up to a maximum 8.7 years [79]. Overall, there was no significant benefit of the prolonged, low-dose maintenance IFN therapy in reducing HCC incidence for those who failed to achieve SVR with the initial Peg-IFN and ribavirin therapy. It is only in a subgroup analysis that a lower HCC rate was observed among those with cirrhosis at baseline who subsequently received the maintenance IFN therapy. These data suggest that IFN maintenance therapy may be beneficial to a subset of patients who have cirrhosis and have failed to achieve SVR. Since significant adverse effects can be associated with IFN therapy, the clinical application of long-term IFN therapy needs to be individualized.

Does IFN treatment have a role in preventing HCC recurrence and improving survival after curative resection or tumor ablation? In a recent systematic review and meta-analysis on ten studies with a total of 645,301 patients who received IFN after HCC resection or ablation, Singal et al. [80] found that IFN significantly reduced HCC recurrence (OR 0.26; 95% CI 0.15–0.45; $P < 0.00001$). Again, the benefit of preventing HCC recurrence was most evident for those with SVR compared to nonresponders (OR 0.19; 95% CI 0.06–0.60; $P = 0.005$).

In summary, there is sufficient evidence that interferon treatment can reduce the rate of HCC in patients with chronic hepatitis C, that is, particularly significant for those who achieved SVR after a definitive course of therapy. Moreover, these observations underscore the importance of eradicating the HCV prior to the development of advanced hepatic fibrosis in preventing HCC occurrence. The combination therapy with the new direct-acting antivirals (DAAs) plus Peg-IFN and ribavirin is anticipated to increase the SVR rates even among the most difficult to treat patient populations. There were promising results from phase III clinical trials that the addition of the protease inhibitor (telaprevir or boceprevir) to Peg-IFN and ribavirin was associated with a SVR rate greater than 70% among HCV genotype-1 patients [81, 82]. With the improved SVR rates, it is conceivable that these new therapeutic regimens would be more effective in reducing the HCC risk in chronic hepatitis C.

Prevention of HCC Related to Hereditary Hemochromatosis (HH)

Early detection and treatment is the key to prevent the development of HCC in this genetic disorder. Every effort should be made to diagnose and start treatment with therapeutic phlebotomy before development of cirrhosis. Patients who achieve adequate iron depletion before the onset of cirrhosis or diabetes have been found to have survival comparable with that of the general population [83, 84]. On the other hand, once cirrhosis is established, the risk of HCC remains despite successful reduction of iron load by phlebotomy [84]. Studies have shown that patients with normal serum aminotransferases, age <40 years, serum ferritin levels < 1,000 µg/l, and absence of splenomegaly are unlikely to have cirrhosis [85, 86] and should undergo aggressive therapeutic phlebotomy to reduce the excessive iron. Those with ferritin >1,000 µg/l or elevated serum aminotransferases should undergo a liver biopsy to rule out significant hepatic fibrosis. If cirrhosis is established, regular

HCC surveillance should be performed to detect early liver tumor. Venesection remains the standard therapy for HH, and phlebotomy should be performed when there is evidence of iron accumulation, such as sustained elevation of serum ferritin and increased transferrin iron saturation. It is important to identify individuals with hemochromatosis gene mutations prior to excessive iron deposition resulting in end organ damage. Generally, one unit of bloodletting every week until the serum ferritin level is less than 50 mcg/l followed by periodic maintenance phlebotomy is optimal for iron depletion and to prevent further iron accumulation. In the initial induction phase, serum ferritin should be monitored at least once or twice a month [87]. Desferrioxamine, an iron-chelating agent, can also be used in patients who are intolerant of venesection due to hypotension, anemia, or cardiac failure [88].

Since HH is a familial disorder, screening of the first-degree relatives should be performed once a proband has been identified. However, the clinical presentations of HH can be variable due to the heterogeneous manifestations of the same genotype [89]. Fasting serum transferrin saturation and ferritin levels are recommended as screening tests for first-degree relatives [89]. Genetic testing for hemochromatosis gene mutations should be reserved for those with elevated serum transferrin saturation. For those confirmed to have HH with elevated serum transferrin saturation, therapeutic phlebotomy should be initiated using the same guidelines as for the proband [86, 90]. In addition, nutritional advice should focus on a balanced diet with low alcohol intake and avoid excessive vitamin C supplementation. Avoidance of iron and mineral supplements and regular consumption of uncooked sea foods are also recommended [84].

HCC risk also increases in other forms of excessive iron conditions such as dietary iron overload among Africans and beta thalassemia with iron overload from repeated blood transfusions. Iron chelators such as desferrioxamine, deferiprone, and deferasirox are the treatment of choice for beta thalassemia or other iron-loading anemias [91]. The effects of these agents on HCC prevention have not yet been documented.

Prevention of HCC Related to Nonalcoholic Fatty Liver Disease

Nonalcoholic fatty liver disease (NAFLD) is a spectrum of disease that ranges from benign steatosis to nonalcoholic steatohepatitis (NASH) [92]. With the obesity epidemic, NAFLD has become the most common cause of chronic liver disease in the United States and other developed countries. The estimated relative risk for HCC in NAFLD is about 18–27 [93–95], but well-designed prospective study is necessary to confirm the NAFLD-related HCC rate.

Complications of NASH, including HCC, are expected to increase with the continuing epidemics of metabolic syndrome. HCC surveillance for patients with NASH-related cirrhosis is important for early diagnosis. Public health preventive measures should focus on mitigation of modifiable risk factors such as obesity, diabetes mellitus, hyperlipidemia, and concomitant alcohol consumption. Lifestyle modifications aimed at reducing body weight, optimizing diabetic control, and improving dyslipidemia are the initial approach in patients with NAFLD. Pharmacologic approach includes insulin-sensitizing agents (metformin, rosiglitazone, pioglitazone), antioxidants, lipid-lowering agents like statins, and cytoprotective agents. However, none of these agents have been shown to be effective in preventing NASH-related disease progression or HCC rate in large-scale randomized controlled studies [96]. Therapeutic surgical options such as bariatric surgery should be considered among patient with morbid obesity who fails to respond the lifestyle modification approaches. There are, however, no controlled studies to demonstrate the impact of such measures in preventing or reducing HCC currently.

Summary

Annually, there is an estimated 750,000 new cases of HCC globally which results in approximately 695,000 deaths [1]. At least 80% of the HCC worldwide are attributed to chronic hepatitis B and C infection. Effective prevention of HBV and HCV infection or their progression from acute to chronic disease progression could therefore prevent as many as 450,000 deaths from HCC each year [97]. The most effective strategy to prevent HBV-related HCC is through HBV vaccination. A vaccine, however, is not available for HCV. Primary prevention of HCV infection and HCV-related HCC depends on public health measures such as universal precaution, screening of blood and blood products, and education. For those who are currently infected with HBV or HCV, antiviral therapy is the only option for secondary HCC prevention. Despite technical, ethical, and logistic limitations, most of the published studies have consistently shown that antiviral treatment leading to persistent viral suppression is correlated to a significant reduction in HCC rates in chronic hepatitis B and C. It is important to note, however, such benefit is most evident among patients who are sustained responders to the therapy and who received treatment in the earlier stages of the disease prior to development of cirrhosis. Moreover, the risk is not entirely eliminated, and HCC can still occur among responders despite therapy. Similarly for other chronic liver diseases such as hereditary hemochromatosis, autoimmune liver diseases, and nonalcoholic fatty liver disease, early diagnosis and management prior to advanced disease progression are the keys to reduce the risk of HCC.

These facts underscore the importance of advocating primary prevention of the underlying liver diseases, early diagnosis, and interventions. For those with advanced hepatic fibrosis, regular HCC surveillance is necessary even after successful therapy. Research efforts should focus on developing effective HCV vaccines, improved diagnostic tests for genetic and metabolic liver diseases, as well as sensitive and specific HCC screening modalities for at-risk patient populations.

References

1. Ferlay J, Shin HR, Bray F, Forman D, Mathers C, Parkin DM. Estimates of worldwide burden of cancer in 2008: GLOBOCAN 2008. Int J Cancer. 2010;127(12):2893–917.
2. El-Serag HB. Hepatocellular carcinoma: recent trends in the United States. Gastroenterology. 2004;127(5 Suppl 1):S27–34.

3. Yang JD, Roberts LR. Hepatocellular carcinoma: A global view. Nat Rev Gastroenterol Hepatol. 2010;7(8):448–58.
4. Sherman M. Epidemiology of hepatocellular carcinoma. Oncology. 2010;78 Suppl 1:7–10.
5. Nordenstedt H, White DL, El-Serag HB. The changing pattern of epidemiology in hepatocellular carcinoma. Dig Liver Dis. 2010;42 Suppl 3:S206–214.
6. Di Bisceglie AM. Hepatitis B and hepatocellular carcinoma. Hepatology. 2009;49(5 Suppl):S56–60.
7. Sherman M. Hepatocellular carcinoma: New and emerging risks. Dig Liver Dis. 2010;42 Suppl 3:S215–222.
8. El-Serag HB. Epidemiology of hepatocellular carcinoma in USA. Hepatol Res. 2007;37 Suppl 2:S88–94.
9. Starley BQ, Calcagno CJ, Harrison SA. Nonalcoholic fatty liver disease and hepatocellular carcinoma: a weighty connection. Hepatology. 2010;51(5):1820–32.
10. Fattovich G, Stroffolini T, Zagni I, Donato F. Hepatocellular carcinoma in cirrhosis: incidence and risk factors. Gastroenterology. 2004;127(5 Suppl 1):S35–50.
11. Dragani TA. Risk of HCC: genetic heterogeneity and complex genetics. J Hepatol. 2010;52(2):252–7.
12. Di Bisceglie AM, Lyra AC, Schwartz M, et al. Hepatitis C-related hepatocellular carcinoma in the United States: influence of ethnic status. Am J Gastroenterol. 2003;98(9):2060–3.
13. Marrero JA, Fontana RJ, Su GL, Conjeevaram HS, Emick DM, Lok AS. NAFLD may be a common underlying liver disease in patients with hepatocellular carcinoma in the United States. Hepatology. 2002;36(6):1349–54.
14. Fattovich G, Bortolotti F, Donato F. Natural history of chronic hepatitis B: special emphasis on disease progression and prognostic factors. J Hepatol. 2008;48(2):335–52.
15. Di Bisceglie AM. Hepatitis C and hepatocellular carcinoma. Hepatology. 1997;26(3 Suppl 1):34S–8S.
16. McMahon BJ. Natural history of chronic hepatitis B. Clin Liver Dis. 2010;14(3):381–96.
17. Wu HC, Wang Q, Yang HI, et al. Aflatoxin B1 exposure, hepatitis B virus infection, and hepatocellular carcinoma in Taiwan. Cancer Epidemiol Biomarkers Prev. 2009;18(3):846–53.
18. Colombo M, Donato MF. Prevention of hepatocellular carcinoma. Semin Liver Dis. 2005;25(2):155–61.
19. Chagas AL, Kikuchi LO, Oliveira CP, et al. Does hepatocellular carcinoma in non-alcoholic steatohepatitis exist in cirrhotic and non-cirrhotic patients? Br J Med Biol Res. 2009;42(10):958–62.
20. Takuma Y, Nouso K. Nonalcoholic steatohepatitis-associated hepatocellular carcinoma: our case series and literature review. World J Gastroenterol. 2010;16(12):1436–41.
21. Madhoun MF, Fazili J, Bright BC, Bader T, Roberts DN, Bronze MS. Hepatitis C prevalence in patients with hepatocellular carcinoma without cirrhosis. Am J Med Sci. 2010;339(2):169–73.
22. Nzeako UC, Goodman ZD, Ishak KG. Hepatocellular carcinoma in cirrhotic and noncirrhotic livers. A clinico-histopathologic study of 804 North American patients. Am J Clin Pathol. 1996;105(1):65–75.
23. Kew MC. Prevention of hepatocellular carcinoma. Ann Hepatol. 2005;9(2):120–32.
24. El-Serag HB. Hepatocellular carcinoma: an epidemiologic view. J Clin Gastroenterol. 2002;35(5 Suppl 2):S72–78.
25. Zhang BH, Yang BH, Tang ZY. Randomized controlled trial of screening for hepatocellular carcinoma. J Cancer Res Clin Oncol. 2004;130(7):417–22.
26. Bruix J, Sherman M. Management of hepatocellular carcinoma: an update. Hepatology. 2011;53(3):1020–2.
27. Lok AS. Prevention of hepatitis B virus-related hepatocellular carcinoma. Gastroenterology. 2004;127(5 Suppl 1):S303–309.
28. Chang MH, You SL, Chen CJ, et al. Decreased incidence of hepatocellular carcinoma in hepatitis B vaccines: a 20-year follow-up study. J Natl Cancer Inst. 2009;101(19):1348–55.
29. Wichajarn K, Kosalaraksa P, Wiangnon S. Incidence of hepatocellular carcinoma in children in Khon Kaen before and after national hepatitis B vaccine program. Asian Pac J Cancer Prev. 2008;9(3):507–9.

30. Lanier AP, Holck P, Ehrsam Day G, Key C. Childhood cancer among Alaska Natives. Pediatrics. 2003;112(5):e396.
31. Yang HI, Lu SN, Liaw YF, et al. Hepatitis B e antigen and the risk of hepatocellular carcinoma. N Engl J Med. 2002;347(3):168–74.
32. Yu MW, Yeh SH, Chen PJ, et al. Hepatitis B virus genotype and DNA level and hepatocellular carcinoma: a prospective study in men. J Natl Cancer Inst. 2005;97(4):265–72.
33. Chen CJ, Yang HI, Su J, et al. Risk of hepatocellular carcinoma across a biological gradient of serum hepatitis B virus DNA level. J Am Med Assoc. 2006;295(1):65–73.
34. Iloeje UH, Yang HI, Su J, Jen CL, You SL, Chen CJ. Predicting cirrhosis risk based on the level of circulating hepatitis B viral load. Gastroenterology. 2006;130(3):678–86.
35. Chen CJ, Iloeje UH, Yang HI. Long-term outcomes in hepatitis B: the REVEAL-HBV study. Clin Liver Dis. 2007;11(4):797–816. viii.
36. Lau DT, Bleibel W. Current status of antiviral therapy for hepatitis B. Ther Adv Gastroenterol. 2008;1(1):61–75.
37. Lin SM, Sheen IS, Chien RN, Chu CM, Liaw YF. Long-term beneficial effect of interferon therapy in patients with chronic hepatitis B virus infection. Hepatology. 1999;29(3):971–5.
38. Ikeda K, Kobayashi M, Saitoh S, et al. Significance of hepatitis B virus DNA clearance and early prediction of hepatocellular carcinogenesis in patients with cirrhosis undergoing interferon therapy: long-term follow up of a pilot study. J Gastroenterol Hepatol. 2005;20(1):95–102.
39. Sung JJ, Tsoi KK, Wong VW, Li KC, Chan HL. Meta-analysis: Treatment of hepatitis B infection reduces risk of hepatocellular carcinoma. Aliment Pharmacol Ther. 2008;28(9):1067–77.
40. Lok AS, McMahon BJ. Chronic hepatitis B: update 2009. Hepatology. 2009;50(3):661–2.
41. Liaw YF. Impact of YMDD mutations during lamivudine therapy in patients with chronic hepatitis B. Antivir Chem Chemother. 2001;12 Suppl 1:67–71.
42. Liaw YF, Sung JJ, Chow WC, et al. Lamivudine for patients with chronic hepatitis B and advanced liver disease. N Engl J Med. 2004;351(15):1521–31.
43. Yuen MF, Seto WK, Chow DH, et al. Long-term lamivudine therapy reduces the risk of long-term complications of chronic hepatitis B infection even in patients without advanced disease. Antivir Ther. 2007;12(8):1295–303.
44. Matsumoto A, Tanaka E, Rokuhara A, et al. Efficacy of lamivudine for preventing hepatocellular carcinoma in chronic hepatitis B: A multicenter retrospective study of 2795 patients. Hepatol Res. 2005;32(3):173–84.
45. Di Marco V, Marzano A, Lampertico P, et al. Clinical outcome of HBeAg-negative chronic hepatitis B in relation to virological response to lamivudine. Hepatology. 2004;40(4):883–91.
46. Papatheodoridis GV, Lampertico P, Manolakopoulos S, Lok A. Incidence of hepatocellular carcinoma in chronic hepatitis B patients receiving nucleos(t)ide therapy: a systematic review. J Hepatol. 2010;53(2):348–56.
47. Kim BK, Park JY, Kim do Y, et al. Persistent hepatitis B viral replication affects recurrence of hepatocellular carcinoma after curative resection. Liver Int. 2008;28(3):393–401.
48. Hung IF, Poon RT, Lai CL, Fung J, Fan ST, Yuen MF. Recurrence of hepatitis B-related hepatocellular carcinoma is associated with high viral load at the time of resection. Am J Gastroenterol. 2008;103(7):1663–73.
49. Williams IT, Bell BP, Kuhnert W, Alter MJ. Incidence and transmission patterns of acute hepatitis C in the United States, 1982–2006. Arch Intern Med. 2011;171(3):242–8.
50. Alter MJ. Healthcare should not be a vehicle for transmission of hepatitis C virus. J Hepatol. 2008;48(1):2–4.
51. Donahue JG, Munoz A, Ness PM, et al. The declining risk of post-transfusion hepatitis C virus infection. N Engl J Med. 1992;327(6):369–73.
52. Seeff LB. Natural history of chronic hepatitis C. Hepatology. 2002;36(5 Suppl 1):S35–46.
53. Poynard T, Moussalli J, Ratziu V, Regimbeau C, Opolon P. Effect of interferon therapy on the natural history of hepatitis C virus-related cirrhosis and hepatocellular carcinoma. Clin Liver Dis. 1999;3(4):869–81.
54. Yoshida H, Tateishi R, Arakawa Y, et al. Benefit of interferon therapy in hepatocellular carcinoma prevention for individual patients with chronic hepatitis C. Gut. 2004;53(3):425–30.

55. Masuzaki R, Yoshida H, Omata M. Interferon reduces the risk of hepatocellular carcinoma in hepatitis C virus-related chronic hepatitis/liver cirrhosis. Oncology. 2010;78 Suppl 1:17–23.
56. Heathcote EJ. Prevention of hepatitis C virus-related hepatocellular carcinoma. Gastroenterology. 2004;127(5 Suppl 1):S294–302.
57. Ueno Y, Sollano JD, Farrell GC. Prevention of hepatocellular carcinoma complicating chronic hepatitis C. J Gastroenterol Hepatol. 2009;24(4):531–6.
58. Nishiguchi S, Kuroki T, Nakatani S, et al. Randomised trial of effects of interferon-alpha on incidence of hepatocellular carcinoma in chronic active hepatitis C with cirrhosis. Lancet. 1995;346(8982):1051–5.
59. Nishiguchi S, Shiomi S, Nakatani S, et al. Prevention of hepatocellular carcinoma in patients with chronic active hepatitis C and cirrhosis. Lancet. 2001;357(9251):196–7.
60. Mazella J, Botto JM, Guillemare E, Coppola T, Sarret P, Vincent JP. Structure, functional expression, and cerebral localization of the levocabastine-sensitive neurotensin/neuromedin N receptor from mouse brain. J Neurosci. 1996;16(18):5613–20.
61. Bruno S, Silini E, Crosignani A, et al. Hepatitis C virus genotypes and risk of hepatocellular carcinoma in cirrhosis: a prospective study. Hepatology. 1997;25(3):754–8.
62. Fattovich G, Giustina G, Degos F, et al. Effectiveness of interferon alfa on incidence of hepatocellular carcinoma and decompensation in cirrhosis type C. European Concerted Action on Viral Hepatitis (EUROHEP). J Hepatol. 1997;27(1):201–5.
63. Effect of interferon-alpha on progression of cirrhosis to hepatocellular carcinoma: a retrospective cohort study. International Interferon-alpha Hepatocellular Carcinoma Study Group. Lancet. 1998;351(9115):1535–39.
64. Imai Y, Kawata S, Tamura S, et al. Relation of interferon therapy and hepatocellular carcinoma in patients with chronic hepatitis C Osaka Hepatocellular Carcinoma Prevention Study Group. Ann Intern Med. 1998;129(2):94–9.
65. Benvegnu L, Chemello L, Noventa F, Fattovich G, Pontisso P, Alberti A. Retrospective analysis of the effect of interferon therapy on the clinical outcome of patients with viral cirrhosis. Cancer. 1998;83(5):901–9.
66. Serfaty L, Aumaitre H, Chazouilleres O, et al. Determinants of outcome of compensated hepatitis C virus-related cirrhosis. Hepatology. 1998;27(5):1435–40.
67. Valla DC, Chevallier M, Marcellin P, et al. Treatment of hepatitis C virus-related cirrhosis: a randomized, controlled trial of interferon alfa-2b versus no treatment. Hepatology. 1999;29(6):1870–5.
68. Okanoue T, Itoh Y, Minami M, et al. Interferon therapy lowers the rate of progression to hepatocellular carcinoma in chronic hepatitis C but not significantly in an advanced stage: a retrospective study in 1148 patients. Viral Hepatitis Therapy Study Group. J Hepatol. 1999;30(4):653–9.
69. Yoshida H, Shiratori Y, Moriyama M, et al. Interferon therapy reduces the risk for hepatocellular carcinoma: national surveillance program of cirrhotic and noncirrhotic patients with chronic hepatitis C in Japan. IHIT Study Group. Inhibition of Hepatocarcinogenesis by Interferon Therapy. Ann Intern Med. 1999;131(3):174–81.
70. Singal AK, Singh A, Jaganmohan S, et al. Antiviral therapy reduces risk of hepatocellular carcinoma in patients with hepatitis C virus-related cirrhosis. Clin Gastroenterol Hepatol. 2009;8(2):192–9.
71. Papatheodoridis GV, Papadimitropoulos VC, Hadziyannis SJ. Effect of interferon therapy on the development of hepatocellular carcinoma in patients with hepatitis C virus-related cirrhosis: a meta-analysis. Aliment Pharmacol Ther. 2001;15(5):689–98.
72. Miyake Y, Iwasaki Y, Yamamoto K. Meta-analysis: reduced incidence of hepatocellular carcinoma in patients not responding to interferon therapy of chronic hepatitis C. Int J Cancer. 2010;127(4):989–96.
73. Morgan TR, Ghany MG, Kim HY, et al. Outcome of sustained virological responders with histologically advanced chronic hepatitis C. Hepatology. 2010;52(3):833–44.
74. Imai Y, Tamura S, Tanaka H, et al. Reduced risk of hepatocellular carcinoma after interferon therapy in aged patients with chronic hepatitis C is limited to sustained virological responders. J Viral Hepat. 2010;17(3):185–91.

75. Yu ML, Lin SM, Chuang WL, et al. A sustained virological response to interferon or interferon/ribavirin reduces hepatocellular carcinoma and improves survival in chronic hepatitis C: a nationwide, multicentre study in Taiwan. Antivir Ther. 2006;11(8):985–94.
76. Di Bisceglie AM, Shiffman ML, Everson GT, et al. Prolonged therapy of advanced chronic hepatitis C with low-dose peginterferon. N Engl J Med. 2008;359(23):2429–41.
77. Afdhal NH, Levine R, Brown Jr R, Freilich B, O'brien M, Brass C. Colchicine versus peg-interferon Alfa 2B long term therapy: results of the 4 year copilot trial. Hepatology. 2008;48:S4.
78. Bruix J, Poynard T, Colombo M, et al. Maintenance therapy with peginterferon alfa-2b does not prevent hepatocellular carcinoma in cirrhotic patients with chronic hepatitis C. Gastroenterology. 2011;140(7):1990–9.
79. Lok AS, Everhart JE, Wright EC, et al. Maintenance Peginterferon therapy and other factors associated with hepatocellular carcinoma in patients with advanced hepatitis C. Gastroenterology. 2011;140(3):840–9.
80. Singal AK, Freeman Jr DH, Anand BS. Meta-analysis: interferon improves outcomes following ablation or resection of hepatocellular carcinoma. Aliment Pharmacol Ther. 2010;32(7):851–8.
81. McHutchison JG, Manns MP, Muir AJ, et al. Telaprevir for previously treated chronic HCV infection. N Engl J Med. 2011;362(14):1292–303.
82. Pawlotsky JM. The Results of Phase III Clinical Trial With Telaprevir and Boceprevir Presented at the Liver Meeting 2010: A New Standard of Care for Hepatitis C Virus Genotype 1 Infection, But With Issues Still Pending. Gastroenterology. 2011;140(3):746–54.
83. Kowdley KV, Tait JF, Bennett RL, Motulsky AG. 1993. In:Pagon RA, Bird TD, Dolan CR, Stephens K, (eds.), GeneReviews. Seattle (WA) University of Washington, Seattle; 1993–2000.
84. Kowdley KV. Iron, hemochromatosis, and hepatocellular carcinoma. Gastroenterology. 2004;127(5 Suppl 1):S79–86.
85. Guyader D, Jacquelinet C, Moirand R, et al. Noninvasive prediction of fibrosis in C282Y homozygous hemochromatosis. Gastroenterology. 1998;115(4):929–36.
86. Harrison SA, Bacon BR. Relation of hemochromatosis with hepatocellular carcinoma: epidemiology, natural history, pathophysiology, screening, treatment, and prevention. Med Clin North Am. 2005;89(2):391–409.
87. Alexander J, Kowdley KV. HFE-associated hereditary hemochromatosis. Genet Med. 2009;11(5):307–13.
88. Nielsen P, Fischer R, Buggisch P, Janka-Schaub G. Effective treatment of hereditary haemochromatosis with desferrioxamine in selected cases. Br J Haematol. 2003;123(5):952–3.
89. Phatak PD, Bonkovsky HL, Kowdley KV. Hereditary hemochromatosis: time for targeted screening. Ann Intern Med. 2008;149(4):270–2.
90. El-Serag HB, Inadomi JM, Kowdley KV. Screening for hereditary hemochromatosis in siblings and children of affected patients. A cost-effectiveness analysis. Ann Intern Med. 2000;132(4):261–9.
91. Bring P, Partovi N, Ford JA, Yoshida EM. Iron overload disorders: treatment options for patients refractory to or intolerant of phlebotomy. Pharmacotherapy. 2008;28(3):331–42.
92. Powell EE, Cooksley WG, Hanson R, Searle J, Halliday JW, Powell LW. The natural history of nonalcoholic steatohepatitis: a follow-up study of forty-two patients for up to 21 years. Hepatology. 1990;11(1):74–80.
93. Adams LA, Lymp JF, St Sauver J, et al. The natural history of nonalcoholic fatty liver disease: a population-based cohort study. Gastroenterology. 2005;129(1):113–21.
94. Ratziu V, Bonyhay L, Di Martino V, et al. Survival, liver failure, and hepatocellular carcinoma in obesity-related cryptogenic cirrhosis. Hepatology. 2002;35(6):1485–93.
95. Starley BQ, Calcagno CJ, Harrison SA. Nonalcoholic fatty liver disease and hepatocellular carcinoma: A weighty connection. Hepatology. 2010;51(5):1820–32.
96. Ratziu V, Caldwell S, Neuschwander-Tetri BA. Therapeutic trials in nonalcoholic steatohepatitis: Insulin sensitizers and related methodological issues. Hepatology. 2010;52(6):2206–15.
97. Lok AS-F. Does antiviral therapy for hepatitis B and C prevent hepatocellular carcinoma? J Gastroenterol Hepatol. 2011;26(2):221–7.

Chapter 13
Emerging Serum Biomarkers of HCC

Anjana A. Pillai and Claus J. Fimmel

Introduction

Hepatocellular carcinoma (HCC) is the third most common cause of cancer-related death worldwide [1] and is associated with poor patient survival. This is largely due to late detection—the majority of patients are diagnosed at advanced stages when curative resection or liver transplantation can no longer be offered. While overall cancer mortality has decreased in the United States, the incidence of HCC continues to rise. In fact, HCC has become the fastest growing cancer in the USA [1]. Two prospective studies have suggested a survival benefit for HCC surveillance with AFP in patients with chronic HBV infection [2, 3]. These reports have been widely quoted as rationale for the continued efforts to identify and validate HCC serum markers for early detection in all patient cohorts. However, until the past year, no comparable studies had been performed in patients with cirrhosis and non-HBV-related liver disease.

Biomarkers are defined as indicators of cellular, biochemical, molecular, or genetic alterations by which normal or abnormal biological processes can be recognized or monitored [4]. A large number of candidate serum biomarkers for HCC have been identified over the last decade. The ideal HCC biomarker should be highly sensitive and specific, cost-effective, reproducible, and user-friendly. The evaluation of candidate markers has been formalized by a landmark report by the Early Detection Research Network (EDRN) of the National Cancer Institute Early Detection Research Network (EDRN). As proposed by the EDRN, five successive phases are required for biomarker validation: preclinical exploratory studies (phase 1),

A.A. Pillai, MD
Emory University Hospital, Division of Digestive Diseases, Emory Transplant Center,
Atlanta, GA, USA

C.J. Fimmel, MD (✉)
Division of Gastroenterology, Hepatology and Nutrition, Loyola University Medical Center,
2160 South First Avenue, Maywood, IL 60153, USA
e-mail: cfimmel@lumc.edu

N. Reau and F.F. Poordad (eds.), *Primary Liver Cancer: Surveillance, Diagnosis and Treatment*, Clinical Gastroenterology, DOI 10.1007/978-1-61779-863-4_13,
© Springer Science+Business Media New York 2012

clinical assay development for disease detection (phase 2), retrospective longitudinal studies to detect preclinical disease (phase 3), prospective screening studies (phase 4), and cancer control studies (phase 5). The majority of HCC serum biomarkers trials have been limited to phases 1–3. The most commonly used HCC serum markers worldwide, serum α-fetoprotein (AFP) and DCP, are not sufficiently sensitive or specific for HCC screening or surveillance purposes. Not surprisingly, the current guidelines by the American Association for the Study of Liver Diseases (AASLD) do not advocate serum marker HCC surveillance for patients with cirrhosis [5].

In this chapter, we review existing and emerging HCC serum markers and grade their performance using the EDRN criteria.

Single Protein Biomarkers

AFP

α-Fetoprotein (AFP) is a single polypeptide chain glycoprotein synthesized by embryonic liver cells of the vitelline sac and fetal intestinal tract under physiologic conditions. AFP was initially discovered in fetal serum by Bergstrand and Czar in 1956 [6] and was first described as a human tumor-associated protein in 1964 by Tatarinov [7]. The first quantitative serum assays for AFP were developed by Ruoslahti and Seppala [8]. The exact function of AFP is not well established. AFP tissue and serum levels are elevated in patients with HCC, during hepatocyte regeneration, in chronic liver disease, and in embryonic carcinomas. The sensitivity and specificity of AFP in HCC screening studies vary according to study design, patient population, and threshold values used for screening. AFP may be modestly elevated in patients with chronic liver disease including hepatitis C (HCV) infection. Serum AFP levels also rise during the regenerative phase of severe liver injury, including acute liver failure [9]. A similar trend has been also noted in chronic liver injury. For example, AFP serum levels decrease in patients without hepatoma who are undergoing HCV antiviral therapy [10].

The sensitivity of AFP for HCC detection is limited since a substantial percentage of HCCs do not overexpress the protein [11–14]. This limitation has been documented in many studies. For example, an earlier case–control study by Trevisani et al. suggested that the optimal AFP threshold for HCC screening should be 20 ng/ml, with resulting sensitivity and specificity of 60% and 90%, respectively [11]. Unfortunately, using this cutoff would result in a false-negative test result in 40% of the cases. Raising the cutoff to 200 ng/ml to increase specificity would further reduce sensitivity to 22%.

A recent study assessed the sensitivity and specificity of serum AFP in cirrhotic patients with established HCC and non-HCC controls. At the optimum cutoff level of 10.9 ng/ml, AFP had a sensitivity of 66% and specificity of 82% [15]. Assuming a 1% prevalence of HCC in a screening population, these performance characteristics would correspond to a positive predictive value of 3.7% and false-positive and false-negative rates of 17.8% and 30%, respectively.

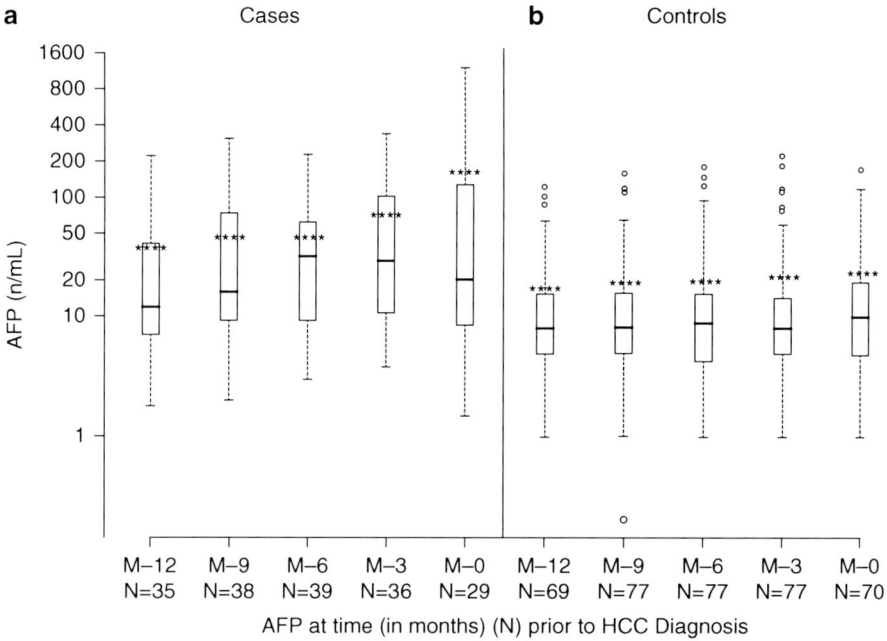

Fig. 13.1 Box plots of AFP values in HCC cases (**a**) and matched controls (**b**) in the HALT-C trial at months -12, -9, -6, -3, and 0 (time of HCC diagnosis). Data are shown as mean ± SD. AFP values increased from 37.0 ± 51.3 ng/ml at month -12 to 157.6 ± 296.6 ng/ml at month 0 in the HCC cases ($p > 0.0001$) (1A), but remained unchanged in the controls (17.4 ± 25.8 and 23.0 ± 34.2 ng/ml (1B), respectively) (Taken from [16], with the authors' permission)

One shortcoming of prior studies on HCC biomarkers has been the lack of prospective studies in well-defined at-risk populations. This limitation was overcome in the recently completed HALT-C ("Hepatitis C Antiviral Long-Term Treatment against Cirrhosis") trial. This trial followed over 1,000 patients with HCV-related cirrhosis for an average of 4.3 years. During the study, 39 new cases of HCC were discovered. Since serum samples were prospectively collected in all patients, the authors had the unique opportunity to evaluate AFP and DCP under realistic surveillance conditions [16]. Not surprisingly, the performance of AFP as an early marker of HCC varied with the time to diagnosis and the chosen cutoff values. Using cutoff values of 20 ng/ml or 200 ng/ml, the sensitivities and specificities of AFP at time of diagnosis were 61% and 81% and 22% and 100%, respectively. The sensitivity increased significantly at lower cutoff levels (<10 ng/ml) but at the expense of decreased specificity (15%–57%). Using a clinically relevant detection interval of 12 months prior to diagnosis and a cutoff value of 20 ng/ml, the sensitivity and specificity of AFP were only 47% and 75%, respectively (Fig. 13.1). These data clearly demonstrate the limitations of AFP as a sole biomarker for HCC surveillance.

The performance of AFP is affected by patient demographics, the etiology of the underlying liver disease, and the degree of fibrosis. In a multicenter, case–control study of patients with HCV, the sensitivity of AFP at a cutoff level of 10 ng/ml was 57.1% in African–Americans, significantly lower than the value of 81.6% in patients of other ethnic groups [17]. A similar decrease in sensitivity in African–American patients was also noted in the HALT-C trial [16]. Furthermore, AFP levels are significantly higher in females as compared to males and increase in parallel with the fibrosis stage in both genders [10].

A recently FDA-approved modification of the AFP assay is based on the detection of a specific Lens culinaris agglutinin glycoform (AFP-L3). This assay is commercially available and simultaneously measures total serum AFP and AFP-L3. A recent study demonstrated a sevenfold increase in the risk of HCC development in patients with an AFP-L3 above 10% as compared to patients with a ratio below 10% [18, 19]. Several subsequent studies have shown variable sensitivity 36–96% and specificity 89–94% for AFP-L3 [20–23].

The performance of AFP-L3 was dependent on the tumor size. In small HCCs (<2 cm), its sensitivity was only 35–45%, whereas it was 80–90% in larger tumors (>5 cm) [18, 24]. Similar to AFP, the low sensitivity of AFP-L3 for the detection of small HCCs is disappointing and limits its clinical utility.

AFP remains useful as a confirmatory test in cirrhotic patients with liver masses. AFP levels exceeding 200 ng/ml in conjunction with characteristic imaging criteria are highly specific for the diagnosis of HCC [11, 17]. Additionally, a persistently elevated AFP level is associated with an increased risk for the future development of HCC [25, 26], suggesting a role for AFP as a "risk indicator." Finally, longitudinal measurements of AFP in patients with AFP-secreting HCCs may be useful to assess tumor growth, response to treatment, or recurrence after treatment.

Because of its limited utility as a screening test, current AASLD practice guidelines do not recommend the use of AFP for HCC surveillance [5]. Therefore, AFP is considered an inadequate screening test for HCC [27, 28].

Des-γ-Carboxy Prothrombin

Des-gamma-carboxy prothrombin (DCP), also known as prothrombin induced by vitamin K absence II (PIVKA II), was first described as a potential HCC marker by Liebman in 1984 [29]. DCP is an abnormal form of prothrombin that is generated by the abnormal undercarboxylation of the prothrombin precursor in HCC cells [30].

The utility of DCP as a surveillance marker for HCC remains limited. Its sensitivity and specificity have been evaluated in several case control studies, with reported values ranging from 28–89% and 87–96%, respectively [31–34]. A recent report by Tsai in Chinese patients demonstrated a sensitivity of <50% for HCCs of less than 3 cm in size [35].

In the HALT-C study, the sensitivity and specificity of DCP at time of diagnosis were, respectively, 74% and 86% at a cutoff of 40 mAU/ml and 43% and 100% at a cutoff of 150 mAU/ml [16], arguing against its use as a surveillance test in this at-risk population (Fig. 13.2).

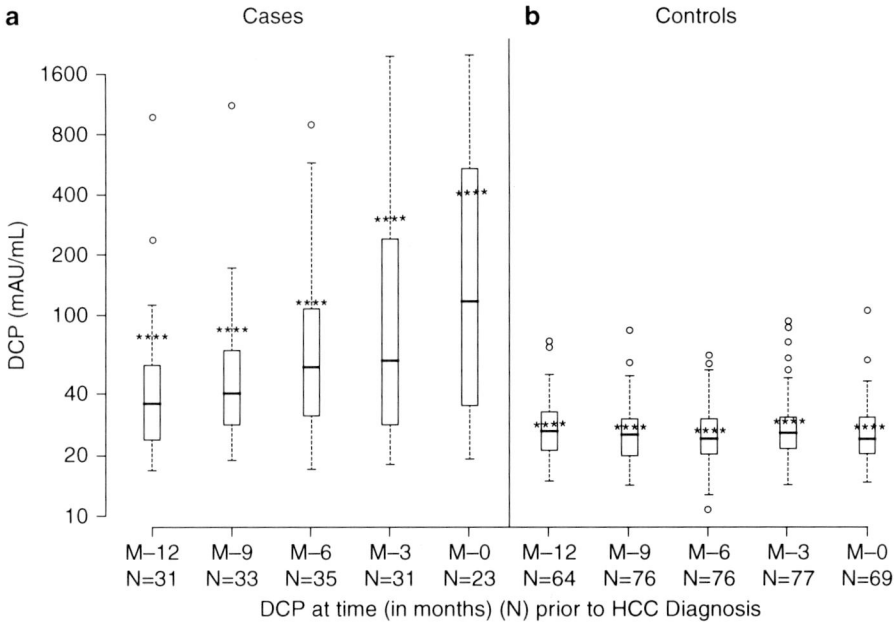

Fig. 13.2 Box plots of DCP values in HCC cases (**a**) and matched controls (**b**) in the HALT-C trial at months -12, -9, -6, -3, and 0 (time of HCC diagnosis). Data are shown as mean $\pm$ SD. DCP values increased from 79.1 ± 172.5 mAU/ml at -12 to 413.4 ± 597.7 mAU/ml at month ($p < .0001$) in the HCC cases (2A). DCP values remained stable in controls (28.8 ± 11.4 and 27.9 ± 13.1 mAU/ml, respectively) (2B) (Taken from [16], with the authors' permission)

Previous studies have clearly demonstrated increased DCP levels in patients with tumor invasion of the portal vein, intrahepatic metastasis, and capsular infiltration [36–38]. These data indicate that DCP may have a value as an indicator of advanced or aggressive HCC rather than as an early disease marker.

Head-to-head comparison studies of DCP and AFP have shown conflicting results. Several studies from Japan [39–42] and one recent study from the USA [34] showed a superior performance of DCP, whereas others found no significant differences. A wide range of DCP (40–100 mAU/ml) and AFP (20–200 ng/ml) cutoff levels were used, which limits the validity of the comparisons.

Combining both markers improves overall sensitivity but predictably decreases specificity [33, 43]. For example, in the HALT-C study population, combining DCP and AFP increased the sensitivity at the 12-month time point from 43% to 47% at the low thresholds (i.e., 40 mAU/ml and 20 ng/ml) to 73%, with a concomitant decrease in specificity to 71% (from 94% to 75%, respectively). In simple terms, a combination of the two markers using the more sensitive thresholds would still miss one in four HCCs. Interestingly, the majority of the 39 HCC cases detected in the HALT-C trial were discovered by imaging modalities (US, CT, or MR). In only nine cases did the doubling of serum AFP result in or contribute to the diagnosis of HCC [16].

Based on the current available data, AFP or DCP—alone or in combination—is of questionable utility for early HCC detection. Despite their continued widespread use worldwide, the appeals to abandon serological surveillance for early HCC detection have been renewed [28, 44].

Alpha-L-Fucosidase

Alpha-L-fucosidase (AFU) is a lysosomal enzyme that catabolizes the fucosidation of multiple serum proteins. Its activity is frequently elevated in patients with HCC and chronic liver disease [45, 46]. In 1998, Giardina and colleagues prospectively followed serum AFU activities in 132 cirrhotic patients. During the 8-year follow-up period, they noted significant increase in serum AFU levels in a subset of patients with HCC. Interestingly, this change preceded the ultrasonographic visualization of the lesions in many cases [47]. However, the overall sensitivity of this test is low, and its specificity is limited due to its elevation in noncancerous extrahepatic diseases such as diabetes, pancreatitis, and hypothyroidism.

Glypican-3

Glypican-3 (GPC3) is a cell-surface glycoprotein that plays a role in regulating cell proliferation and survival during embryonic development by modulating the activity of various growth factors. It is absent in the hepatocytes of healthy subjects and patients with chronic hepatitis, but is highly expressed in hepatocellular cancer [48, 49] and malignant melanoma cells [50]. An initial report demonstrated GPC3 protein expression in 72% of HCCs and increased GPC3 serum levels in 53% of HCC patients [51]. No correlation was noted between GPC3 and AFP levels, suggesting a potential utility for GPC3 as a serum marker for AFP-negative tumors. Similarly promising findings were reported in several recent studies [52, 53]. Despite favorable initial reports, GPC 3 has not gained acceptance or diagnostic use. This is due to disappointing results in several recent studies [54, 55] and to ongoing concerns regarding the specificity of the antibody reactivities in different ELISAs [54].

Golgi Protein 73

GP73 (Golm1, Golph2) is a 73-kDa Golgi glycoprotein that is expressed at minimal levels in normal hepatocytes under normal physiologic conditions [56]. Increased expression of GP73 was first described in hepatocytes of patients with adult giant-cell hepatitis [56]. Further studies demonstrated that hepatocyte expression of GP73 was upregulated in patients with a variety of acute or chronic forms of liver disease,

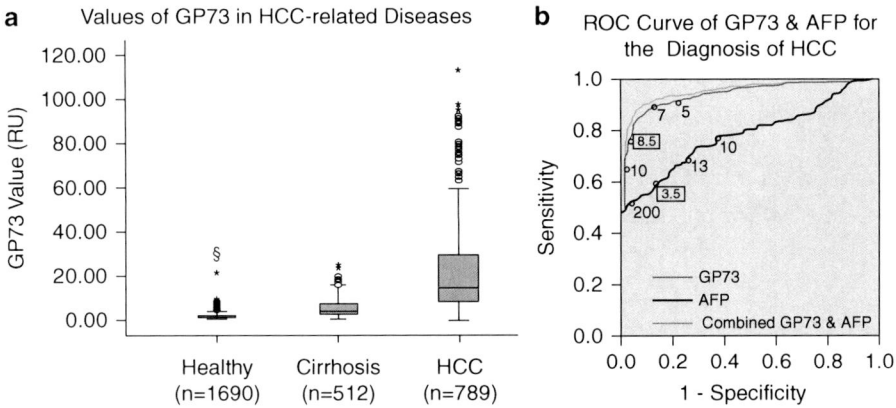

a Values of GP73 in HCC-related Diseases

b ROC Curve of GP73 & AFP for the Diagnosis of HCC

Fig. 13.3 Comparison of serum GP73 and AFP values in patients with hepatocellular carcinoma (HCC). 3A: GP73 values of healthy subjects, liver cirrhosis, and HCC were measured by semiquantitative Western blotting and expressed as relative units (RU). Mean levels and ranges were 1.2 (0.9–1.7) in normal subjects, 4.7 (2.6–8.0) in patients with cirrhosis, and 14.7 (8.4–29.4) in patients with HCC. Outliers (*open circles*) and extremes (*asterisks*) are marked. The increase in serum GP73 in patients with HCC as compared to cirrhotic patients was statistically significant ($p<0.001$). 3B. Comparison of GP73 and AFP for the diagnosis of HCC. Receiver operating characteristics (ROC) curves for AFP, GP73, and the combination of both markers for the diagnosis of HCC, using optimal cutoff levels of 8.5 RU (GP73) and 35 ng/ml (AFP), respectively. The area under the ROC curve for GP73 was significantly different from that of AFP ($p<0.001$), whereas no difference was detected between the GP73 as a single marker and its combination with AFP (Taken from [62], with the authors' permission)

regardless of specific disease etiology [57, 58]. Block and colleagues first reported increased serum GP73 (sGP73) levels in patients with HBV-related HCC [59]. Similarly findings were subsequently obtained in patients with HCV-related HCC [60]. sGP73 levels were found to be significantly higher in patients with HCC compared to cirrhotic controls without HCC. The sensitivity and specificity of sGP73 for the presence of HCC were 69% and 75%, respectively.

Since these promising initial reports, the performance of sGP73 has been studied in a variety of patient populations, using Western blotting- or ELISA-based assay techniques (reviewed in [61]). Overall, excellent sensitivities and specificities have been reported in patient populations with less advanced fibrosis, especially in HBV-infected patients. In a recent cross-sectional study of more than 4,000 Chinese subjects, the performance characteristics of sGP73 were dramatically superior to those of AFP [62] (Fig. 13.3). Similar trends were observed in other, smaller HBV cohorts [63–65]. In contrast, several recent studies have shown poor HCC specificity in patients with advanced cirrhosis [66–71]. These discrepant results may be due to the severity of the underlying liver disease on hepatocyte GP73 expression. Early studies had demonstrated a progressive upregulation of GP73 hepatocyte expression with increasing fibrosis stage [57, 58]. A proportionate increase in sGP73 secretion might lead to the stage-dependent performance as a marker of HCC. A recent study by Yamoto [68] and colleagues provides indirect support for this hypothesis.

The authors demonstrated that sGP73 serum levels were not significantly lowered after HCC resection in cirrhotic patients, suggesting that noncancerous hepatocytes may be a major source of sGP73 in a cirrhotic liver. This lack of tumor specificity will likely limit the overall utility of sGP73 as a global HCC serum marker.

Other Candidate Markers

Vascular endothelial growth factor (VEGF), a known marker of tumor angiogenesis, was found to be elevated in livers and sera of subjects with advanced HCC, notably in those with portal vein emboli, microscopic vein invasion, poorly encapsulated tumors, and recurrent HCC [72, 73]. Other serum markers, such as chromogranin A [74], squamous cell carcinoma antigen (SCCA) [75], transforming growth factor B1 (TGFB1) [76], hepatocyte growth factor (HGF) [77], human cervical cancer oncogene (HCCR) [78], insulin-like growth factor-II (IGF-II) [79], and KL-6 [80] have also been evaluated with respect to HCC serum diagnostics. These markers have not been validated in adequately powered, prospective studies, and many of them are limited by their lack of HCC specificity. Future studies are needed to confirm their utility in HCC screening.

Tumor-Derived Autoantibodies

The occurrence of tumor-derived autoantibodies (TAAs) in patients with HCC has been documented in several prior studies [81–85]. TAAs are considered markers of malignant transformation since their occurrence is triggered by the abnormal processing of cellular proteins during carcinogenesis which results in autoantigenicity [86, 87]. Unfortunately, the sensitivity of TAAs for HCC is low, and they lack liver specificity since they have been described in a wide range of malignancies. One approach to overcome this problem is to combine panels of TAAs and non-TAA markers such as AFP, as recently described in a study by Chen and colleagues [88]. In their study, a panel of 10 HCC-associated TAAs had a combined sensitivity of 66.2%, which was further increased by the inclusion of AFP. The specificity of the TAA panel for HCC vs. liver cirrhosis was not impressive (66.7%). To date, no prospective studies have been published to demonstrate the utility of TAAs in HCC.

Proteomics and Glycoproteomics

Serum proteomics have long been touted as a potential breakthrough technology for the identification of cancer markers, including HCC. This technology allows the detection and quantitation of thousands of protein and their fragments in serum or plasma. The resolution of proteomic assays has continuously risen over the past decade due to novel mass spectrometric methods such as surface-enhanced laser desorption ionization time-of-flight mass spectrometry (SELDI-TOF MS).

In a widely quoted study from 2003, Poon and colleagues used SELDI-TOF serum analysis in 38 Chinese patients with HCC and 20 control patients with chronic hepatitis [89]. They identified 250 serum proteomic features which separated the two groups with a specificity of 90% and sensitivity of 92%. This study has not been reproduced.

Schwegler and colleagues combined serum proteomics with individual HCC serum markers to study 170 subjects that included subjects without liver disease, patients with chronic hepatitis but without cirrhosis, cirrhotics, and cirrhotic patients with HCC [90]. Thirty-eight proteomic features were identified that distinguished cirrhotics with and without cancer with a sensitivity and specificity of 61% and 76%, respectively. When measurements of AFP, DCP, and GP73 were combined with the proteomics data, the sensitivity and specificity improved to 75% and 92%, respectively.

Paradis et al. compared protein expression profiles in the sera of 82 cirrhotic patients with and without HCC to define an optimum discriminator protein profile in patients with HCC [91]. The authors discovered the intensity of 30 protein peaks significantly differed between cirrhotic patients with and without HCC. An algorithm including the six highest-scoring peaks allowed the correct classification (HCC present or absent) in 92.5% of patients in the discovery set and 90% in the validation set. The most informative protein fragment (8,900 Da) was purified and identified as a C-terminal vitronectin fragment. The authors went on to show that serum measurements of this fragment were predictive of HCC, suggesting potential diagnostic utility for this protein.

The initial excitement for serum proteomics approaches to cancer diagnosis has subsided due to several well-publicized limitations and failures of the method. Key unresolved issues include the extreme biological noisiness of the method, its lack of reproducibility within sample sets and between different laboratories, its prohibitive costs, and the lack of standardization. As a result, none of the published HCC proteomics studies have surpassed the minimal level (level 1) of the EDRN criteria (see Table 13.1).

A related approach is based on the long-known changes in the glycosylation patterns of serum proteins in cancer patients. This concept has already been exploited in the case of AFP-L3, a hyperfucosylated form of AFP (see above). Increases in serum protein fucosylation in patients with chronic liver disease and HCC have been demonstrated by several authors. In a recent study, Communale identified 56 proteins that were hyperfucosylated in HCC patients and developed lectin-ELISAs for two particularly promising candidates, hemopexin and fetuin-A. Increased levels of fucosylated hemopexin (1.4-fold) and fetuin-A (2.5-fold) were present in HCC patients. Despite this modest difference, both markers performed respectably in a diagnostic pilot study of over 300 patients [92, 93]. On the other hand, a recent study by Morota did not confirm the promising results for fucosylated hemopexin [66].

One potential confounding factor in the study by Communale was the difference in the degree of cirrhosis in HCC patients and cirrhotic controls since. In the HCC

Table 13.1 Evaluation of HCC serum markers

Marker	Serum quantitation method	EDRN level
AFP	ELISA[a]	4
AFP-L3	Liquid-phase antibody assay[a]	2
DCP	ELISA[b]	3
α-L-fucosidase	Enzymatic assay	3
Glypican-3	ELISA	2
GP73	ELISA[b]	2
TAAs	ELISA, Western blotting	1
Serum proteomics	2DE, SELDI-TOF, MS	2
miRNAs	qPCR	1

[a]Commercially available and FDA-approved
[b]Assays commercially available outside the USA

group, the underlying cirrhosis tended to be more severe, as reflected in a higher percentage of patients with Child B or C disease, whereas the majority of the cirrhotic control patients had Child A disease. Subtle differences in the degree of underlying cirrhosis could potentially confound the data by attributing changes in serum marker levels to the presence of cancer rather than to differences in the cirrhosis stage. This consideration applies to many of the published studies in the field. The best way to avoid this bias is to perform prospective studies in patients at risk for HCC, as exemplified by the HALT-C trial (see above).

Despite many promising leads, the diagnostic utility of glycoproteomics remains unclear. Methodological refinements—including the use of nanotechnology approaches—may result in the identification of additional marker candidates [94].

MicroRNAs

MicroRNAs (miRNAs) are small, noncoding RNAs that regulate gene expression, cell differentiation, stem cell maintenance, and epithelial–mesenchymal transition [95, 96]. Deregulation of miRNAs commonly occurs in malignancy and depending on the genes targeted, miRNAs can act as tumor suppressors or oncogenes [97]. Several recent studies have shown changes in the levels of miRNAs in HCC tissues [98–105].

Recent studies suggest that miRNAs are stable in serum and that quantitative real-time (qRT)-PCR reactions can be used to measure their abundance. Work in a variety of cancers has suggested that serum miRNA measurements are of potential diagnostic utility.

To date, there are three published reports on the abundance of miRNAs in serum of HCC patients. In the first study, Li and colleagues identified several miRNAs in serum that showed elevated levels in patients with HBV infection [106]. Two miRNAs (miR-10a and miR-125 b) were predictive of HBV-related HCC.

Using a similar approach in a cohort of patients with predominantly HCV-related liver disease, Qu and colleagues identified two miRNAs (miR-16, miR-199a) with significantly reduced serum levels in HCC patients [107]. Closer inspection of their data reveals considerable overlap between HCC and "chronic liver disease" patients. Furthermore, more than 50% of the control patients did not have advanced cirrhosis, a feature that might magnify the differences between cancer patients and control. A third study published by Xu and colleagues provides a clear example of three circulating miRNAs (miR-21, miR-122, and miR-223) that are present at increased levels in HBV-infected HCC patients as compared to normal controls [108]. However, even higher levels were found in HBV-infected patients without HCC. The authors hypothesized that miRNAs upregulation may be due to liver injury rather than carcinogenesis, which will limit their usefulness as a biomarker of HCC. It will remain to be seen whether truly HCC-specific miRNAs can be identified and validated.

One important methodological issue is the lack of validated internal reference standards for the quantification of serum miRNAs. Given the large number of miRNAs that are dysregulated in HCC, we anticipate a growing number of further studies on this subject in the future. At this stage, however, the work on this promising class of potential biomarkers should be considered at the "proof-of-concept" stage.

Summary and Conclusions

Few cancer biomarkers survive the arduous journey from bench to bedside, and hepatocellular cancer is no exception to this trend. To put the issue in perspective, there are currently only nine FDA-approved biomarkers for cancers in the USA. None of these markers can claim absolute cancer specificity, and most of them are used to monitor patients with known disease for recurrences or responses to antitumor therapy [109]

Proteomics—despite its conceptual promise—has yet to deliver clinically useful tests [110]. In a recent review, only 3% (41 of 1,261) of proteins with reported cancer-related differential expression were clinically utilized for serum diagnostics in some form [111].

The results of the HALT-C trial have provided perhaps the most unequivocal documentation of the limitations of AFP and DCP, the two leading HCC serum biomarkers. This unique trial achieved an impressive sample size and follow-up duration and failed to demonstrate any particular utility for AFP, DCP, or their combination. One major advantage of the HALT-C trials was its prospective design. This minimized the confounding effect of the underlying liver disease on marker levels—an important issue in traditional comparative studies. The HALT-C serum bank provides an ideal sample repository for the evaluation of any new candidate markers in the future.

References

1. Kamangar F, Dores GM, Anderson WF. Patterns of cancer incidence, mortality, and prevalence across five continents: defining priorities to reduce cancer disparities in different geographic regions of the world. J Clin Oncol. 2006;24(14):2137–50.
2. Zhang BH, Yang BH, Tang ZY. Randomized controlled trial of screening for hepatocellular carcinoma. J Cancer Res Clin Oncol. 2004;130(7):417–22.
3. McMahon BJ, et al. Screening for hepatocellular carcinoma in Alaska natives infected with chronic hepatitis B: a 16-year population-based study. Hepatology. 2000;32(4 Pt 1): 842–6.
4. Srivastava S, Gopal-Srivastava R. Biomarkers in cancer screening: a public health perspective. J Nutr. 2002;132(8 Suppl):2471S–5S.
5. Bruix J, Sherman M. Management of hepatocellular carcinoma: an update. Hepatology. 2010;53(3):1020–2.
6. Bergstrand CG, Czar B. Demonstration of a new protein fraction in serum from the human fetus. Scand J Clin Lab Invest. 1956;8(2):174.
7. IuS T. Detection of embryo-specific alpha-globulin in the blood serum of a patient with primary liver cancer. Vopr Med Khim. 1964;10:90–1.
8. Ruoslahti E, Seppala M. Studies of carcino-fetal proteins. 3. Development of a radioimmunoassay for -fetoprotein. Demonstration of -fetoprotein in serum of healthy human adults. Int J Cancer. 1971;8(3):374–83.
9. Schmidt LE, Dalhoff K. Alpha-fetoprotein is a predictor of outcome in acetaminophen-induced liver injury. Hepatology. 2005;41(1):26–31.
10. Di Bisceglie AM, et al. Serum alpha-fetoprotein levels in patients with advanced hepatitis C: results from the HALT-C Trial. J Hepatol. 2005;43(3):434–41.
11. Trevisani F, et al. Serum alpha-fetoprotein for diagnosis of hepatocellular carcinoma in patients with chronic liver disease: influence of HBsAg and anti-HCV status. J Hepatol. 2001;34(4):570–5.
12. Pateron D, et al. Prospective study of screening for hepatocellular carcinoma in Caucasian patients with cirrhosis. J Hepatol. 1994;20(1):65–71.
13. Zoli M, et al. Efficacy of a surveillance program for early detection of hepatocellular carcinoma. Cancer. 1996;78(5):977–85.
14. Izuno K, et al. Early detection of hepatocellular carcinoma associated with cirrhosis by combined assay of des-gamma-carboxy prothrombin and alpha-fetoprotein: a prospective study. Hepatogastroenterology. 1995;42(4):387–93.
15. Marrero JA, et al. Alpha-fetoprotein, des-gamma carboxyprothrombin, and lectin-bound alpha-fetoprotein in early hepatocellular carcinoma. Gastroenterology. 2009;137(1):110–8.
16. Lok AS, et al. Des-gamma-carboxy prothrombin and alpha-fetoprotein as biomarkers for the early detection of hepatocellular carcinoma. Gastroenterology. 2010;138(2):493–502.
17. Nguyen MH, et al. Racial differences in effectiveness of alpha-fetoprotein for diagnosis of hepatocellular carcinoma in hepatitis C virus cirrhosis. Hepatology. 2002;36(2):410–7.
18. Li D, Mallory T, Satomura S. AFP-L3: a new generation of tumor marker for hepatocellular carcinoma. Clin Chim Acta. 2001;313(1–2):15–9.
19. Yamagata Y, et al. Simultaneous determination of percentage of Lens culinaris agglutinin-reactive alpha-fetoprotein and alpha-fetoprotein concentration using the LiBASys clinical auto-analyzer. Clin Chim Acta. 2003;327(1–2):59–67.
20. Wang SS, et al. Utility of lentil lectin affinity of alpha-fetoprotein in the diagnosis of hepatocellular carcinoma. J Hepatol. 1996;25(2):166–71.
21. Oka H, et al. Multicenter prospective analysis of newly diagnosed hepatocellular carcinoma with respect to the percentage of Lens culinaris agglutinin-reactive alpha-fetoprotein. J Gastroenterol Hepatol. 2001;16(12):1378–83.
22. Khien VV, et al. Clinical evaluation of lentil lectin-reactive alpha-fetoprotein-L3 in histology-proven hepatocellular carcinoma. Int J Biol Markers. 2001;16(2):105–11.

23. Taketa K, et al. A collaborative study for the evaluation of lectin-reactive alpha-fetoproteins in early detection of hepatocellular carcinoma. Cancer Res. 1993;53(22):5419–23.
24. Taketa K. Alpha-fetoprotein: reevaluation in hepatology. Hepatology. 1990;12(6):1420–32.
25. Oka H, et al. Prospective study of alpha-fetoprotein in cirrhotic patients monitored for development of hepatocellular carcinoma. Hepatology. 1994;19(1):61–6.
26. Zhang JY, et al. A case-control study of risk factors for hepatocellular carcinoma in Henan, China. Am J Trop Med Hyg. 1998;59(6):947–51.
27. Sherman M. Alphafetoprotein: an obituary. J Hepatol. 2001;34(4):603–5.
28. Forner A, Reig M, Bruix J. Alpha-fetoprotein for hepatocellular carcinoma diagnosis: the demise of a brilliant star. Gastroenterology. 2009;137(1):26–9.
29. Liebman HA, et al. Des-gamma-carboxy (abnormal) prothrombin as a serum marker of primary hepatocellular carcinoma. N Engl J Med. 1984;310(22):1427–31.
30. Ono M, et al. Measurement of immunoreactive prothrombin precursor and vitamin-K-dependent gamma-carboxylation in human hepatocellular carcinoma tissues: decreased carboxylation of prothrombin precursor as a cause of des-gamma-carboxyprothrombin synthesis. Tumour Biol. 1990;11(6):319–26.
31. Aoyagi Y, et al. Clinical significance of simultaneous determinations of alpha-fetoprotein and des-gamma-carboxy prothrombin in monitoring recurrence in patients with hepatocellular carcinoma. Cancer. 1996;77(9):1781–6.
32. Nomura F, et al. Serum des-gamma-carboxy prothrombin levels determined by a new generation of sensitive immunoassays in patients with small-sized hepatocellular carcinoma. Am J Gastroenterol. 1999;94(3):650–4.
33. Grazi GL, et al. The role of tumor markers in the diagnosis of hepatocellular carcinoma, with special reference to the des-gamma-carboxy prothrombin. Liver Transplant Surg. 1995;1(4):249–55.
34. Marrero JA, et al. Des-gamma carboxyprothrombin can differentiate hepatocellular carcinoma from nonmalignant chronic liver disease in American patients. Hepatology. 2003;37(5):1114–21.
35. Tsai SL, et al. Plasma des-gamma-carboxyprothrombin in the early stage of hepatocellular carcinoma. Hepatology. 1990;11(3):481–8.
36. Suehiro T, et al. Protein induced by vitamin K absence or antagonist II as a prognostic marker in hepatocellular carcinoma. Comparison with alpha-fetoprotein. Cancer. 1994;73(10):2464–71.
37. Toyosaka A, et al. Intrahepatic metastases in hepatocellular carcinoma: evidence for spread via the portal vein as an efferent vessel. Am J Gastroenterol. 1996;91(8):1610–5.
38. Koike Y, et al. Des-gamma-carboxy prothrombin as a useful predisposing factor for the development of portal venous invasion in patients with hepatocellular carcinoma: a prospective analysis of 227 patients. Cancer. 2001;91(3):561–9.
39. Kasahara A, et al. Clinical evaluation of plasma des-gamma-carboxy prothrombin as a marker protein of hepatocellular carcinoma in patients with tumors of various sizes. Dig Dis Sci. 1993;38(12):2170–6.
40. Mita Y, et al. The usefulness of determining des-gamma-carboxy prothrombin by sensitive enzyme immunoassay in the early diagnosis of patients with hepatocellular carcinoma. Cancer. 1998;82(9):1643–8.
41. Nakagawa T, et al. Clinicopathologic significance of protein induced vitamin K absence or antagonist II and alpha-fetoprotein in hepatocellular carcinoma. Int J Oncol. 1999;14(2):281–6.
42. Takikawa Y, et al. Plasma abnormal prothrombin (PIVKA-II): a new and reliable marker for the detection of hepatocellular carcinoma. J Gastroenterol Hepatol. 1992;7(1):1–6.
43. Ishii M, et al. Simultaneous measurements of serum alpha-fetoprotein and protein induced by vitamin K absence for detecting hepatocellular carcinoma. South Tohoku District Study Group. Am J Gastroenterol. 2000;95(4):1036–40.
44. Sherman M. Serological surveillance for hepatocellular carcinoma: time to quit. J Hepatol. 2010;52(4):614–5.

45. Deugnier Y, et al. Serum alpha-L-fucosidase: a new marker for the diagnosis of primary hepatic carcinoma? Hepatology. 1984;4(5):889–92.
46. Ishizuka H, et al. Prediction of the development of hepato-cellular-carcinoma in patients with liver cirrhosis by the serial determinations of serum alpha-L-fucosidase activity. Intern Med. 1999;38(12):927–31.
47. Giardina MG, et al. Serum alpha-L-fucosidase activity and early detection of hepatocellular carcinoma: a prospective study of patients with cirrhosis. Cancer. 1998;83(12):2468–74.
48. Hsu HC, Cheng W, Lai PL. Cloning and expression of a developmentally regulated transcript MXR7 in hepatocellular carcinoma: biological significance and temporospatial distribution. Cancer Res. 1997;57(22):5179–84.
49. Zhu ZW, et al. Enhanced glypican-3 expression differentiates the majority of hepatocellular carcinomas from benign hepatic disorders. Gut. 2001;48(4):558–64.
50. Nakatsura T, et al. Identification of glypican-3 as a novel tumor marker for melanoma. Clin Cancer Res. 2004;10(19):6612–21.
51. Capurro M, et al. Glypican-3: a novel serum and histochemical marker for hepatocellular carcinoma. Gastroenterology. 2003;125(1):89–97.
52. Nakatsura T, et al. Glypican-3, overexpressed specifically in human hepatocellular carcinoma, is a novel tumor marker. Biochem Biophys Res Commun. 2003;306(1):16–25.
53. Tangkijvanich P, et al. Diagnostic role of serum glypican-3 in differentiating hepatocellular carcinoma from non-malignant chronic liver disease and other liver cancers. J Gastroenterol Hepatol. 2010;25(1):129–37.
54. Yasuda E, et al. Evaluation for clinical utility of GPC3, measured by a commercially available ELISA kit with Glypican-3 (GPC3) antibody, as a serological and histological marker for hepatocellular carcinoma. Hepatol Res. 2010;40(5):477–85.
55. Beale G, et al. AFP, PIVKAII, GP3, SCCA-1 and follisatin as surveillance biomarkers for hepatocellular cancer in non-alcoholic and alcoholic fatty liver disease. BMC Cancer. 2008;8:200.
56. Kladney RD, et al. GP73, a novel Golgi-localized protein upregulated by viral infection. Gene. 2000;249(1–2):53–65.
57. Kladney RD, et al. Expression of GP73, a resident Golgi membrane protein, in viral and nonviral liver disease. Hepatology. 2002;35(6):1431–40.
58. Iftikhar R, et al. Disease- and cell-specific expression of GP73 in human liver disease. Am J Gastroenterol. 2004;99(6):1087–95.
59. Block TM, et al. Use of targeted glycoproteomics to identify serum glycoproteins that correlate with liver cancer in woodchucks and humans. Proc Natl Acad Sci USA. 2005;102(3):779–84.
60. Marrero JA, et al. GP73, a resident Golgi glycoprotein, is a novel serum marker for hepatocellular carcinoma. J Hepatol. 2005;43(6):1007–12.
61. Wright LM, et al. In gastroenterology & hepatology. Curr Res. 2010;4:1–24.
62. Mao Y, et al. Golgi protein 73 (GOLPH2) is a valuable serum marker for hepatocellular carcinoma. Gut. 2010;59(12):1687–93.
63. Zhao XY, et al. [Detection and evaluation of serum GP73, a resident Golgi glycoprotein, as a marker in diagnosis of hepatocellular carcinoma]. Zhonghua Zhong Liu Za Zhi. 2010;32(12):943–5.
64. Hu JS, et al. GP73, a resident Golgi glycoprotein, is sensibility and specificity for hepatocellular carcinoma of diagnosis in a hepatitis B-endemic Asian population. Med Oncol. 2010;27(2):339–45.
65. Li X, Wu K, Fan D. Serum Golgi Phosphoprotein 2 level: a better marker than alpha-fetoprotein for diagnosing early hepatocellular carcinoma. Hepatology. 2009;50(1):325.
66. Morota K, et al. A comparative evaluation of Golgi protein-73, fucosylated hemopexin, alpha-fetoprotein, and PIVKA-II in the serum of patients with chronic hepatitis, cirrhosis, and hepatocellular carcinoma. Clin Chem Lab Med. 2011;49(4):711–8.
67. Ozkan H, et al. Diagnostic and prognostic validity of Golgi protein 73 in hepatocellular carcinoma. Digestion. 2011;83(1–2):83–8.

68. Yamamoto K, et al. AFP, AFP-L3, DCP, and GP73 as markers for monitoring treatment response and recurrence and as surrogate markers of clinicopathological variables of HCC. J Gastroenterol. 2010;45(12):1272–82.
69. Tian L, et al. Serological AFP/golgi protein 73 could be a new diagnostic parameter of hepatic diseases. Int J Cancer. 2010 Dec 7. PMID: 21140449.
70. Riener MO, et al. Golgi phosphoprotein 2 (GOLPH2) expression in liver tumors and its value as a serum marker in hepatocellular carcinomas. Hepatology. 2009;49(5):1602–9.
71. Gu Y, et al. Quantitative analysis of elevated serum Golgi protein-73 expression in patients with liver diseases. Ann Clin Biochem. 2009;46(Pt 1):38–43.
72. Mise M, et al. Clinical significance of vascular endothelial growth factor and basic fibroblast growth factor gene expression in liver tumor. Hepatology. 1996;23(3):455–64.
73. Li XM, et al. Serum vascular endothelial growth factor is a predictor of invasion and metastasis in hepatocellular carcinoma. J Exp Clin Cancer Res. 1999;18(4):511–7.
74. Leone N, et al. Elevated serum chromogranin A in patients with hepatocellular carcinoma. Clin Exp Med. 2002;2(3):119–23.
75. Giannelli G, et al. SCCA antigen combined with alpha-fetoprotein as serologic markers of HCC. Int J Cancer. 2005;117(3):506–9.
76. Bedossa P, et al. Transforming growth factor-beta 1 (TGF-beta 1) and TGF-beta 1 receptors in normal, cirrhotic, and neoplastic human livers. Hepatology. 1995;21(3):760–6.
77. Yamagamim H, et al. Serum concentrations of human hepatocyte growth factor is a useful indicator for predicting the occurrence of hepatocellular carcinomas in C-viral chronic liver diseases. Cancer. 2002;95(4):824–34.
78. Yoon SK, et al. The human cervical cancer oncogene protein is a biomarker for human hepatocellular carcinoma. Cancer Res. 2004;64(15):5434–41.
79. Tsai JF, et al. Serum insulin-like growth factor-II and alpha-fetoprotein as tumor markers of hepatocellular carcinoma. Tumour Biol. 2003;24(6):291–8.
80. Moriyama M, et al. Detection of serum and intrahepatic KL-6 in anti-HCV positive patients with hepatocellular carcinoma. Hepatol Res. 2004;30(1):24–33.
81. Wright LM, Kreikemeier JT, Fimmel CJ. A concise review of serum markers for hepatocellular cancer. Cancer Detect Prev. 2007;31(1):35–44.
82. Wang Y, et al. Large scale identification of human hepatocellular carcinoma-associated antigens by autoantibodies. J Immunol. 2002;169(2):1102–9.
83. Le Naour F, et al. A distinct repertoire of autoantibodies in hepatocellular carcinoma identified by proteomic analysis. Mol Cell Proteomics. 2002;1(3):197–203.
84. Koziol JA, et al. Recursive partitioning as an approach to selection of immune markers for tumor diagnosis. Clin Cancer Res. 2003;9(14):5120–6.
85. Himoto T, et al. Analyses of autoantibodies against tumor-associated antigens in patients with hepatocellular carcinoma. Int J Oncol. 2005;27(4):1079–85.
86. Zhang JY, et al. De-novo humoral immune responses to cancer-associated autoantigens during transition from chronic liver disease to hepatocellular carcinoma. Clin Exp Immunol. 2001;125(1):3–9.
87. Ulanet DB, et al. Unique conformation of cancer autoantigen B23 in hepatoma: a mechanism for specificity in the autoimmune response. Proc Natl Acad Sci USA. 2003;100(21):12361–6.
88. Chen Y, et al. Autoantibodies to tumor-associated antigens combined with abnormal alpha-fetoprotein enhance immunodiagnosis of hepatocellular carcinoma. Cancer Lett. 2010;289(1):32–9.
89. Poon TC, et al. Comprehensive proteomic profiling identifies serum proteomic signatures for detection of hepatocellular carcinoma and its subtypes. Clin Chem. 2003;49(5):752–60.
90. Schwegler EE, et al. SELDI-TOF MS profiling of serum for detection of the progression of chronic hepatitis C to hepatocellular carcinoma. Hepatology. 2005;41(3):634–42.
91. Paradis V, et al. Identification of a new marker of hepatocellular carcinoma by serum protein profiling of patients with chronic liver diseases. Hepatology. 2005;41(1):40–7.
92. Comunale MA, et al. Identification and development of fucosylated glycoproteins as biomarkers of primary hepatocellular carcinoma. J Proteome Res. 2009;8(2):595–602.

93. Wang M, et al. Novel fucosylated biomarkers for the early detection of hepatocellular carcinoma. Cancer Epidemiol Biomarkers Prev. 2009;18(6):1914–21.

94. Tang J, et al. Concanavalin A-immobilized magnetic nanoparticles for selective enrichment of glycoproteins and application to glycoproteomics in hepatocellular carcinoma cell line. Proteomics. 2010;10(10):2000–14.

95. Bartel DP. MicroRNAs: genomics, biogenesis, mechanism, and function. Cell. 2004;116(2): 281–97.

96. Lewis BP, et al. Prediction of mammalian microRNA targets. Cell. 2003;115(7):787–98.

97. Chen CZ. MicroRNAs as oncogenes and tumor suppressors. N Engl J Med. 2005; 353(17):1768–71.

98. Ji J, et al. MicroRNA expression, survival, and response to interferon in liver cancer. N Engl J Med. 2009;361(15):1437–47.

99. Toffanin S, et al. MicroRNA-based classification of hepatocellular carcinoma and oncogenic role of miR-517a. Gastroenterology. 2011;140(5):1618–28. e16.

100. Meng F, et al. MicroRNA-21 regulates expression of the PTEN tumor suppressor gene in human hepatocellular cancer. Gastroenterology. 2007;133(2):647–58.

101. Pineau P, et al. miR-221 overexpression contributes to liver tumorigenesis. Proc Natl Acad Sci USA. 2010;107(1):264–9.

102. Ding J, et al. Gain of miR-151 on chromosome 8q24.3 facilitates tumour cell migration and spreading through downregulating RhoGDIA. Nat Cell Biol. 2010;12(4):390–9.

103. Viswanathan SR, et al. Lin28 promotes transformation and is associated with advanced human malignancies. Nat Genet. 2009;41(7):843–8.

104. Xiong Y, et al. Effects of microRNA-29 on apoptosis, tumorigenicity, and prognosis of hepatocellular carcinoma. Hepatology. 2010;51(3):836–45.

105. Coulouarn C, et al. Loss of miR-122 expression in liver cancer correlates with suppression of the hepatic phenotype and gain of metastatic properties. Oncogene. 2009;28(40):3526–36.

106. Li LM, et al. Serum microRNA profiles serve as novel biomarkers for HBV infection and diagnosis of HBV-positive hepatocarcinoma. Cancer Res. 2010;70(23):9798–807.

107. Qu KZ, et al. Circulating microRNAs as biomarkers for hepatocellular carcinoma. J Clin Gastroenterol. 2011;45(4):355–60.

108. Xu J, et al. Circulating microRNAs, miR-21, miR-122, and miR-223, in patients with hepatocellular carcinoma or chronic hepatitis. Mol Carcinog. 2011;50(2):136–42.

109. Rhea JM, Molinaro RJ. Cancer biomarkers: surviving the journey from bench to bedside. MLO Med Lab Obs. 2011;43(3):10–2. 16, 18; quiz 20, 22.

110. Diamandis EP. Cancer biomarkers: can we turn recent failures into success? J Natl Cancer Inst. 2010;102(19):1462–7.

111. Polanski M, Anderson NL. A list of candidate cancer biomarkers for targeted proteomics. Biomark Insights. 2007;1:1–48.

Chapter 14
Emerging Therapies for Hepatocellular Carcinoma

Renumathy Dhanasekaran and Roniel Cabrera

Introduction

Hepatocellular carcinoma (HCC) is a global health problem due to its increasing incidence and high lethality [1]. In fact, HCC is the third most common cause of cancer deaths and the leading complication in patients with cirrhosis [2]. The rising incidence poses challenges to the clinician since the majority of patients present with advanced disease when they are no longer candidates for a definitive cure. Further, the coexistence of cirrhosis and HCC adds two competing causes of death, each one critical to consider since both influence management. Unfortunately, only 5–37% of HCC patients are actually eligible for curative treatments with orthotopic liver transplantation (LT) or surgical resection [3, 4]. When curative treatments are no longer options due to advanced-stage disease, the treatment options are limited. However, we have had some recent advances in the treatment of unresectable HCC with the advent of novel locoregional and targeted systemic therapy [5–7]. The clinical success of the oral multikinase inhibitor sorafenib, showing a survival benefit in the management of advanced HCC, has opened the floodgates of research in the field of molecular-targeted therapies for HCC. These recent advances in treatment, along with surveillance programs, will lead to improved overall survival for our patients with HCC [8]. In this chapter, we review the major recent advancements and emerging therapies being evaluated for the treatment of HCC.

R. Dhanasekaran, MD
Department of Medicine, University of Florida, Gainsville, FL, USA

R. Cabrera, MD, MS (✉)
Division of Gastroenterology, Hepatology and Nutrition, Section of Hepatobiliary Diseases,
University of Florida, Gainsville, FL, USA
e-mail: cabrer@medicine.ufl.edu

N. Reau and F.F. Poordad (eds.), *Primary Liver Cancer: Surveillance, Diagnosis and Treatment*, Clinical Gastroenterology, DOI 10.1007/978-1-61779-863-4_14,
© Springer Science+Business Media New York 2012

Table 14.1 BCLC staging

	Performance status	Tumor burden	Liver function
Stage A			
A1	0	Single <5 cm	No PHT
A2	0	Single <5 cm	PHT, normal bilirubin
A3	0	Single <5 cm	PHT, elevated bilirubin
A4	0	Up to 3, <3 cm	Child class A–B
Stage B	0	Large multinodular	Child class A–B
Stage C	1–2	Vascular invasion or extrahepatic disease	Child class A–B
Stage D	3–4	Any	Child class C

Stages of HCC

HCC is more complex than most solid malignancies. HCC typically arises in a liver with cirrhosis, and the coexistence of these two conditions—cirrhosis and tumor—along with the patient performance status independently influence prognosis and eligibility for the different treatment modalities [9]. For these reasons, any staging system for HCC has to take into account these prognostic factors such as the extent of tumor burden, the degree of hepatic dysfunction, and the performance status of the patient. A number of staging systems have been proposed like Okuda, CLIP (Cancer of the Liver Italian Program), and AJCC (American Joint Committee on Cancer). However, the staging system that has emerged as the most clinically useful is the BCLC (Barcelona-Clinic Liver Cancer) staging classification by linking stage with treatment algorithms (Table 14.1). The BCLC has been independently validated by US and European studies and is also endorsed by major liver societies such as EASL and AASLD (American Association for the Study of Liver Diseases). Further, the staging system is currently a critical element to stage and stratify patients for clinical trials. In this review, we will discuss the various emerging therapies in the context of the BCLC staging classification (Table 14.2).

Early Stage of HCC

The current treatment strategy for early-stage HCC involves surgical resection, LT, or ablation depending on the eligibility criteria. In general, patients with preserved liver function who do not have portal hypertension undergo surgical resection. If there is portal hypertension alone or with liver dysfunction, due to a significant risk of poor outcome with resection, LT is the treatment of choice. If they are not eligible for resection or LT, then ablation techniques like radiofrequency ablation (RFA) are used. Some of the recent advances in the management of early-stage HCC include laparoscopic resection, adjuvant therapy to prevent recurrence after resection, pre-LT bridging locoregional therapy, and newer ablation techniques.

Table 14.2 Emerging therapies and future challenges based on stage of tumor

Stage of tumor	Group characteristics	Established therapy	Emerging therapy	Future challenges
Early stage	• Single tumor<5 cm or 2–3 tumors each <3 cm • ECOG performance status 0 • Child–Pugh class A–B	• No portal hypertension-resection • Portal hypertension-transplantation • Ineligible for surgery—PEI, RFA	Resection • Laparoscopic resection • Preventing recurrence-TACE, immunotherapy, retinoin, interferon Transplantation • Expansion of criteria • Pre transplant TACE • Molecular profiling Ablation therapy • Newer modalities (IRE, Microwave) • Combination therapy (with TACE, with Sorafenib)	Resection • Resect larger tumors • Predict recurrence • Prevent recurrence • Decrease morbidity/mortality • Transplant advanced stages • Keep people on the list longer • Downstage tumors with TACE • Predict recurrence • Predict/prevent recurrence • Improve outcome with adjuvant therapy
Intermediate stage	• Multinodular tumor beyond Milan criteria • ECOG PS 0 • No vascular invasion • No extrahepatic spread	Chemoembolization	• Drug-eluting beads • Y-90 radioembolization • Combination sorafenib + TACE • Sorafenib alone • Image-guided nanoembolization	• Improve efficacy • Combining approaches to improve outcome • Chemo vs. radioembolization • Role for sorafenib
Advanced stage	• ECOG PS 1-2 • Portal invasion • N1,M1	Sorafenib	Drugs with molecular targets like • Bevacizumab • Sunitinib • Brivanib • Erlotinib	• New drug better than sorafenib • Molecular profiling of tumors • Combination chemotherapy

Resection

Surgical resection is the treatment of choice for early HCC without portal hypertension, which can result in a 5-year survival rate of up to 50% [10]. Resection can be associated with high morbidity and a complicated postoperative course, particularly in patients with underlying cirrhosis. This increased risk has sparked interests in less invasive approaches like laparoscopic resection.

Laparoscopic Resection

The safety and feasibility of laparoscopic resection in appropriately selected patients is being increasingly reported in the literature [11–15]. A recent cohort experience with minimally invasive surgery for hepatic tumors that included 210 patients with HCC demonstrated excellent interim survival rates and lower local recurrence rates when compared to RFA alone [16]. Another single-center series reported shorter average length of hospital stay and improved postoperative quality of life among patients who received laparoscopic resection [17]. However, this study did not directly compare the two groups for survival or recurrence rates. In a study that directly compared laparoscopic and open resection, there was no difference in the postoperative 2-year survival between the two treatments [18]. However, the mean hospital stay and postoperative complication rates were lower with laparoscopic resection. Apart from the lower postoperative complications associated with laparoscopic resection, another attractive aspect of this approach is the ability to spare abdominal collateral venous circulation and avoidance of peritoneal adhesions [15]. If hepatic recurrence occurs, then these aspects have a major advantage during the potential repeat operations or salvage transplantation. Despite several reports on the safety and feasibility of laparoscopic resection, robust data on long-term survival are scant, with most studies being retrospective and nonrandomized. As the clinical experience grows, laparoscopic resection could potentially play a larger role in patients with early HCC.

Resection as Bridge to Transplant

Recent studies have suggested a role for resection as a bridge to LT [19, 20]. Given the worsening shortage of available donors and the progressively increasing waiting list time on the LT list, this strategy might become a reality in patients with early HCC. This approach proposes resection as a bridge treatment to prevent tumor progression during the waiting period and to further consider only the patients who develop recurrence for salvage transplantation. Belghiti et al. compared patients who underwent primary LT vs. patients who underwent LT after resection and found that the post-LT survival rates were similar—5-year survival of 59% vs. 61%. But the decision to resect patients with potentially transplantable disease is a difficult one. The potential risks for decompensation of hepatic function after resection and the fact that transplant surgery will be more challenging in a patient who has already undergone a resection does raise concerns regarding this approach. These concerns have been communicated in a study by Adam et al. that reported that transplantation after bridging liver resection was associated with a higher operative mortality, an increased risk of recurrence, and a poorer outcome when compared to primary LT [21]. Given the current evidence, using resection as a bridge to transplantation remains a gray area in the management of early-stage HCC, but it may potentially play a significant role if future studies show more encouraging results.

Recurrence After Resection

The most common complication of resection is recurrence. Recurrence is the main cause of death and can exceed 70% at 5 years [10, 22, 23]. Most of the recurrences are from intrahepatic dissemination of primary lesion (60–70%) and less commonly from de novo (metachronous) tumors (30–40%). Such high recurrence rates are the major drawbacks of surgical resection, particularly in patients with cirrhosis. Presently, therapeutic strategies to prevent and treat recurrence are limited.

If the tumor recurs and the tumor burden is within the Milan criteria, then salvage LT has been reported as a potential therapeutic strategy [24, 25]. Poon et al. reported that when recurrence occurs after resection in early HCC, up to 79% of patients were within the Milan criteria and hence eligible for LT [20]. A number of strategies to prevent recurrence have been studies including alpha interferon, adoptive immunotherapy, peretinoin, and thalidomide therapy [26–29]. However, none of these treatments to date have shown increased survival for HCC and only limited evidence to suggest improvement in disease-free survival [30].

Options for adjuvant therapy in HCC are very limited, and clinical trial results have been disappointing. Currently, we have no adjuvant therapy available for early HCC. New research evaluating adjuvant therapy in HCC using a xenograft animal model of HCC showed sorafenib was effective in suppressing postsurgical HCC recurrence and abdominal metastasis [31]. These findings in animal models of HCC along with the proven clinical benefit of sorafenib in advanced HCC have paved the way for the STORM trial [32]. This trial is an ongoing phase III, randomized, double-blind, placebo-controlled trial of adjuvant sorafenib in early HCC patients who have undergone surgical resection or local ablation with the goal to prevent recurrence. The results of the STORM trial are eagerly awaited given the recent finding with anti-VEGF therapy not showing a survival benefit in the adjuvant setting in colorectal cancer, despite its efficacy in metastatic colorectal disease [33].

Transplantation

LT is considered the best curative option for HCC since it offers a solution for both the cancer and the underlying cirrhosis. But each transplantation entails significant resource utilization, and supply-to-demand ratio is currently unfavorable due to the limited availability of donor organs [34]. Given this, currently, LT is reserved only for patients with early-stage HCC that satisfy the Milan criteria—no evidence of extrahepatic tumor and unifocal tumor mass ≤5 cm in diameter or multifocal tumors ≤3 in number (each one ≤3 cm in diameter) [35]. LT for HCC within the Milan criteria is associated with a 5-year survival rate of ≥70% and a low tumor recurrence rate of <15%. The rationale behind implementing these restrictive criteria is to achieve comparable post-transplant outcomes between patients with cirrhosis without HCC and cirrhosis with HCC. Recently, a national conference reviewed the existing literature on the policy of increased priority for candidates with early-stage HCC on the transplant waiting list in the USA and the treatments received [36]. After examining the existing literature, a consensus recommendation was made that there should be no change in the current national policy regarding HCC criteria and simultaneously encouraged regional agreements to explore expanding the Milan criteria.

Expansion Beyond Milan Criteria

The increasing demand for LT is causing a growing interest in expanding the transplant criteria [37 40]. However, the potential downside with this approach is that the post-LT outcomes can worsen as the criteria are made more liberal. The idea of expanding the criteria has been compared to the European Metro system and has been called the "Metro ticket" concept, with the possibility that "the further the distance, the greater the price." Mazzaferro et al. analyzed data on patients who underwent transplantation for HCC with tumor burden exceeding Milan criteria in a multicenter study [41]. Of the 1,556 patients studied, 1,112 (71.4%) patients had HCC exceeding Milan criteria on explant pathology. These patients had a 5-year overall survival of 53.6%, while those who met the criteria had a 5-year survival of 73.3%. They were able to calculate hazard ratios for survival based on morphological and biological characteristics of the tumor-like size of the nodules, size of the largest nodule, and presence of vascular invasion. Based on this study, a "metroticket calculator" was developed and made available online which will give an estimation of post-LT survival on entering data regarding tumor characteristics (http://www. hcc-olt-metroticket.org/).

The transplant center at UCSF (University of California, San Francisco) suggested an expansion of transplant criteria to include solitary tumor ≤6.5 cm, or ≤3 nodules with the largest lesion ≤4.5 cm and total tumor diameter ≤8 cm (UCSF criteria). Yao et al. initially reported that patients with HCC meeting the UCSF criteria had excellent survival rates of 90% at 1 year and 75.2% at 5 years [38]. These criteria were later independently validated in a study by Duffy et al. who reported a 22-year single-center experience from UCLA. They showed that patients meeting Milan criteria had similar 5-year posttransplant survival to patients meeting UCSF criteria by preoperative imaging (79% vs. 64%; $P=0.061$) and explant pathology [42]. Another set of criteria from the Pittsburgh Medical Center involves classification into six different stages (I, II, IIIA, IIIB, IVA, and IVB) based on vascular invasion, lobar distribution, size of the largest nodule, lymph node status, and metastatic disease [43]. Chen et al. suggested that since these criteria provided more accurate prognostic classification, it would be reasonable to combine these with the Milan criteria for recipient selection [44]. A further study comparing the Milan, UCSF, and UPMC criteria found that the UCSF criteria better predicted post-LT outcome than the Milan criteria [45]. The investigators also concluded that the Pittsburgh criteria were at a disadvantage since it required information on microvascular invasion which is difficult to ascertain preoperatively without a biopsy. Since biopsies are not routinely performed and most clinicians only have imaging data prior to listing, Toso et al. proposed using total tumor volume assessed radiologically as criteria for LT listing [46]. In this study, tumor volume criteria enhanced the accuracy of pretransplant radiological assessment without worsening post-LT outcomes when compared to Milan and UCSF classifications, despite broadening the inclusion criteria.

But the safety of expanding the Milan criteria has not been established. An intention-to-treat analysis of LT for HCC using organ procurement transplant network (OPTN) data showed worse post-LT survival if tumor burden exceeded the Milan criteria [47]. Overall, there has been no consensus on the expansion of criteria for recipient selection. Lack of robust supporting data, requirement of pathologic data which are unavailable preoperatively, and current limitations of imaging studies all argue against presently expanding criteria.

Downstaging Tumors

Given the current strict adherence to Milan criteria, another approach that groups have used to increase availability of transplantation is to downstage tumors using pre-LT locoregional therapies [48–50]. Most of these studies involve small number of patients or are designed poorly. Yao et al. conducted the first prospective study to examine the effect of downstaging tumors prior to LT [51]. Among the 30 patients enrolled, 70% met criteria for successful downstaging. Over a follow-up period of 16 months, no post-LT recurrences were reported in those downstaged. This study did demonstrate the feasibility of downstaging, but the follow-up duration was not long enough for meaningful conclusions regarding survival and recurrence.

Pretransplant Locoregional Therapy

In the year 2006 alone, 746 patients with a diagnosis of HCC were placed on the liver transplant waiting list in the USA, and the dropout rate among them was significant, at 272 per 1,000 patient years [52]. Hence, several centers routinely use pre-LT bridging locoregional therapies to maintain the tumor burden within Milan criteria in patients on the transplant list in order to prevent dropouts. But the potential of these procedures to worsen liver function does raise questions regarding the justification for their use, and the concern that treatments may be translating tumors with aggressive biology into recurrences remains. Studies have actually not shown a survival benefit in employing these interventions [53, 54]. In a recent study from our center examining the role of pre-LT TACE in patients with hepatitis C-related-HCC, we similarly found that it had no benefit on post-transplant survival or tumor recurrence [55]. But few studies have demonstrated the efficacy of pre-LT TACE in preventing tumor progression and hence decreasing dropout rates from the transplant list [56, 57]. Based on this, current guidelines recommend the use of locoregional therapy for bridging to transplant only if the anticipated time on the waiting list is longer than 6 months [58]. Newer approaches to maintain tumor burden with the adjuvant use of sorafenib are also being explored. HeiLivCa (Heidelberg Liver Cancer Study) is an ongoing phase III randomized, double-blind, multicenter study on using sorafenib in patients with HCC on the transplant list. The lack of robust data due to insurmountable variables like controlling for the various wait times across regions and the various modalities that vary across centers come in the way recommending a broader role for pre-LT locoregional therapy.

Tumor Ablation

Percutaneous ablation offers the best treatment option for patients with early-stage HCC who are not eligible for resection or LT. Radiofrequency ablation (RFA) and percutaneous ethanol injection (PEI) are the two most commonly employed ablative techniques. RFA was shown to be superior to PEI in a recent meta-analysis and randomized comparison in terms of local disease control, recurrence-free survival, and survival [59, 60]. Hence, RFA is currently the first-line therapy employed in this patient group. However, RFA has significant associated adverse events like pain, intraperitoneal bleeding, tumor seeding, hepatic abscess formation, bile duct injury, and hepatic decompensation. Further, RFA also has limitations in terms of tumor location where it may be contraindicated in certain areas of the liver due to the potential damage to adjacent tissues and loss of efficacy due to large blood vessels causing the heat-sink phenomena. For these reasons, newer and improved ablation techniques are being investigated.

A new technique for local ablation is using microwave technology and producing thermal coagulation of tissues with the use of microwaves to induce an ultrahigh-speed alternating electric field. Most of the literature using microwave ablation is from Japan. A recent study reviewed all the literature on microwave ablation for HCC from 1990 to 2007 [61]. Microwave ablation was reported to have several advantages, including high thermal efficiency, higher capability of coagulating blood vessels, and faster ablation times while having a reasonable safety profile. Further studies are needed to determine its potential applicability and incorporation into current treatment paradigms for early HCC.

Irreversible electroporation (IRE, Angiodynamics) is another new tissue ablation technique in which micro- to millisecond electrical pulses are delivered to cancer tissue leading to necrosis through irreversible cell membrane permeabilization.

The advantages of this technique over RFA include its potential to spare adjacent vasculature, lack of detrimental effects on surrounding architecture, and the ability to control and monitor the affected area with electrical impedance tomography [62]. Animal studies have confirmed the feasibility and efficacy of this technique in the treatment of HCC [63]. There are concerns regarding potential cardiac arrhythmias with the use of electrical pulses, and synchronization of the treatment delivery with the refractory period of the cardiac cycle has been advised. Currently, IRE is being evaluated for the treatment of early HCC by a prospective multicenter clinical trial. The results of this study can hopefully pave the way for a wider use of this technology.

New drug delivery methods with exciting potential in oncology include tumor-targeted nanomedicine. ThermoDox (Celsion) is a temperature-sensitive version of liposomal doxorubicin, which after intravenous administration rapidly releases the drug upon heating. Employing RFA along with ThermoDox should lead to targeted release of the drug into the tumor, thus improving local tumor control by leading to enhanced necrosis. Results of phase I study of ThermoDox on HCC established its safety in patients undergoing RFA for HCC, and Celsion has been granted FDA (Food and Drug Administration) Orphan Drug designation. A phase III multicenter trial, ThermoDox® clinical study (HEAT Study), is currently under way [64]. Recently, data from 294 patients enrolled were reviewed by the Data Monitoring Committee, which provided continued support for the phase III study.

Intermediate-Stage HCC

The liver has a dual blood supply from the hepatic artery and portal vein, which normally is mainly from the portal vein. During the development and progression of HCC, the blood supply to the tumor becomes increasingly arterialized while the nontumorous liver retains its predominant portal venous supply. The dual blood supply of the liver and arterialization of HCC provides the rationale for the use of transarterial chemoembolization (TACE) as a treatment for HCC. TACE is recommended as the standard of care for patients with multinodular HCC that have progressed beyond curative treatments with resection and transplantation. Two randomized controlled trials demonstrated the benefit of TACE over supportive care in patients with unresectable, multifocal HCC with adequate liver function compatible with Child A cirrhosis, absence of extrahepatic disease or vascular invasion, and a lack of cancer-related symptoms. These studies and subsequent meta-analysis which show improvement in the 3-year survival rates (from 10% to 40–50%) and the median survival (from 16 to 20 months) have established TACE as standard practice for asymptomatic multinodular HCC [65–68]. From these studies, we learn that the optimal candidates for TACE are patients with Child A cirrhosis and multifocal noninvasive HCC with an excellent performance status. Thus, the main contraindications for TACE are decompensated Child B or C cirrhosis, portal vein invasion, or thrombosis since treatment increases the risk of liver failure. However, other investigators have found no notable increase in TACE-related complications and similar treatment-related benefits in HCC patients with portal vein thrombosis using highly selective TACE [69].

Conventional TACE

The procedure of TACE contains a number of variables that are applied in a hetero-geneous manner across centers. These variables include the type of anticancer drugs and dose, the use of Lipiodol, the choice of embolic agent, delivery, timing, selectivity, the treatment schedule (on demand based on residual tumor enhancement or fixed schedule), and whether embolization is done to complete or near stasis. An important point to recognize is that all these variables have the potential to lead to different outcomes, and the optimal treatment strategy with respect to all these variable remains to be determined. Typically, conventional TACE involves administering chemotherapeutic agents such as doxorubicin, cisplatin, or epirubicin mixed with iodized poppy seed oil (Lipiodol) directly into the arteries that supply the tumor. The blood flow to the supplying artery is then blocked off with embolization. The embolization can be achieved with various agents such as gelfoam, polyvinyl alcohol, or microspheres. Thus, TACE achieves tumor necrosis both by the ensuing ischemia and by the anticancer effect of the drugs. But TACE offers only a moderate survival benefit in intermediate HCC and can lead to decompensation of the liver function. The future challenges with TACE include identifying methods to improve efficacy and consistency of the procedure while minimizing adverse effects.

TACE with Drug-Eluting Beads

A new strategy in the way TACE is performed with unique properties is the drug-eluting beads (Precision TACE or LC/DC bead™ TACE, Biocompatibles, UK). These LC beads are made of a polyvinyl alcohol monomer that has been modified with negatively charged sulfonate groups. The negatively charged deformable beads allow them to absorb positively charged chemotherapeutic agents such as doxorubicin when they are mixed together. The beads absorb a predictable concentration of the doxorubicin and upon reaching the tumor, vascular bed slowly releases the drug [70–72]. This strategy ensures local controlled delivery and high intratumoral retention of doxorubicin in a predictable fashion with minimal systemic toxicity. The simultaneous release of drug with induction of ischemia as the intra-arterially delivered beads embolize the tumor allows the technique to be performed in a more homogenous and reproducible manner.

The initial clinical experience with LC bead TACE in single-arm phase II studies reported rates of objective responses that ranged between 66% and 85% with a 1-year survival of 92–97% and a 2-year survival of 88–91%, with a sharp reduction in chemotherapy-related systemic side effects [72–74]. Further, the development of biliary abscess in the initial study was not observed in the two subsequent cohort studies. The efficacy and safety of LC bead TACE was directly compared with conventional TACE in a randomized phase II trial called the PRECISION V study with a total of 212 patients [75]. The LC bead group showed higher rates of complete response, objective response, and disease control compared with the conventional TACE group. But there was no significant difference in the primary endpoint of 6-month tumor response as assessed by EASL criteria (LC bead 63% vs. conventional TACE 52%; $P = 0.11$). However, drug-eluting beads were associated with improved tolerability marked by significant reduction in doxorubicin-related side effects and serious liver toxicity. In addition, patients with more advanced characteristics (Child B cirrhosis, worse performance status, bilobar disease) demonstrated significantly higher tumor response rates with LC bead TACE with improved safety. Thus, given that the current AASLD guidelines do not recommend chemoembolization for Child B cirrhosis, these findings suggest that LC bead TACE can be safely used in these patients. A subsequent observational study also demonstrated a survival benefit of drug-eluting beads over conventional TACE [76]. To clarify and confirm the clinical benefits of one treatment over another, a phase III randomized controlled trial is needed. In the meantime, new modes of drug delivery will continue development. Recent examples are hepaspheres (HepaSphere™ Microspheres, Merit Medical Systems, Utah, USA) which are superabsorbent polymer microspheres undergoing early-stage evaluation [77].

Radioembolization

Another new technique for treating HCC is transarterial brachytherapy or transarterial radioembolization (TARE). TARE involves hepatic arterial injection of yttrium-90 microspheres (Y-90) that is available as glass (TheraSpheres, MDS Nordion) or resin (Sirtex, Sirtex Medical) and can be delivered to single or multiple segments based on selective arterial cannulation. In contrast to the drug-eluting beads, Y-90 microspheres are smaller measuring 20–60 µm in size. While chemoembolization leads to tumor ischemia with undesired angiogenesis that can lead to tumor progression, the small size of Y-90 microspheres results in preferential trapping in the tumor capillary bed with little macroembolic effect that does not result in significant angiogenesis. These spheres can safely deliver up to 150 Gy of β-radiation to induce tumor necrosis by radiation and microscopic embolization once they obstruct in the tumor capillary bed. Their trapping in the tumor capillary bed limits radiation exposure to adjacent healthy tissue given its radius of action of up to 1 cm and half-life of 62 h [78]. Further advantages of Y-90 microspheres over TACE are its applicability in patients with portal vein thrombosis due to lack of a macroembolic effect, and it also eliminates the adverse effects of chemotherapeutic drugs and the need for post-procedure hospitalization [79]. A critical aspect of treatment with Y-90 microspheres is the need for pretreatment evaluation to clearly define aberrant vascular anatomy with angiogram to perform prophylactic embolization. One of the serious complications of radioembolization is the potential development of severe gastroduodenal ulcerations. To minimize the incidence of this adverse outcome, it is required to selectively block the gastroduodenal artery with metal coils prophylactically prior to the actual radioembolization. Though this approach has been successful, it does potentially complicate the cost and logistics of performing this procedure. Pretreatment procedures should also include a macroaggregated albumin (MAA) scan to confirm that hepatic-artery-to-lung shunting is <16% to prevent lung injury [80]. Additional nontarget delivery of Y-90 radiation can cause pancreatitis, pneumonitis, and cholecystitis.

Presently, our current clinical experience for the use of Y-90 microspheres in HCC lacks controlled data directly comparing TARE to TACE and comes largely from uncontrolled, single-center experiences. One of the largest single-center, longitudinal cohort experience using Y-90 microspheres (TheraSpheres, MDS Nordion) included nearly 300 HCC patients with the majority having multifocal disease (73%) and with a large percentage having portal vein thrombosis (43%) [81]. This series reported an overall time to progression of 7.9 months and an overall tumor response rate of 57% by EASL criteria. As expected, the survival differed significantly by the dual competing risks of HCC stage and Child–Pugh status. Patients with Child A cirrhosis and intermediate-stage (BCLC B) HCC benefited the most with a median survival of 17.2 months, while patients with Child B cirrhosis had the worse outcomes with a median survival of 7.7 months. The most common treatment-related adverse effects were fatigue, vague abdominal pain, and nausea/vomiting. Another recent study from the same group retrospectively compared Y-90 ($n=122$) with chemoembolization ($n=123$) and showed statistically similar survival (20.5 months vs. 17.4 months, $P=0.23$) [82]. But Y-90 radioembolization resulted in longer time to progression and was associated with less toxicity than chemoembolization. One of the limitations of this study is their comparison of Y-90 to conventional TACE which is a Lipiodol-based embolization and is known to be associated with more adverse effects than the currently preferred drug-eluting LC bead TACE [75]. In this study, the authors clearly communicate the major barriers of a randomized trial comparing TARE vs. TACE to determine which intervention is superior. One of the main concerns over such a study is that the number of patients needed based on power calculation to demonstrate equivalency between TACE and TARE treatments in intermediate-stage HCC is a sample size of more than 1,000 patients [83].

As Y-90 treatment moves from initial investigations to larger, multicenter series, it continues to show consistent data and thus a lot of promise as a treatment in HCC. In light of the lack of options for treatment, Y-90 does have a role in the treatment of HCC. Patients with HCC and portal vein thrombosis are a challenging subgroup to treat since their hepatic blood flow is already significantly compromised. TARE has been reported to be a relatively safe option to attain disease control in this population [79, 84]. However, prior to full integration into the current treatment paradigms and acceptance into the BCLC staging classification, Y-90 needs further study with randomized trials directly comparing its use to current standards or used in combination with current treatments.

Combination TACE and Sorafenib

HCC is a highly vascular tumor, and tumor angioneogenesis plays a significant role in its progression. The hypoxia and tumor ischemia resulting from chemoembolization have been shown to significantly increase proangiogenic growth factors such as VEGF that induce angiogenesis in the peripheral parts of the tumor, thereby offsetting the desired antitumor effects of TACE [85]. These proangiogenic factors are targeted by systemic targeted therapies like sorafenib. In addition, in a phase II study, when sorafenib was combined with doxorubicin, a greater antitumor activity and overall survival (13.7 months for sorafenib plus doxorubicin vs. 6.5 months for doxorubicin and placebo) were observed suggesting synergy when these two agents are combined [86]. These findings form the basis behind combining locoregional therapy like TACE with doxorubicin and systemic antiangiogenic drugs like sorafenib. Thus, the rationale for administering sorafenib without pause during treatment with TACE is to prevent tumor growth in response to increased levels of VEGF as a result of the hypoxia elicited by TACE.

Our center has examined the safety, tolerance, and efficacy of combining TACE and sorafenib with a protocol that uses concomitant TACE with doxorubicin-eluting beads and sorafenib [87]. In this protocol, sorafenib is administered continuously without stopping as the patients undergo TACE. Our results show the combination to be tolerable but with a high rate of adverse events similar to when sorafenib is used alone. In addition, the combination did not adversely affect the ability to perform TACE. Further, this initial clinical experience with combination yielded encouraging efficacy results with a disease control rate of 68% and overall median survival of 18.5 months given that 20% of the 47 patients had stage C HCC and Child–Pugh B cirrhosis. Additional single-arm studies have presented interim results in abstract form using the combination of TACE and sorafenib and also show early promise for this novel approach. [88], [89–91]. In particular, one of these early studies showed that sorafenib is able to prevent an increase in the circulating levels of this growth factor in response to TACE and may therefore prevent tumor growth after TACE, which may translate into greater survival benefits than with TACE monotherapy. Currently, this combination regimen of TACE specifically with doxorubicin-eluting beads and sorafenib is undergoing evaluation as part of a multinational, randomized, double-blind, placebo-controlled study (SPACE). The SPACE study evaluates the combination TACE and sorafenib for intermediate-stage HCC with Child–Pugh A cirrhosis [75]. While the preliminary results of this approach are promising, if the current research with a randomized design confirms these results, combination TACE-sorafenib could become incorporated into clinical practice. Apart from sorafenib, bevacizumab, another antiangiogenic VEGF inhibitor, has also been studied in a single-arm study in combination with TACE [92]. Results from this early experience demonstrated a 100% disease control rate and a median overall survival of 13.5 months, but deaths from gastrointestinal bleeding were reported in this abstract presentation raising safety concern for this particular combination.

Advanced-Stage HCC

Even with current screening and surveillance strategies, a majority of patients with HCC continue to be diagnosed at an advanced stage. The management of advanced HCC is a challenge to clinicians since these patients have limited options since they are not eligible for resection, transplantation, ablation, or TACE. A major advancement in the management of advanced HCC has been the clinical development of the oral multikinase inhibitor sorafenib. The evaluation of sorafenib in two pivotal studies—SHARP and Asian Pacific trials—showing a consistent survival benefit led to the regulatory approval of sorafenib as the first systemic treatment in advanced HCC [93, 94]. This approval has ushered in a new era of research in molecular-targeted therapy for HCC. The clinical success of sorafenib showed that targeting signaling pathways involved in HCC using molecular therapies are rational new treatment options deserving continued development [95]. While our knowledge of the molecular pathways driving the progression of HCC continues to evolve, a number of potential targets have been identified. The pathways identified as potential targets include the tyrosine kinase receptor EGFR, RAS/MAPK, PI3K-Akt-mTOR, angiogenesis inhibitors, enhancing apoptosis, and telomerase inhibitors. More than a dozen drugs are under evaluation at various phases of clinical development. Several targeted agents are in different phases of clinical development such as EGFR inhibitors (erlotinib, cetuximab, lapatinib), VEGF/VEGFR inhibitors (bevacizumab, vandetanib, AZD2171, sunitinib), Ras/Raf/MEK inhibitors (lonafarnib, AZD6244), PI3K/Akt/mTOR/PTEN inhibitors (sirolimus, everolimus), apoptosis inducers (mapatumumab), proteasome inhibitors (bortezomib), and HDAC inhibitors (LBH589, vorinostat). An overview of these emerging molecular agents is discussed below. Tables 14.3 and 14.4 summarize the clinical trials further along with development for advanced HCC.

Molecular Targets for HCC

Sorafenib

Sorafenib (Nexavar, Bayer and Onyx) is a multitargeted receptor tyrosine kinase inhibitor (TKI) that blocks tumor cell proliferation by targeting the Raf/MEK/ERK signaling pathway and exerts an antiangiogenic effect by targeting the receptor kinases of vascular endothelial growth factor receptor (VEGFR)-2, VEGFR-3, and platelet-derived growth factor receptor-beta (PDGFR-beta). In addition, recent studies show that sorafenib may have other beneficial mechanisms of action by influencing regulatory immune pathways involved in tumor immunity such as myeloid-derived suppressor cells and effector T-lymphocyte responses. The clinical success and approval of sorafenib monotherapy for advanced HCC has created a strong interest to evaluate for possible synergy by combining sorafenib with other chemotherapeutic agents.

Table 14.3 Phase II trials on molecular targeted therapies for HCC

Drug	Company	Study (year)	N	Design	Overall survival	Toxicity profile
Multikinase inhibitors						
Sorafenib + doxorubicin	Bayer	Abou-Alfa et al. (2008) [97]	96	Phase II randomized, double blind	13.7 months Sor+D and 6.5 months for D	Toxicity profiles were similar to those for the single agents
Sunitinib	Pfizer	Zhu et al. (2009) [108]	34	Phase II, two stage	9.8 months	Leukopenia/neutropenia, thrombocytopenia, elevation of aminotransferases, and fatigue
Sunitinib	Pfizer	Faivre et al. (2009) [110]	37	Phase II, open label, two stage	Pronounced toxicities and low response rate	Four deaths (10.8%)
VEGF inhibitors						
Bevacizumab	Genentech	Siegel et al. (2008) [104]	46	Phase II, single arm	3-year survival 23%.	Grade 3 or higher hemorrhage occurred in 11% of patients
Bevacizumab + gemcitabine + oxaliplatin	Genentech	Zhu et al. (2006) [105]	33	Phase II, single arm	9.6 months	Leukopenia/neutropenia, transient elevation of aminotransferases, hypertension, and fatigue
Bevacizumab + erlotinib	Genentech	Thomas et al. (2009) [106]	40	Phase II, single arm	15.65 months	Fatigue ($n=8$; 20%), hypertension ($n=6$; 15%), diarrhea ($n=4$; 10%) elevated transaminases ($n=4$; 10%), gastrointestinal hemorrhage ($n=5$; 12.5%),
Brivanib	Bristol-Myers Squibb	Raoul et al. (2009) [114]	55	Phase II, single arm, two cohorts	10.0 months	Fatigue (16%), AST elevation (19%), and hyponatremia (41%) in Cohort A and hypertension (7.3%), diarrhea (4.9%), and headache (4.9%) in Cohort B

(continued)

Table 14.3 (continued)

Drug	Company	Study (year)	N	Design	Overall survival	Toxicity profile
EGFR antagonists						
Erlotinib	Genentech	Thomas et al. (2007) [118]	40	Phase II, single arm	10.75 months	No patients required dose reductions of erlotinib
Erlotinib	Genentech	Philip et al. (2005) [117]	38	Phase II, single arm	13 months	Ten patients (26%) had toxicity-related dose reductions of erlotinib
Lapatinib	GlaxoSmithKline	Ramanathan et al. (2009) [119]	57	Phase II, single arm	6.2 months	Well tolerated
Lapatinib	GlaxoSmithKline	Bekaii-Saab et al. (2009) [120]	25	Phase II, single arm	12.6 months	Diarrhea (73%), nausea (54%), and rash (42%)
Cetuximab	Bristol-Myers Squibb	Zhu et al. (2007) [121]	30	Phase II, single arm	9.6 months	No Grade 4 toxicity. Grade 3 toxicity-1 patient
Cetuximab + gemcitabine	Bristol-Myers Squibb	Asnacios et al. (2008) [122]	45	Phase II, single arm	9.5 months	Thrombocytopenia (24%), neutropenia (20%), and anemia (4%).
mTOR inhibitor						
Everolimus	Novartis	Blaszkowsky et al. (2010) [128]	28	Phase I–II, two stage	8.4 months	Lymphopenia (12%), SGOT (12%), hyponatremia (8%), and one pt (4%) each with anemia, SGPT, hyperglycemia, proteinuria, and rash

VEGF vascular endothelial growth factor, *PDGF* platelet derived growth factor, *EGFR* epidermal growth factor receptor, *VEGFR* vascular endothelial growth factor receptor, *PDGFR* platelet-derived growth factor receptor, and *FGFR* fibroblast growth factor receptor

Table 14.4 Ongoing trials on emerging therapies for HCC

Trial name (ID)	Title	Sponsor	Phase	Design	Primary end point
STORM (NCT00692770)	Sorafenib as adjuvant treatment in the prevention of recurrence of HCC	Bayer	III	Allocation: randomized Control: active Intervention model: parallel assignment Masking: double blind	Recurrence-free survival
HeiLivCa (ISRCTN24081794)	TACE combined with sorafenib vs. TACE plus placebo in patients HCC before	Bayer	III	Allocation: randomized Control: active intervention Masking: double blind	Time to progression
HEAT (NCT00441376)	A Study of ThermoDox™ in combination With RFA in primary and metastatic tumors of the liver	Celsion	III	Allocation: nonrandomized Control: uncontrolled Assignment Masking: open label	Maximum tolerated dose, timing, safety, pharmacokinetics
SEARCH (NCT00901901)	Nexavar–Tarceva Combination therapy for first line treatment of patients diagnosed with HCC	Bayer	III	Allocation: randomized Intervention model: parallel assignment Masking: open label	Safety/efficacy study
SUN1170 (NCT00699374)	Phase 3 open-label study of sutent in advanced hepatocellular carcinoma	Pfizer	III	Allocation: randomized Model: parallel assignment Masking: open label	Overall survival. Study discontinued
RAMP-UP (NCT01203787)	Sorafenib dose ramp-up in hepatocellular carcinoma (HCC)	University of Florida	II	Allocation: randomized Control: dose comparison Model: parallel assignment Masking: open label	Total (cumulative) dose delivery of sorafenib
SOCRATES (NCT00618384)	TACE and Sorafenib for advanced HCC	Heinrich-Heine University Duesseldorf	II	Allocation: nonrandomized Intervention model: single group assignment Masking: open label	Time to progression
SPACE (NCT00855218)	A Phase II randomized, double-blind, placebo-controlled study of sorafenib or placebo in combination with TACE performed with DC bead and Doxorubicin for intermediate stage HCC	Bayer	II	Allocation: randomized Intervention model: parallel assignment Masking: double blind	Time to progression

The synergistic effect of combining sorafenib plus doxorubicin has been demonstrated for other solid tumors, and a phase I extension trial reported similar results for HCC [96]. A recent double-blind, phase II, randomized study comparing the safety and efficacy of sorafenib plus doxorubicin ($n=47$) vs. placebo plus doxorubicin ($n=49$) in patients with advanced HCC showed promise with the combination of sorafenib and doxorubicin. The study reported significantly greater median time to progression (8.6 months vs. 4.8 months, $P=0.02$) and median overall survival (13.7 months vs. 6.5 months, $P=0.006$) in patients on sorafenib than on placebo [97]. In general, the safety profile of combination therapy vs. monotherapy appeared similar. However, an increased incidence of left ventricular dysfunction occurred with the combination than with monotherapy that will require further careful monitoring in future studies. The potential synergism between sorafenib plus doxorubicin is being evaluated in ongoing phase III trials where sorafenib alone is being compared to sorafenib plus doxorubicin [98].

Combination of sorafenib with other molecular-targeted therapies is also being explored. A clinical, phase III, multicenter, randomized controlled trial testing of sorafenib plus erlotinib vs. sorafenib plus placebo as first-line treatment in advanced HCC (SEARCH trial) is ongoing [99]. Other potential sorafenib-based combinations being studied include combination with mTOR inhibitors and insulin growth factor receptor (IGF-R) inhibitors. The role of sorafenib in combination with transarterial therapies such as TACE is also being studied as discussed in the intermediate HCC stage section.

Despite the enthusiasm surrounding the survival benefit found with sorafenib in the registration trial, there remains uncertainty on whether sorafenib will be efficacious and an appropriate therapy for the majority of patients with HCC and cirrhosis in clinical practice. There are several differences between the patients in the pivotal SHARP trial and the majority of patients with advanced HCC in clinical practice. One is that HCV was the cause of liver disease in approximately 30% of patients, which is usually the cause of liver disease in more than 60%–70% of patients in the United States and Western Europe [100]. While the SHARP trial was not designed to assess the efficacy of sorafenib based on the etiology of liver disease, a subgroup analysis in abstract form of 178 patients with HCV-associated HCC showed a superior overall survival in patients receiving sorafenib (14 months) vs. placebo (7.9 months) [101]. This finding has generated interest at evaluating the potential antiviral activity and/or anti-portal hypertension properties of sorafenib within clinical studies. Secondly, the majority of patients seen in clinical practice fall outside the enrollment criteria studied in the SHARP trial by the degree of underlying liver function impairment and do not have Child A cirrhosis as the study population within the trial. Thus, the clinical question remains if the safety and tolerability of sorafenib can hold up in clinical practice in patients with more compromised cirrhosis and still provide a survival benefit. Currently, there are limited data on the use of sorafenib in Child B cirrhosis, and use needs to be individualized with close monitoring and assessment of risk-benefit profile. Thirdly, in real-life clinical practice, when this drug is used in patients with cirrhosis, full dosing of sorafenib can be challenging. The majority of patients experience adverse reactions related to sorafenib which are problematic and very often require dose reduction and permanent or intermittent drug interruptions. Data from the ongoing phase 4 GIDEON registry study, a global prospective, noninterventional study of patients with unresectable HCC assigned to sorafenib, may provide much needed safety/toxicity profile and efficacy in patients treated with sorafenib outside of the clinical trial setting [102]. Presently, our center is evaluating in an open-label randomized study if increasing the dose of sorafenib slowly over several weeks vs. starting standard full dose can improve tolerance and drug delivery [103]. We are testing if the use of a dose escalation strategy for sorafenib will improve the tolerability and allow a greater percentage of patients to remain on this drug.

The most common sorafenib-related adverse events are fatigue, weight loss, hypertension, rash, hand-foot skin reaction (HFSR), alopecia, diarrhea, anorexia, nausea, and abdominal pain. Generally, adverse reactions develop during the first 4–6 weeks of treatment, particularly the hypertension and dermatologic reactions. Patients require very close monitoring after start of therapy to assess for these side effects and institute prompt dose reduction and/or interruption. This early and frequent clinical evaluation for adverse events with dose modifications that is responsive to the severity is critical in maintaining patients on treatment. Overall, once the adverse event has resolved or come under reasonable control, it is often possible to escalate back to full dosing. Further, the complexity in the management of the underlying cirrhosis of the HCC patients also requires close monitoring of potential complications related to cirrhosis, which is most successful with a multidisciplinary approach.

Bevacizumab

Bevacizumab (Avastin, Genentech/Roche) is a recombinant humanized monoclonal antibody that targets VEGF. This agent has currently been approved in the management of metastatic colorectal cancer and non-small cell lung cancer. Its role in the management of HCC has been investigated as a single agent or in combination with cytotoxic chemotherapy or targeted therapy in single-arm studies. A recent phase II study of bevacizumab monotherapy in unresectable HCC observed a median progression-free survival (PFS) of 6.9 months and median overall survival of 12.4 months [104]. But serious bleeding complications were reported in 11% of the HCC patients. Another single-arm phase II study using bevacizumab combined with gemcitabine and oxaliplatin chemotherapy (GEMOX-B) showed a median PFS of 5.3 months and median overall survival of 9.6 months in patients with advanced HCC [105]. A third phase II study combining the two targeted therapies of bevacizumab and erlotinib reported encouraging clinically meaningful antitumor activity in advanced HCC with a median PFS of 9 months and a median overall survival of 15 months [106]. While these studies suggest potential biologic activity for bevacizumab, presently, there no major phase III studies planned with this agent.

Sunitinib

Sunitinib (Sutent, Pfizer) is an oral TKI that targets receptor kinases that include VEGFR-1, VEGFR-2, PDGFR-a/b, c-KIT, FLT3, and RET kinases [107]. In contrast to sorafenib, sunitinib has more potent TKI activity against VEGFR-1 and VEGFR-2. This agent is currently approved in the management of renal cell carcinoma and metastatic neuroendocrine tumors. Initial single-arm phase II trials with sunitinib in advanced HCC showed modest antitumor activity [108, 109], but there were concerns regarding toxicities and tolerability, particularly with the higher 50 mg dose [110, 111]. Recently, the phase III study (SUN 1170) directly comparing sunitinib with sorafenib was terminated early following an independent data monitoring committee review finding higher incidence of serious adverse events in the sunitinib arm and failure of sunitinib to demonstrate superiority to sorafenib [112, 113]. Based on these findings, further development of sunitinib in HCC is very unlikely.

Brivanib

Brivanib (Bristol-Myers Squibb) is an oral agent that is a dual inhibitor of VEGFR and fibroblast growth factor receptor (FGFR)-signaling pathways. In a single-arm phase II trial studying the safety and efficacy of brivanib in 96 patients with advanced HCC, brivanib demonstrated a median overall survival of 10 months and tolerable adverse effects [114]. Brivanib demonstrated activity as both first-line and second-line agent in sorafenib-refractory treatment in HCC. This agent is currently under investigation in phase III studies as a first-line treatment vs. the clinical standard of sorafenib and as a second-line agent in patients with sorafenib-refractory advanced HCC.

Erlotinib

Epidermal growth factor (EGF) receptors have been found to be overexpressed on hepatocytes in patients with HCC [115, 116]. Erlotinib (Tarceva, Genentech/Roceh) is an EGFR TKI, and it is currently used in the treatment of non-small cell lung cancer and pancreatic cancer. In a single-arm phase II trial of erlotinib monotherapy for 38 patients with advanced HCC, a benefit was observed for EGFR/HER1 blockade with erlotinib [117]. This study demonstrated a benefit with a 59% disease control rate and a median overall survival of 13 months. A second single-arm phase II study using single-agent erlotinib in 40 patients with advanced HCC also reported tolerable adverse events and a modest disease-control benefit. The benefit was manifested as modestly prolonged PFS and a median overall survival of 10.75 months [118]. A phase III study evaluating the combination of erlotinib with sorafenib vs. single-agent sorafenib is ongoing (SEARCH trial).

Other Drugs

Lapatinib (Tykerb, GSK) is another inhibitor of EGFR. This TKI also blocks Her-2/Neu pathways. Phase II trials with lapatinib for advanced HCC showed that this agent was well tolerated and there was evidence of activity in HCC, but therapy did not meet the predefined efficacy rate [119, 120]. Cetuximab is a chimeric monoclonal antibody against EGFR currently being used in metastatic colorectal cancer and head and neck cancer. Studies on cetuximab monotherapy in HCC did not demonstrate significant antitumor activity [121]. But combination of cetuximab with gemcitabine and oxaliplatin appeared to be active in a subgroup of poor-prognosis patients with progressive advanced-stage HCC [122]. Other drugs targeting various molecular pathways involved in the molecular pathogenesis of HCC which have shown promise in the treatment of advanced HCC in early uncontrolled clinical trials include vatalinib (PTK787, Novartis) not undergoing further development [123]; linifanib (ABT-869, Abbot) in a phase III study being compared with sorafenib [124]; MEK inhibitors (BAY86-9766, Bayer) in phase II study in combination with sorafenib [125]; mapatumumab (HGS1012, Human Genome Sciences), a human agonist monoclonal antibody to the tumor necrosis factor-related apoptosis-inducing ligand receptor 1 (TRAIL-R1) in phase I–II evaluation in combination with sorafenib [126]; and everolimus (Afinitor, Novartis), an oral mTOR inhibitor in phase I–II evaluation for the treatment of advanced HCC [127, 128].

Conclusion

HCC is a challenging malignancy to treat. Each patient's unique genetic background contributes significantly to tumor behavior, treatment response, and prognosis. Advances in molecular profiling studies using DNA microarray-based gene-expression profiling will elucidate the key regulatory networks affected and provide insight of the tumor and its microenvironment. As more hepatic carcinogenetic pathways are described, the possibility of identifying them as targets for therapy also looks promising. As we improve our knowledge of the relevant expression profiles and molecular pathways, we also need to develop biomarkers that can predict response and anticipate resistance. The wave of molecular-targeted agents that are being evaluated will certainly change the current landscape of treatment to one where targeted therapies will be used in the adjuvant setting, combined with locoregional treatments, or with each other. An important key to the success of future treatments will be our ability to incorporate the individual's genetic/epigenetic background, molecular profile of tumors, and predictive biomarkers in the design of clinical trials. Designing trials where treatment is tailored to clearly defined patients will be critical to expedite discovery and clinical development of new treatment approaches in a cost-effective manner.

References

1. Parkin DM, Bray F, Ferlay J, Pisani P. Estimating the world cancer burden: Globocan 2000. Int J Cancer. 2001;94(2):153–6.
2. El-Serag HB. Hepatocellular carcinoma: recent trends in the United States. Gastroenterology. 2004;127(5):S27–34.
3. Kassahun WT, Fangmann J, Harms J, Hauss J, Bartels M. Liver resection and transplantation in the management of hepatocellular carcinoma: a review. Exp Clin Transplant. 2006; 4(2):549–58.
4. Guan YS, Liu Y. Interventional treatments for hepatocellular carcinoma. Hepatobiliary Pancreat Dis Int. 2006;5(4):495–500.
5. Schwartz M, Roayaie S, Konstadoulakis M. Strategies for the management of hepatocellular carcinoma. Nat Clin Pract Oncol. 2007;4(7):424–32.
6. El-Serag HB, Marrero JA, Rudolph L, Reddy KR. Diagnosis and treatment of hepatocellular carcinoma. Gastroenterology. 2008;134(6):1752–63.
7. Christos SG, Douglas ER, Stephen S, Jean-Francois HG. New nonsurgical therapies in the treatment of hepatocellular carcinoma. Tech Vasc Interv Radiol. 2001;4(3):193–9.
8. Altekruse SF, Kosary CL, Krapcho M, Neyman N, Aminou R, Waldron W, Ruhl J, Howlader N, Tatalovich Z, Cho H, Mariotto A, Eisner MP, Lewis DR, Cronin K, Chen HS, Feuer EJ. In: Stinchcomb DG, Edwards BK, editors. SEER cancer statistics review. Bethesda, MD: National Cancer Institute; 1975–2007. http://seer.cancer.gov/csr/1975_2007/, based on November 2009 SEER data submission, posted to the SEER web site, 2010. Accessed 16 Apr 2011.
9. Bruix J, Sherman M. Management of hepatocellular carcinoma. Hepatology. 2005; 42(5):1208–36.
10. Llovet JM, Fuster J, Bruix J. Intention-to-treat analysis of surgical treatment for early hepatocellular carcinoma: resection versus transplantation. Hepatology. 1999;30(6):1434–40.
11. Cho JY, Han HS, Yoon YS, Shin SH. Experiences of laparoscopic liver resection including lesions in the posterosuperior segments of the liver. Surg Endosc. 2008;22(11):2344–9.
12. Dagher I, Lainas P, Carloni A, Caillard C, Champault A, Smadja C, et al. Laparoscopic liver resection for hepatocellular carcinoma. Surg Endosc. 2008;22(2):372–8.
13. Vibert E, Perniceni T, Levard H, Denet C, Shahri NK, Gayet B. Laparoscopic liver resection. Br J Surg. 2006;93(1):67–72.
14. Dagher I, O'Rourke N, Geller DA, Cherqui D, Belli G, Gamblin TC, et al. Laparoscopic major hepatectomy: an evolution in standard of care. Ann Surg. 2009;250(5):856–60.
15. Cherqui D, Laurent A, Tayar C, Chang S, Van Nhieu JT, Loriau J, et al. Laparoscopic liver resection for peripheral hepatocellular carcinoma in patients with chronic liver disease: mid-term results and perspectives. Ann Surg. 2006;243(4):499–506.
16. Buell JF, Thomas MT, Rudich S, Marvin M, Nagubandi R, Ravindra KV, et al. Experience with more than 500 minimally invasive hepatic procedures. Ann Surg. 2008;248(3):475–86.
17. Chen HY, Juan CC, Ker CG. Laparoscopic liver surgery for patients with hepatocellular carcinoma. Ann Surg Oncol. 2008;15(3):800–6.
18. Belli G, Fantini C, D'Agostino A, Cioffi L, Langella S, Russolillo N, et al. Laparoscopic versus open liver resection for hepatocellular carcinoma in patients with histologically proven cirrhosis: short- and middle-term results. Surg Endosc. 2007;21(11):2004–11.
19. Belghiti J, Cortes A, Abdalla EK, Regimbeau JM, Prakash K, Durand F, et al. Resection prior to liver transplantation for hepatocellular carcinoma. Ann Surg. 2003;238(6):885–92. discussion 92–3.
20. Poon RT, Fan ST, Lo CM, Liu CL, Wong J. Long-term survival and pattern of recurrence after resection of small hepatocellular carcinoma in patients with preserved liver function: implications for a strategy of salvage transplantation. Ann Surg. 2002;235(3):373–82.
21. Adam R, Azoulay D, Castaing D, Eshkenazy R, Pascal G, Hashizume K, et al. Liver resection as a bridge to transplantation for hepatocellular carcinoma on cirrhosis: a reasonable strategy? Ann Surg. 2003;238(4):508–18. discussion 18–9.

22. Tang ZY, Yu YQ, Zhou XD, Ma ZC, Wu ZQ. Progress and prospects in hepatocellular carcinoma surgery. Ann Chir. 1998;52(6):558–63.
23. Takayama T, Sekine T, Makuuchi M, Yamasaki S, Kosuge T, Yamamoto J, et al. Adoptive immunotherapy to lower postsurgical recurrence rates of hepatocellular carcinoma: a randomised trial. Lancet. 2000;356(9232):802–7.
24. Sala M, Fuster J, Llovet JM, Navasa M, Sole M, Varela M, et al. High pathological risk of recurrence after surgical resection for hepatocellular carcinoma: an indication for salvage liver transplantation. Liver Transpl. 2004;10(10):1294–300.
25. Del Gaudio M, Ercolani G, Ravaioli M, Cescon M, Lauro A, Vivarelli M, et al. Liver transplantation for recurrent hepatocellular carcinoma on cirrhosis after liver resection: University of Bologna experience. Am J Transplant. 2008;8(6):1177–85.
26. Muto Y, Moriwaki H, Saito A. Prevention of second primary tumors by an acyclic retinoid in patients with hepatocellular carcinoma. N Engl J Med. 1999;340(13):1046–7.
27. Mazzaferro V, Romito R, Schiavo M, Mariani L, Camerini T, Bhoori S, et al. Prevention of hepatocellular carcinoma recurrence with alpha-interferon after liver resection in HCV cirrhosis. Hepatology. 2006;44(6):1543–54.
28. Sun HC, Tang ZY. Preventive treatments for recurrence after curative resection of hepatocellular carcinoma—a literature review of randomized control trials. World J Gastroenterol. 2003;9(4):635–40.
29. Ho M-C, et al. A randomized pilot phase II study of thalidomide as adjuvant therapy in patient with high recurrence risk hepatocellular carcinoma. Abstract presented at The International Liver Congress™, 2011.
30. Samuel M, Chow PK, Chan Shih-Yen E, Machin D, Soo Kc. Neoadjuvant and adjuvant therapy for surgical resection of hepatocellular carcinoma. Cochrane Database Syst Rev. 2009;1:CD001199.
31. Feng YX, Wang T, Deng YZ, Yang P, Li JJ, Guan DX, et al. Sorafenib suppresses postsurgical recurrence and metastasis of hepatocellular carcinoma in an orthotopic mouse model. Hepatology. 2011;53(2):483–92.
32. Sorafenib as adjuvant treatment in the prevention of recurrence of hepatocellular carcinoma. NIH clinical trials web page. http://clinicaltrials.gov/ct2/show/NCT00692770?term=STORM&rank=1. Accessed 16 Apr 2011.
33. Allegra CJ, Yothers G, O'Connell MJ, Sharif S, Petrelli NJ, Colangelo LH, et al. Phase III trial assessing bevacizumab in stages II and III carcinoma of the colon: results of NSABP protocol C-08. J Clin Oncol. 2011;29(1):11–6.
34. Mazzaferro V, Chun YS, Poon RT, Schwartz ME, Yao FY, Marsh JW, et al. Liver transplantation for hepatocellular carcinoma. Ann Surg Oncol. 2008;15(4):1001–7.
35. Mazzaferro V, Regalia E, Doci R, Andreola S, Pulvirenti A, Bozzetti F, et al. Liver transplantation for the treatment of small hepatocellular carcinomas in patients with cirrhosis. N Engl J Med. 1996;334(11):693–9.
36. Pomfret EA, Washburn K, Wald C, Nalesnik MA, Douglas D, Russo M, et al. Report of a national conference on liver allocation in patients with hepatocellular carcinoma in the United States. Liver Transpl. 2010;16(3):262–78.
37. Herrero JI, Sangro B, Quiroga J, Pardo F, Herraiz M, Cienfuegos JA, et al. Influence of tumor characteristics on the outcome of liver transplantation among patients with liver cirrhosis and hepatocellular carcinoma. Liver Transpl. 2001;7(7):631–6.
38. Yao FY, Ferrell L, Bass NM, Watson JJ, Bacchetti P, Venook A, et al. Liver transplantation for hepatocellular carcinoma: expansion of the tumor size limits does not adversely impact survival. Hepatology. 2001;33(6):1394–403.
39. Roayaie S, Frischer JS, Emre SH, Fishbein TM, Sheiner PA, Sung M, et al. Long-term results with multimodal adjuvant therapy and liver transplantation for the treatment of hepatocellular carcinomas larger than 5 centimeters. Ann Surg. 2002;235(4):533–9.
40. Kneteman NM, Oberholzer J, Al Saghier M, Meeberg GA, Blitz M, Ma MM, et al. Sirolimus-based immunosuppression for liver transplantation in the presence of extended criteria for hepatocellular carcinoma. Liver Transpl. 2004;10(10):1301–11.

41. Mazzaferro V, Llovet JM, Miceli R, Bhoori S, Schiavo M, Mariani L, et al. Predicting survival after liver transplantation in patients with hepatocellular carcinoma beyond the Milan criteria: a retrospective, exploratory analysis. Lancet Oncol. 2009;10(1):35–43.
42. Duffy JP, Vardanian A, Benjamin E, Watson M, Farmer DG, Ghobrial RM, et al. Liver transplantation criteria for hepatocellular carcinoma should be expanded: a 22-year experience with 467 patients at UCLA. Ann Surg. 2007;246(3):502–9. discussion 9–11.
43. Marsh JW, Dvorchik I, Bonham CA, Iwatsuki S. Is the pathologic TNM staging system for patients with hepatoma predictive of outcome? Cancer. 2000;88(3):538–43.
44. Chen J, Xu X, Ling Q, Wu J, Zheng SS. Role of Pittsburgh modified TNM criteria in prognosis prediction of liver transplantation for hepatocellular carcinoma. Chin Med J (Engl). 2007;120(24):2200–3.
45. Yao FY, Ferrell L, Bass NM, Bacchetti P, Ascher NL, Roberts JP. Liver transplantation for hepatocellular carcinoma: comparison of the proposed UCSF criteria with the Milan criteria and the Pittsburgh modified TNM criteria. Liver Transpl. 2002;8(9):765–74.
46. Toso C, Trotter J, Wei A, Bigam DL, Shah S, Lancaster J, et al. Total tumor volume predicts risk of recurrence following liver transplantation in patients with hepatocellular carcinoma. Liver Transpl. 2008;14(8):1107–15.
47. Pelletier SJ, Fu S, Thyagarajan V, Romero-Marrero C, Batheja MJ, Punch JD, et al. An intention-to-treat analysis of liver transplantation for hepatocellular carcinoma using organ procurement transplant network data. Liver Transpl. 2009;15(8):859–68.
48. Otto G, Herber S, Heise M, Lohse AW, Mönch C, Bittinger F, et al. Response to transarterial chemoembolization as a biological selection criterion for liver transplantation in hepatocellular carcinoma. Liver Transpl. 2006;12(8):1260–7.
49. Majno PE, Adam R, Bismuth H, Castaing D, Ariche A, Krissat J, et al. Influence of preoperative transarterial lipiodol chemoembolization on resection and transplantation for hepatocellular carcinoma in patients with cirrhosis. Ann Surg. 1997;226(6):688–701. discussion-3.
50. Millonig G, Graziadei IW, Freund MC, Jaschke W, Stadlmann S, Ladurner R, et al. Response to preoperative chemoembolization correlates with outcome after liver transplantation in patients with hepatocellular carcinoma. Liver Transpl. 2007;13(2):272–9.
51. Yao FY, Hirose R, LaBerge JM, Davern TJ, Bass NM, Kerlan RK, et al. A prospective study on downstaging of hepatocellular carcinoma prior to liver transplantation. Liver Transpl. 2005;11(12):1505–14.
52. 2007 Annual Report of the US organ procurement and transplantation network and the scientific registry of transplant recipients: transplant data 1997–2006. In: Health Resources and Services Administration.
53. Eguchi S, Hidaka M, Tomonaga T, Miyazaki K, Inokuma T, Takatsuki M, et al. Actual therapeutic efficacy of pre-transplant treatment on hepatocellular carcinoma and its impact on survival after salvage living donor liver transplantation. J Gastroenterol. 2009;44(6):624–9.
54. Heckman J, deVera M, Marsh J, Fontes P, Amesur N, Holloway S, et al. Bridging locoregional therapy for hepatocellular carcinoma prior to liver transplantation. Ann Surg Oncol. 2008;15(11):3169–77.
55. Cabrera R, Dhanasekaran R, Caridi J, Clark V, Morelli G, Soldevila-Pico C, Magglioca J, Nelson D, Firpi RJ. Impact of transarterial therapy in hepatitis C-related hepatocellular carcinoma on long-term outcomes after liver transplantation. Am J Clin Oncol. 2011 [Epub ahead of print].
56. Graziadei IW, Sandmueller H, Waldenberger P, Koenigsrainer A, Nachbaur K, Jaschke W, et al. Chemoembolization followed by liver transplantation for hepatocellular carcinoma impedes tumor progression while on the waiting list and leads to excellent outcome. Liver Transpl. 2003;9(6):557–63.
57. Maddala YK, Stadheim L, Andrews JC, Burgart LJ, Rosen CB, Kremers WK, et al. Drop-out rates of patients with hepatocellular cancer listed for liver transplantation: outcome with chemoembolization. Liver Transpl. 2004;10(3):449–55.

58. Bruix J, Sherman M. Management of hepatocellular carcinoma: an update. Alexandria (VA): American Association for the Study of Liver Diseases; 2010. p. 35.
59. Bouza C, Lopez-Cuadrado T, Alcazar R, Saz-Parkinson Z, Amate J. Meta-analysis of percutaneous radiofrequency ablation versus ethanol injection in hepatocellular carcinoma. BMC Gastroenterol. 2009;9(1):31.
60. Lencioni RA, Allgaier H-P, Cioni D, Olschewski M, Deibert P, Crocetti L, et al. Small hepatocellular carcinoma in cirrhosis: randomized comparison of radio-frequency thermal ablation versus percutaneous ethanol injection1. Radiology. 2003;228(1):235–40.
61. Liang P, Wang Y. Microwave ablation of hepatocellular carcinoma. Oncology. 2007;72 Suppl 1:124–31.
62. Davalos RV, Mir IL, Rubinsky B. Tissue ablation with irreversible electroporation. Ann Biomed Eng. 2005;33(2):223–31.
63. Guo Y, Zhang Y, Klein R, Nijm GM, Sahakian AV, Omary RA, et al. Irreversible electroporation therapy in the liver: longitudinal efficacy studies in a rat model of hepatocellular carcinoma. Cancer Res. 2010;70(4):1555–63.
64. NIH clinical trials web page. http://clinicaltrials.gov/ct2/show/NCT00441376?term=thermo dox&rank=1. Accessed 16 Apr 2011.
65. Llovet JM, Real MI, Montana X, Planas R, Coll S, Aponte J, et al. Arterial embolisation or chemoembolisation versus symptomatic treatment in patients with unresectable hepatocellular carcinoma: a randomised controlled trial. Lancet. 2002;359(9319):1734–9.
66. Lo CM, Ngan H, Tso WK, Liu CL, Lam CM, Poon RT, et al. Randomized controlled trial of transarterial lipiodol chemoembolization for unresectable hepatocellular carcinoma. Hepatology. 2002;35(5):1164–71.
67. Marelli L, Stigliano R, Triantos C, Senzolo M, Cholongitas E, Davies N, et al. Transarterial therapy for hepatocellular carcinoma: which technique is more effective? A systematic review of cohort and randomized studies. Cardiovasc Intervent Radiol. 2007;30(1):6–25.
68. Llovet JM, Bruix J. Systematic review of randomized trials for unresectable hepatocellular carcinoma: Chemoembolization improves survival. Hepatology. 2003;37(2):429–42.
69. Georgiades CS, Hong K, D'Angelo M, Geschwind JF. Safety and efficacy of transarterial chemoembolization in patients with unresectable hepatocellular carcinoma and portal vein thrombosis. J Vasc Interv Radiol. 2005;16(12):1653–9.
70. Lewis AL, Taylor RR, Hall B, Gonzalez MV, Willis SL, Stratford PW. Pharmacokinetic and safety study of doxorubicin-eluting beads in a porcine model of hepatic arterial embolization. J Vasc Interv Radiol. 2006;17(8):1335–43.
71. Hong K, Khwaja A, Liapi E, Torbenson MS, Georgiades CS, Geschwind JF. New intra-arterial drug delivery system for the treatment of liver cancer: preclinical assessment in a rabbit model of liver cancer. Clin Cancer Res. 2006;12(8):2563–7.
72. Varela M, Real MI, Burrel M, Forner A, Sala M, Brunet M, et al. Chemoembolization of hepatocellular carcinoma with drug eluting beads: efficacy and doxorubicin pharmacokinetics. J Hepatol. 2007;46(3):474–81.
73. Poon RT, Tso WK, Pang RW, Ng KK, Woo R, Tai KS, et al. A phase I/II trial of chemoembolization for hepatocellular carcinoma using a novel intra-arterial drug-eluting bead. Clin Gastroenterol Hepatol. 2007;5(9):1100–8.
74. Malagari K, Chatzimichael K, Alexopoulou E, Kelekis A, Hall B, Dourakis S, et al. Transarterial chemoembolization of unresectable hepatocellular carcinoma with drug eluting beads: results of an open-label study of 62 patients. Cardiovasc Intervent Radiol. 2008;31(2):269–80.
75. Lammer J, Malagari K, Vogl T, Pilleul F, Denys A, Watkinson A, et al. Prospective randomized study of doxorubicin-eluting-bead embolization in the treatment of hepatocellular carcinoma: results of the PRECISION V study. Cardiovasc Intervent Radiol. 2010;33(1):41–52.
76. Dhanasekaran R, Kooby DA, Staley CA, Kauh JS, Khanna V, Kim HS. Comparison of conventional transarterial chemoembolization (TACE) and chemoembolization with doxorubicin drug eluting beads (DEB) for unresectable hepatocelluar carcinoma (HCC). J Surg Oncol. 2010;101(6):476–80.

77. Bilbao JI, de Luis E, Garcia de Jalon JA, de Martino A, Lozano MD, de la Cuesta AM, et al. Comparative study of four different spherical embolic particles in an animal model: a morphologic and histologic evaluation. J Vasc Interv Radiol. 2008;19(11):1625–38.

78. Kulik LM, Atassi B, van Holsbeeck L, Souman T, Lewandowski RJ, Mulcahy MF, et al. Yttrium-90 microspheres (TheraSphere) treatment of unresectable hepatocellular carcinoma: downstaging to resection, RFA and bridge to transplantation. J Surg Oncol. 2006; 94(7):572–86.

79. Salem R, Lewandowski R, Roberts C, Goin J, Thurston K, Abouljoud M, et al. Use of Yttrium-90 glass microspheres (TheraSphere) for the treatment of unresectable hepatocellular carcinoma in patients with portal vein thrombosis. J Vasc Interv Radiol. 2004;15(4): 335–45.

80. Carr BI. Hepatic arterial 90Yttrium glass microspheres (Therasphere) for unresectable hepatocellular carcinoma: interim safety and survival data on 65 patients. Liver Transpl. 2004;10(2 Suppl 1):S107–10.

81. Salem R, Lewandowski RJ, Mulcahy MF, Riaz A, Ryu RK, Ibrahim S, et al. Radioembolization for hepatocellular carcinoma using Yttrium-90 microspheres: a comprehensive report of long-term outcomes. Gastroenterology. 2010;138(1):52–64.

82. Salem R, Lewandowski RJ, Kulik L, Wang E, Riaz A, Ryu RK, et al. Radioembolization results in longer time-to-progression and reduced toxicity compared with chemoembolization in patients with hepatocellular carcinoma. Gastroenterology. 2011;140(2):497–507.e2.

83. Kulik L. Is radioembolization ready for the barcelona clinic liver cancer staging system? Hepatology. 2010;52(5):1528–30.

84. Inarrairaegui M, Thurston KG, Bilbao JI, D'Avola D, Rodriguez M, Arbizu J, et al. Radioembolization with use of yttrium-90 resin microspheres in patients with hepatocellular carcinoma and portal vein thrombosis. J Vasc Interv Radiol. 2010;21(8):1205–12.

85. Li X, Feng GS, Zheng CS, Zhuo CK, Liu X. Expression of plasma vascular endothelial growth factor in patients with hepatocellular carcinoma and effect of transcatheter arterial chemoembolization therapy on plasma vascular endothelial growth factor level. World J Gastroenterol. 2004;10(19):2878–82.

86. Abou-Alfa GK, Johnson P, Knox JJ, Capanu M, Davidenko I, Lacava J, et al. Doxorubicin plus sorafenib vs doxorubicin alone in patients with advanced hepatocellular carcinoma: a randomized trial. J Am Med Assoc. 2010;304(19):2154–60.

87. Cabrera R, Pannu D, Caridi J, et al. Combination of sorafenib with transarterial chemoembolization for hepatocellular carcinoma. Alim Phar Ther. 2011;34(2):205–13.

88. Chao Y, Yoon J, Li C, Kim B, Lee R, Chang C, et al. START: Study in Asia of the combination of TACE (transcatheter arterial chemoembolization) with sorafenib in patients with hepatocellular carcinoma trial. Abstract no. 211, 2010 Gastrointestinal Cancers Symposium.

89. Reyes DK, Azad NS, Koteish A, Hamilton J, et al. Prospective phase II trial of sorafenib combined with doxorubicin eluting bead-transarterial chemoembolization for patients with unresectable hepatocellular carcinoma: interim analysis. Abstract 1820, The Liver Meeting 2010 AASLD.

90. NIH clinical trials web page. http://clinicaltrials.gov/ct2/show/NCT00618384?term=Socrates+trial+sorafenib&rank=1. Accessed 16 Apr 2011.

91. Dufour JF, Hoppe H, Heim MH, Helbling B, Maurhofer O, Szucs-Farkas Z, et al. Continuous administration of sorafenib in combination with transarterial chemoembolization in patients with hepatocellular carcinoma: results of a phase I study. Oncologist. 2010;15(11):1198–204.

92. Reyes DK, Vossen J, Kamel IR, et al. Phase II trial of bevacizumab combined with transarterial chemoembolization (TACE) for hepatocellular carcinoma: initial experience at two institutions. Abstract presented at ASCO Gastrointestinal Cancers Symposium, January 2010, Orlando, FL.

93. Llovet JM, Ricci S, Mazzaferro V, Hilgard P, Gane E, Blanc JF, et al. Sorafenib in advanced hepatocellular carcinoma. N Engl J Med. 2008;359(4):378–90.

94. Cheng AL, Kang YK, Chen Z, Tsao CJ, Qin S, Kim JS, et al. Efficacy and safety of sorafenib in patients in the Asia-Pacific region with advanced hepatocellular carcinoma: a phase III randomised, double-blind, placebo-controlled trial. Lancet Oncol. 2009;10(1):25–34.

95. Newell P, Villanueva A, Llovet JM. Molecular targeted therapies in hepatocellular carcinoma: from pre-clinical models to clinical trials. J Hepatol. 2008;49(1):1–5.
96. Richly H, Schultheis B, Adamietz IA, Kupsch P, Grubert M, Hilger RA, et al. Combination of sorafenib and doxorubicin in patients with advanced hepatocellular carcinoma: results from a phase I extension trial. Eur J Cancer. 2009;45(4):579–87.
97. Abou-Alfa GK, Johnson P, Knox J, et al. Final results from a phase II (PhII), randomized, double-blind study of sorafenib plus doxorubicin (S + D) versus placebo plus doxorubicin (P + D) in patients (pts) with advanced hepatocellular carcinoma (AHCC) (abstract 128). Presented at 2008 Gastrointestinal Cancers Symposium, Orlando, FL.
98. NIH clinical trials web page. http://www.clinicaltrials.gov/ct2/show/NCT01015833?term=p hase+III+randomized+sorafenib+with+doxorubicin&rank=1. Accessed 16 Apr 2011.
99. NIH clinical trials web page. http://clinicaltrials.gov/ct2/show/NCT00901901?term=sorafen ib+plus+erlotinib+AND+sorafenib+plus+placebo+AND+advanced+AND+SEARCH+trial &rank=1. Accessed 16 Apr 2011.
100. Gomaa AI, Khan SA, Toledano MB, Waked I, Taylor-Robinson SD. Hepatocellular carcinoma: epidemiology, risk factors and pathogenesis. World J Gastroenterol. 2008; 14(27):4300–8.
101. Bolondi L, Caspary W, Bennouna J, et al. Clinical benefit of sorafenib in hepatitis C patients with hepatocellular carcinoma (HCC): subgroup analysis of the SHARP trial, 2008. Presented at Gastrointestinal Cancers Symposium, 25–27 Jan 2008, Orlando, FL
102. Venook AP, Lencioni R, Marrero JA, Kudo M, Nakajima K, Ye S. First interim results of the global investigation of therapeutic decisions in hepatocellular carcinoma (HCC) and of its treatment with sorafenib (GIDEON) study: use of sorafenib (Sor) by oncologists and nononcologists in the management of HCC. #157 Presented at the 2011 Gastrointestinal Cancers Symposium, 20–22 Jan 2011, San Francisco.
103. NIH clinical trials web page. http://www.clinicaltrials.gov/ct2/show/NCT01203787?term= sorafenib+ramp-up&rank=1. Accessed 16 Apr 2011.
104. Siegel AB, Cohen EI, Ocean A, Lehrer D, Goldenberg A, Knox JJ, et al. Phase II trial evaluating the clinical and biologic effects of bevacizumab in unresectable hepatocellular carcinoma. J Clin Oncol. 2008;26(18):2992–8.
105. Zhu AX, Blaszkowsky LS, Ryan DP, Clark JW, Muzikansky A, Horgan K, et al. Phase II study of gemcitabine and oxaliplatin in combination with bevacizumab in patients with advanced hepatocellular carcinoma. J Clin Oncol. 2006;24(12):1898–903.
106. Thomas MB, Morris JS, Chadha R, Iwasaki M, Kaur H, Lin E, et al. Phase II trial of the combination of bevacizumab and erlotinib in patients who have advanced hepatocellular carcinoma. J Clin Oncol. 2009;27(6):843–50.
107. Arora A, Scholar EM. Role of tyrosine kinase inhibitors in cancer therapy. J Pharmacol Exp Ther. 2005;315(3):971–9.
108. Zhu AX, Raymond E. Early development of sunitinib in hepatocellular carcinoma. Expert Rev Anticancer Ther. 2009;9(1):143–50.
109. Zhu AX, Duda DG, Sahani DV, Jain RK. Development of sunitinib in hepatocellular carcinoma: rationale, early clinical experience, and correlative studies. Cancer J. 2009; 15(4):263–8.
110. Faivre S, Raymond E, Boucher E, Douillard J, Lim HY, Kim JS, et al. Safety and efficacy of sunitinib in patients with advanced hepatocellular carcinoma: an open-label, multicentre, phase II study. Lancet Oncol. 2009;10(8):794–800.
111. Faivre SJ, Bouattour M, Dreyer C, Raymond E. Sunitinib in hepatocellular carcinoma: redefining appropriate dosing, schedule, and activity end points. J Clin Oncol. 2009;27(35): e248–50. author reply e51–2.
112. Pfizer Halts Phase 3 Trial of Sutent in Advanced Hepatocellular Carcinoma. Wireless News. 2010.
113. NIH clinical trials web page. http://www.clinicaltrials.gov/ct2/show/NCT00699374. Accessed 16 Apr 2011.

114. Raoul JL, Finn RS, Kang YK, et al. An open-label phase II study of first- and second-line treatment with brivanib in patients with hepatocellular carcinoma (HCC). J Clin Oncol. 2009;27(Suppl):4577.
115. Ito Y, Takeda T, Higashiyama S, Sakon M, Wakasa KI, Tsujimoto M, et al. Expression of heparin binding epidermal growth factor-like growth factor in hepatocellular carcinoma: an immunohistochemical study. Oncol Rep. 2001;8(4):903–7.
116. Carlin CR, Simon D, Mattison J, Knowles BB. Expression and biosynthetic variation of the epidermal growth factor receptor in human hepatocellular carcinoma-derived cell lines. Mol Cell Biol. 1988;8(1):25–34.
117. Philip PA, Mahoney MR, Allmer C, Thomas J, Pitot HC, Kim G, et al. Phase II study of Erlotinib (OSI-774) in patients with advanced hepatocellular cancer. J Clin Oncol. 2005;23(27):6657–63.
118. Thomas MB, Chadha R, Glover K, Wang X, Morris J, Brown T, et al. Phase 2 study of erlotinib in patients with unresectable hepatocellular carcinoma. Cancer. 2007;110(5):1059–67.
119. Ramanathan RK, Belani CP, Singh DA, Tanaka M, Lenz HJ, Yen Y, et al. A phase II study of lapatinib in patients with advanced biliary tree and hepatocellular cancer. Cancer Chemother Pharmacol. 2009;64(4):777–83.
120. Bekaii-Saab T, Markowitz J, Prescott N, Sadee W, Heerema N, Wei L, et al. A multi-institutional phase II study of the efficacy and tolerability of lapatinib in patients with advanced hepatocellular carcinomas. Clin Cancer Res. 2009;15(18):5895–901.
121. Zhu AX, Stuart K, Blaszkowsky LS, Muzikansky A, Reitberg DP, Clark JW, et al. Phase 2 study of cetuximab in patients with advanced hepatocellular carcinoma. Cancer. 2007;110(3):581–9.
122. Asnacios A, Fartoux L, Romano O, Tesmoingt C, Louafi SS, Mansoubakht T, et al. Gemcitabine plus oxaliplatin (GEMOX) combined with cetuximab in patients with progressive advanced stage hepatocellular carcinoma: results of a multicenter phase 2 study. Cancer. 2008;112(12):2733–9.
123. Koch I, Baron A, Roberts S, et al. Influence of hepatic dysfunction on safety, tolerability, and pharmacokinetics (PK) of PTK787/ZK 222584 in patients (pts) with unresectable hepatocellular carcinoma (HCC). J Clin Oncol. 2007;23(Suppl):4134.
124. Jasinghe VJ, Xie Z, Zhou J, Khng J, Poon LF, Senthilnathan P, et al. ABT-869, a multi-targeted tyrosine kinase inhibitor, in combination with rapamycin is effective for subcutaneous hepatocellular carcinoma xenograft. J Hepatol. 2008;49(6):985–97.
125. O'Neil BH, Williams-Goff LW, Kauh J, et al. A phase II study of AZD6244 in advanced or metastatic hepatocellular carcinoma. J Clin Oncol. 2009;27(Suppl):e15574.
126. Sun W, Nelson D, Alberts SR, Poordad F, Leong S, Teitelbaum UR, Woods L, Fox N, O'Neil BH. Phase Ib study of mapatumumab in combination with sorafenib in patients with advanced hepatocellular carcinoma (HCC) and chronic viral hepatitis. J Clin Oncol. 2011;29(Suppl 4) (abstract 261).
127. Chen L, Shiah HS, Chen CY, et al. Randomized, phase I, and pharmacokinetic (PK) study of RAD001, an mTOR inhibitor, in patients (pts) with advanced hepatocellular carcinoma (HCC). J Clin Oncol. 2009;27(Suppl):4587.
128. Blaszkowsky LS, Abrams TA, Miksad RA, Zheng H, Meyerhardt JA, Schrag D, Kwak EL, Fuchs C, Ryan DP, Zh AX. Phase I/II study of everolimus in patients with advanced hepatocellular carcinoma (HCC). J Clin Oncol. 2010 ASCO Annual Meeting proceedings (Post-Meeting Edition), 2010, vol 28, No. 15_suppl (May 20 Supplement).

Index

A

Acanthosis nigricans, 131–132
Acrokeratosis paraneoplastica, 134
Aflatoxin, 7
Alcoholic liver disease, 21–22
Alpha-1-antitrypsin (α1-AT), 145–146
Alpha-fetoprotein (AFP), 104–105,
    248–250
Alpha-L-fucosidase (AFU), 252
Antitumor adjuvant therapy, 225

B

Barcelona Clinic of liver cancer (BCLC)
    staging
    BCLC 0-A, 200–203
    BCLC B
      TACE, 204–206
      TARE, 206–209
    BCLC C, 209–210
    BCLC D, 210
    classification, 200
    system, 168–170
Bazex's syndrome. *See* Acrokeratosis
    paraneoplastica

C

Cancer of the liver Italian program (CLIP)
    scoring system, 164–166
Chemotherapy, 153–154
Children with HCC
    clinical presentation, 148–149
    differential diagnosis
      AFP, 149
      bloodwork, 149–151
      imaging modalities, 151

liver diseases, 150
role of biopsy, 151
staging, 151–153
epidemiology
    alpha-1-antitrypsin, 145–146
    biology, 147–148
    cirrhosis, 146
    environmental toxins, 147
    familial adematous polyposis, 146
    glycogen storage disease type 1, 146
    and HBV, 144–145
    and HCV, 145
    hereditary tyrosinemia type 1, 145
    incidence and prevalence, 144
    progressive familial intrahepatic
      cholestasis, 146
prognosis, 155
treatment
    alternative therapies, 155
    chemotherapy, 153–154
    transplantation, 154–155
Chinese University prognostic index (CUPI),
    167–168
Cholangiocarcinoma
    acrokeratosis paraneoplastica, 134
    hypercalcemia, 133–134
    Sweet's syndrome, 134
    venous thromboembolic events, 135
Chronic hepatitis B infection, 19–21
Chronic hepatitis C infection, 21
Chronic inflammatory demyelinating
    polyradiculoneuropathy
    (CIDP), 133
Cirrhosis
    causes, 23
    children with HCC, 146
    etiology and risk factors, 4

N. Reau and F.F. Poordad (eds.), *Primary Liver Cancer: Surveillance, Diagnosis and Treatment*, Clinical Gastroenterology, DOI 10.1007/978-1-61779-863-4,
© Springer Science+Business Media New York 2012

Printed by Publishers' Graphics LLC
JCIMO131217.15.21.26